Date Due

OCT 23 2001			
7/3/02			
MAR 11 2003			
APR 03 2003			
MAY 06 2004			
DEC 01 2005			
OCT 14 2009			
FEB 17 2014			

BRODART, CO. Cat. No. 23-233-003 Printed in U.S.A.

Quality of Life in Epilepsy

Quality of Life in Epilepsy

Beyond seizure counts in assessment and treatment

Edited by

Gus A. Baker
and
Ann Jacoby
University of Liverpool, UK

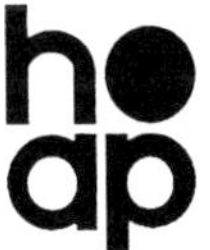

harwood academic publishers
Australia • Canada • France • Germany • India
Japan • Luxembourg • Malaysia • The Netherlands
Russia • Singapore • Switzerland

Published by license under the Harwood Academic Publishers imprint, part of The Gordon and Breach Publishing Group.

 Printed in Singapore.

Amsteldijk 166
1st Floor
1079 LH Amsterdam
The Netherlands

British Library Cataloguing in Publication Data

A catalogue record for this book is available from the British Library.
ISBN: 90-5823-121-6

To our children: Alex, Kate, Bethan and Joshua

CONTENTS

TABLES, ILLUSTRATIONS AND BOXES

FOREWORD

Epilepsy, perhaps more than any other medical disorder, is associated with profound deleterious psychological and sociological consequences that are not directly related to the actual disease process. Rather, severe disabilities result from the fear that an epileptic seizure might occur at some time in the future, and the negative public image associated with the diagnosis itself. Persons with epilepsy, who may be perfectly normal apart from the fact that epileptic seizures do, or might, occur from time to time, are commonly subjected to stringent limitations on their daily activities, ostensibly to protect them or others from injury or death. They may not be allowed to drive an automobile, an essential requirement for a satisfying social, if not vocational, life in most industrialised countries; they are often forbidden to take up certain types of employment or pursue some professional careers; and in many societies opportunities to marry and have a family are reduced or abolished if the condition becomes known. The fact that seizures occur without warning fosters a sense of insecurity that adversely affects healthy social development. Opportunities for satisfying interpersonal relationships are further compromised when seizures begin in childhood and parents adopt an overprotective attitude that prevents acquisition of skills required for a full independent life. Finally, persons with epilepsy have been reviled throughout the ages in most cultures as possessed by demons, insane, infectious, or pitiless sinners undergoing righteous punishment. Such stigmas persist to some degree throughout the world, including the industrialised countries, and continue to sufficiently plague persons with epilepsy to the extent that they prefer not to admit to their disorder if they can at all avoid detection.

Persons with epilepsy seek medical help not because they have seizures, but because their seizures interfere with their potential for a full and satisfying life. Until recently, the primary, or sole, focus of the medical profession towards persons with epilepsy has been their seizures, with the assumption that drugs, surgery, or other interventions that reduce or eliminate the offending ictal events will suffice in resolving their patient's unacceptable predicament. There is now abundant evidence that this is in fact untrue; many persons with epilepsy who no longer have seizures continue to be significantly disabled due to some or all of the negative psychological and sociological consequences cited previously. These disabilities can often be reduced or eliminated by appropriate type and timing of antiepileptic intervention; psychological, psychiatric, and social counselling; and public education. Happily, research in this area of epilepsy care has burgeoned in the past decade, and progress has been greatly enhanced by the creation of instruments to quantitatively measure health-related quality of life. Consequently, in most major epilepsy centres today, effectiveness of treatment is no longer measured only by frequency of seizures, but also by the impact treatment has had on the patients' perception of improvements in their predicament, and ultimately by their capacity to live independent, fulfilling lives. This book summarises the tremendous progress that has been made in this field of epilepsy research over the past few years, and testifies to the importance of the concept of quality of life outcomes when designing new approaches to help persons with epilepsy in the future.

Jerome Engel Jr.

PREFACE

Our interest in the subject matter of this book began more than a decade ago, when one of our co-authors, Professor David Chadwick, recruited us to work with him on studies of the impact of epilepsy and its treatment. We would like to thank him for recognising that social scientists have an important contribution to make to understanding this complex condition and for giving us the opportunity to develop a research programme around it. Our thanks also to Cath Brennand at the Centre for Health Services Research in the University of Newcastle and Jayne Brooks in the Department of Neurosciences at the Walton Centre, Liverpool, for their excellent editorial skills and support; to Harwood Academic Publishers for their commitment to the project and enduring support; and all those people with epilepsy who have contributed to our various studies over the years.

Since we began working in this field, the science of quality of life has developed enormously. There is now a much clearer understanding of the concept, how quality of life can be measured and how such measures can be applied to answering important clinical questions. These developments have been as significant for epilepsy as for other chronic conditions. The topic of quality of life is now a regular feature at national and international meetings on epilepsy and increasing numbers of publications focus on it.

This volume seeks to draw together current knowledge and understanding of quality of life issues in epilepsy, both substantive and methodological. We are fortunate that over the years we have developed a network of colleagues who are experts in this field. We are privileged that they have agreed to be our co-authors. Their diverse backgrounds testify to the importance of a multidisciplinary approach to this topic. We are sure their contributions will inform, educate, stimulate and occasionally provoke.

At the heart of this volume and our research is the conviction that patients have an important role to play in clinical decision-making and that their perspectives must be heard. We hope this volume will contribute to that process.

LIST OF CONTRIBUTORS

Albert P. Aldenkamp
Head of Behavioural Research, Head of Child Neurologic Programme for Children with Learning Disabilities and Professor of Neuropsychological Aspects of Learning Disabilities, Department of Behavioural Science and Psychological Services Epilepsy Centre, Kempenhaeghe and Faculty of Social and Behavioural Sciences, University of Amsterdam, The Netherlands

Joan K. Austin
Distinguished Professor, Indiana University School of Nursing, Indianapolis, IN, USA

Kathy Bairstow
Advice and Information Officer, British Epilepsy Association, Leeds, UK

Gus A. Baker
Senior Lecturer in Clinical Neuropsychology, University Department of Neurosciences, Walton Centre for Neurology and Neurosurgery, Liverpool, UK

Tim Betts
Reader in Psychiatry and Clinical Director, Birmingham University Seizure Clinic, Queen Elizabeth Psychiatric Hospital, Birmingham, UK

Malachy Bishop
Doctoral Fellow, Department of Rehabilitation Psychology, University of Wisconsin, USA

Monika Bullinger
Professor of Medical Psychology, Institute for Medical Psychology, Hamburg, Germany

David Chadwick
Professor of Neurology, University Department of Neurosciences, Walton Centre for Neurology and Neurosurgery, Liverpool, UK

Simon J. De Groot
General Practitioner, St John's Group Practice, Doncaster, UK

David W. Dunn
Associate Professor of Psychiatry and Neurology, Division of Child and Adolescent Psychiatry, Indiana University School of Medicine, Indianapolis, IN, USA

Colin A. Espie
Professor of Clinical Psychology and Head of Department of Psychological Medicine, University of Glasgow, Glasgow, UK

Janet Follett
Member, Council of Management, British Epilepsy Association, Leeds, UK

Dennis D. Gagnon
Assistant Director, ICOM Health Economics, Johnson and Johnson, Raritan, NJ, USA

Patricia A. Gibson
Associate Professor and Director, Epilepsy Information Service, Department of Neurology, Wake Forest University School of Medicine, Winston-Salem, NC, USA

Laura H. Goldstein
Reader in Neuropsychology, Institute of Psychiatry, London
and Honorary Consultant Clinical Psychologist, Lishman Neuropsychiatry Unit, Maudsley Hospital, London, UK

Sabine Heel
Doctoral Student, Institute for Medical Psychology, Ludwig-Maximilians-Universität, Munich, Germany

Marc Hendriks
Neuropsychologist and Senior Researcher, Epilepsy Centre, Breda
and Nijmegen Institute of Cognition and Information, University of Nijmegen, The Netherlands

Bruce Hermann
Professor of Neuropsychology, Department of Neurology, University of Wisconsin, Madison, WI, USA

Ann Jacoby
Professor of Medical Sociology, Department of Primary Care, University of Liverpool, Liverpool, UK

Mike Kerr
Senior Lecturer in Neuropsychiatry, Welsh Centre for Learning Disabilities, University of Wales College of Medicine, Cardiff, UK

John-Paul Leach
Specialist Registrar in Neurology and Neurophysiology, University Department of Neurosciences, Walton Centre for Neurology and Neurosurgery, Liverpool, UK

Veronica Leach
Research Registrar in Neurology, University Department of Neurosciences, Walton Centre for Neurology and Neurosurgery, Liverpool, UK

Philip Lee
Chief Executive, British Epilepsy Association, Leeds, UK

Harry W. McConnell
Locum Consultant, The Centre for Epilepsy, Maudsley Hospital, London, UK

Pauline McNulty
Senior Director, ICOM Health Economics, Johnson and Johnson, Raritan, NJ, USA

Stefan K.F. Schwabe
Senior Director and Global Product Leader, The RW Johnson Pharmaceutical Research Institute, Raritan, NJ, USA

Peter J. Snyder
Associate Director, Outcomes Research Group, Pfizer Central Research, Hartford, CT, USA

Anne Sweeney
CNS Paediatric Epilepsy, Alder Hey Children's Hospital, Liverpool, UK

Raymond C. Tallis
Professor of Geriatric Medicine, Department of Geriatric Medicine, Hope Hospital, Salford, UK

Nicole von Steinbüchel
Professor of Psychology, Institute for Medical Psychology, Ludwig-Maximilians-Universität, Munich, Germany

Chapter 1

THE PROBLEM OF EPILEPSY

Ann Jacoby and Gus A. Baker

Though known as 'the sacred disease' to the ancient Greeks, epilepsy has much more often been associated with negative and pejorative imagery. Across time and different cultures, it has variously been viewed as the outcome of sin, as the product of demonic possession and as a form of madness, and consequently as a condition to be feared and rejected. The treatment of people with epilepsy throughout history has been a reflection of this. Legal and statutory restrictions on people with epilepsy are centuries old and universal and surveys of public opinion carried out during this century suggest that the ancient myths and superstitions about the nature of epilepsy still linger (Dell, 1986). Given the historical reality of epilepsy, it is not surprising that people with epilepsy continue to regard their condition as potentially, if not actually, stigmatising and to report that it has a fundamental impact on their quality of life.

Another defining quality of epilepsy is uncertainty. A person with epilepsy faces a whole range of clinical uncertainties, over the diagnosis, over whether and when seizures will occur, over the nature of seizures and how best they can be controlled and over whether or not they will ultimately remit. Living with a diagnosis of epilepsy involves managing that clinical uncertainty by balancing available options and possible choices, including over the matter of treatment. The unpredictability of the nature and course of epilepsy is a key factor that impacts on the quality of life of people who develop it.

There is a substantial literature documenting the various ways in which the socio-historical and clinical realities of epilepsy affect the lives of those living with it. Epilepsy is known to be associated with increased mortality and morbidity, impaired psychological functioning and reduced social functioning. The diverse ways in which the impact of epilepsy is felt means that people with epilepsy find themselves in 'a particular predicament' (Taylor, 1989) to which they must somehow adapt and adjust. The diagnosis of epilepsy involves learning to cope with the physical impact of seizures and the medications prescribed to control them; with the limitations imposed by statute, which may have major implications for social functioning and employment; with the limitations imposed by prejudice, fear and lack of understanding by others; and with the impact on the psyche. Not surprisingly, this challenge proves easier for some people than others.

THE CLINICAL REALITY OF EPILEPSY

Epilepsy is one of the most common neurological disorders, with an age-adjusted incidence of between 20 and 70 per 100,000 and a prevalence of 4 to 10 per 1000. It is estimated that around 50 million people have epilepsy world-wide, with rates somewhat higher in the developing than in the developed world (Bharucha and Shorvon, 1997). Epilepsy is no longer seen as a single disorder, but a group of disorders in which seizures recur. Understanding that this is the case has led neurologists to develop a classification of epileptic syndromes (ILAE, 1989) in which a range of factors including seizure type, neurological history, family history, age of seizure onset and aetiology are considered. The most important subdivision of the epileptic syndromes is between those with a recognisable cause, the 'symptomatic' epilepsies and those without, the so-called cryptogenic or idiopathic epilepsies. It is often a cause of considerable frustration and distress to people with epilepsy that in around 60–70% of cases, there is no identifiable cause for epilepsy (though a number of main causes have been identified for both children and adults). On a more positive note, they can take comfort in evidence from recent epidemiological studies that suggest that for most people with epilepsy, the outlook is excellent. Around 70–80% of those newly diagnosed with epilepsy will enter remission shortly after embarking on antiepileptic treatment (Sander, 1993).

Another aspect of epilepsy which surprises many lay people, both with and without epilepsy, is that there are many different types of epileptic seizure. The classification discussed by Leach and colleagues in Chapter 2 divides seizures into two groups: partial seizures, in which only one hemisphere of the brain is involved; and generalised seizures, where there is no evidence of localised onset. Seizures can also be differentiated according to whether or not they involve any alteration or impairment of consciousness. Because different seizures manifest themselves so differently, they also vary in the degree to which they present a risk to physical safety, their predictability, their responsiveness to treatment and their stigma potential; and so in relation to the views of those experiencing them about the degree of their severity.

For clinicians treating individuals who present with possible seizures or epilepsy, there are a number of fundamental definitional difficulties. These include: what constitutes a seizure; which seizures should be considered in the diagnosis of epilepsy; whether or not a first or single seizure constitutes epilepsy; whether someone whose seizures recur only rarely should be considered as having epilepsy; and whether a person whose seizures are in long term remission still has epilepsy. All these questions are debated at some length in the key medical texts on epilepsy. The important point here from the viewpoint of the person concerned is that these definitional uncertainties mean that clinicians decide under what circumstances the label 'epilepsy' should be applied largely on the basis of clinical observation and interpretation.

Historically, treatment for seizures and epilepsy has included exorcism and the invoking of the gods, blood letting, purging, dietary restrictions, herbal remedies and surgery. It could be argued that therapy reached a somewhat more sophisticated level after the use of bromides was introduced in the mid-1850s. The first 'modern' antiepileptic agent was developed in the last century, called phenobarbitone because it was first synthesised on St Barbara's Day in 1864 (Scott, 1993). Currently antiepileptics constitute the major treatment approach, with four novel agents licensed for use in the UK over the last eight years. The advent of the new antiepileptics has shifted neurological thinking away from the view that polytherapy is almost always undesirable to one of the possibility of drug combinations with 'synergistic properties' (Chadwick, 1994). The vexed questions of whether and when to start antiepileptic drug treatment are considered by Leach and his colleagues in Chapter 2. Available evidence suggests that following an initial unprovoked seizure, as many as 61% of affected individuals will experience a recurrence, with most second seizures occurring within a year of the first (Hauser and Hesdorffer, 1990). Reynolds (1995) has argued the case for early treatment on the grounds that epilepsy is a process with the potential to become intractable and early treatment reduces the likelihood of this happening. The counter-argument is that studies of specific epileptic syndromes suggest that antiepileptics may not have any real effect on clinical outcome (Chadwick, 1995). Given that there is a considerable body of research (presented in Chapters 2 and 3) into the adverse cognitive, behavioural other systemic and teratogenic effects of antiepileptics, it is important that people with epilepsy are given adequate information about them. They can then more realistically balance the costs of such effects against the possible psychosocial consequences of continuing seizures when deciding whether to start or stop treatment (Jacoby *et al.*, 1992, 1993).

Recent developments in brain imaging mean that surgery is increasingly seen as a viable treatment option. It has been estimated that surgery could reasonably be offered to between five and 10% of people with focal epilepsy unresponsive to antiepileptic medications (CSAG, 2000). The clinical outcome for epilepsy surgery is good, with success rates approaching 70% (Engel *et al.*, 1993). Successful surgery can also result in spectacular improvements in quality of life (CSAG, 2000 and see Chapter 6). However, it is clear that the one does not automatically follow from the other and the matter of surgical candidates' expectations of their surgery figures large in the likely quality of life outcome (Wilson *et al.*, 1998).

THE SOCIAL REALITY OF EPILEPSY

The view of epilepsy as first and foremost a social label, rather than a medical or organic certainty, is firmly routed in the work of writers such as Falk and Gorman (1972), Schneider and Conrad (1981, 1983), Scambler (1984, 1989) and West (1979, 1986). Central to the work of all these authors is the emphasis on the stigmatising nature of epilepsy and the status role of being an 'epileptic'. The person with epilepsy is required to take on the whole history of its stigma, such that having epilepsy is seen as far worse than simply having seizures (Schneider and Conrad, 1983). In all these studies, beliefs about the social meaning of epilepsy impinged not just on the attitudes to its diagnosis of those affected, but also on their subsequent behaviour. Scambler (1989) reports that many people try to capitalise on the clinical uncertainty surrounding their condition to deny or renegotiate the diagnosis; and where unable to do so, opt to conceal it from others. Schneider and Conrad reported that the people in their study developed both preventive strategies to combat the likelihood of them having seizures and defensive strategies for occasions when they did so. Other family members too appear to make assumptions about the stigmatising nature of epilepsy (West, 1979) and may even take on the role of 'stigma coaches' to their relative with epilepsy.

Recent studies in the developed world have tended to present a less than favourable picture of lay attitudes to epilepsy. People with epilepsy are characterised in such studies as antisocial, excitable, aggressive and potentially violent, weak and physically unattractive (Vinson, 1975;

Harrison and West, 1977; Scambler, 1983). Surveys in the developing world demonstrate that such negative views are held even more strongly and with more devastating effect (Adamolekun, 1999). Encouragingly, there is also evidence that public attitudes, in the developed world at least, are improving (Caveness and Gallup, 1980; Canger and Cornaggia, 1985; Jensen and Dam, 1992). Nonetheless, many people with epilepsy appear unconvinced and continue to hold the view that their condition is one against which prejudice persists (Scambler, 1989). This perception of the way they are viewed by others can, not surprisingly, have important implications for the psychological well-being of people with epilepsy. A number of studies have found a relationship between the degree to which those affected feel stigmatised by their epilepsy and reported problems such as anxiety, depression, self-esteem and life satisfaction (Arnston *et al.*, 1986; Jacoby *et al.*, 1996; Baker *et al.*, 1997). Even among people whose epilepsy is in remission, feelings of stigma can persist (Jacoby, 1994), supporting Friedson's (1970) view of stigma as ineradicable and irreversible. The finding that feelings of stigma are largely unrelated to any clinical features of epilepsy (Westbrook *et al.*, 1992; Jacoby, 1994) only serves to emphasise the power of its social reality.

THE IMPACT OF EPILEPSY ON QUALITY OF LIFE

From the discussion so far, it should be clear that for the person so diagnosed, the problem of epilepsy is one with the potential to have a significant impact on quality of life. Some of the ways in which epilepsy impacts are common to all chronic illnesses (Turk, 1979; Bury, 1982, 1988; Conrad, 1990); others are the product of epilepsy *per se*. In Chapter 6, Hermann provides a detailed review of the many and diverse ways in which epilepsy has been shown to affect the quality of life of adults with the condition, at the level of their physical, psychological and social functioning. Chapters 7 by Dunn and Austin, 8 by Tallis and 9 by Espie and Kerr address quality of life issues as they pertain to children and adolescents, older people and people with complex epilepsy accompanied by learning disability. Among the most significant effects are, first, that it is associated with increased mortality, particularly among people with symptomatic epilepsy and those who have generalised seizures (Hauser and Hesdorffer, 1990). Second, epilepsy is associated with increased morbidity, both as a result of seizure-related accidents and injuries (Buck *et al.*, 1997) and as an outcome of the adverse effects of antiepileptic medication (Shorvon,

1987; Aldenkamp, 1995). The prevalence of psychological morbidity has been shown to be substantially higher among people with epilepsy than those without (Fenwick, 1987), particularly of anxiety and depression, which frequently co-exist, but also of rather more rare psychiatric disorders (see the reviews by Aldenkamp and Hendriks in Chapter 3 and Hermann in Chapter 6). Reduced self-esteem has been reported among people with epilepsy (Collings, 1990), as has reduced sense of mastery (Matthews and Barabas, 1986). Social withdrawal and consequent social isolation have been documented for people with epilepsy (Lechtenberg, 1984), in part explaining the reported reduced rates of marriage and fertility among them. Reduced educational achievement, under and unemployment have all been shown to be more common among people with epilepsy than their non-epileptic peers (Hauser and Hesdorffer, 1990). What is clear from studies that have sought to disentangle the various contributory factors to these different impacts is that the clinical and social realities of epilepsy are often inextricably entwined. To focus on the former while disregarding the latter represents an over simplistic approach to an extremely complex subject.

MEASURING QUALITY OF LIFE

Though recognition of the effects epilepsy can have on quality of life is not new, attempts to quantify those effects are. The stimuli for this activity are political, philosophical and economic. Within the sphere of medicine, interest in quality of life measurement can be attributed to cultural and philosophical developments in western societies that have prompted criticism of the biomedical model and placed emphasis on a holistic approach to patient care (Levine, 1988). At the same time, a philosophy of 'enlightened consumerism' (Wenger, 1988) has permeated western health care systems. Financial constraints have also precipitated interest in the measurement of quality of life, which is now seen as representing an important element in the economic evaluation of any new health technology or intervention (Brazier *et al.*, 1999). Despite agreement in principle that measuring quality of life to assess the benefits of novel technologies is a good thing, there are still significant concerns about the reality of doing so. This reflects current conceptual and theoretical confusion and methodological difficulties, as outlined in Chapter 4. Despite the concerns, research activity in the area of epilepsy quality of life has burgeoned and a number of validated measures are now available. The current armoury of measures includes ones developed for use with specific subgroups of people with epilepsy, such as those who are newly diagnosed and those undergoing surgery, thus acknowledging that quality of life issues may vary across the disease trajectory and at different life stages. Measures for use in adults are examined in Chapter 5 by von Steinbuchel and colleagues, whose rigorous assessment of their psychometric properties and robustness should make choosing one an easier task for the reader.

As the science of quality of life advances, so does the use of quality of life measures in different settings. In Chapter 12, Baker describes the growing application of such measures to assess treatment outcomes in epilepsy, a development supported by all the major international funding bodies. Appreciation of the current political agenda and the market potential of quality of life measurement means that the pharmaceutical industry is also showing intense interest in this area, as documented by McNulty and colleagues in Chapter 13. One other rather more contentious area of interest described in Chapter 11 is the possible application of quality of life measures to everyday clinical practice. While not a substitute for good clinical care, their use, McDonnell and Snyder argue, can facilitate patient-professional interactions and so enhance understanding of the problem of epilepsy from the patient's viewpoint. However, as in all things, their unquestioned application can never be justified and it is incumbent on those who advocate them to acknowledge their limitations. Chapter 10 by Betts will, hopefully, encourage potential users to judge carefully their value within the context of the clinical encounter. Since quality of life measures are, in the main, validated only for use in groups of people with epilepsy, they may be of limited relevance and inappropriate in managing individual patients.

IMPROVING QUALITY OF LIFE FOR PEOPLE WITH EPILEPSY

At the heart of this book are the personal accounts from Follett (Chapter 14) and Bairstow (Chapter 15) of what it means to be living with epilepsy. Though honest about the difficulties, they are nonetheless optimistic about the ability of people with epilepsy to cope with their condition. The ways in which the various health professionals involved in epilepsy care can help them do so and so contribute to an improved quality of life is eloquently addressed in Chapters 16–19. Management of chronic conditions such as epilepsy is now seen as primarily the responsibility of primary care. De Groot examines the important role the primary care practitioner can play in Chapter 16. The nurse specialist represents another important care initiative and though epilepsy has been slow to emulate the experience of conditions such as asthma and diabetes, the concept of the epilepsy nurse specialist is gaining considerable support (see Chapter 18). The complementary roles of the clinical psychologist and social worker are described in Chapters 17 and 19. One other source of support, and an increasingly vociferous voice for epilepsy, is the patient support group. There is now a world-wide network of such groups, the International Bureau for Epilepsy. In Chapter 20, its current president draws on his own experience as Chief Executive of the British Branch to write about the contribution such pressure groups can make to improving the quality of life of people with epilepsy.

THE CHALLENGE OF QUALITY OF LIFE RESEARCH

We hope that the limitations of focussing only on the clinical aspects of epilepsy will be sufficiently well highlighted in the chapters that follow and that our readers will acknowledge the need for wider assessments of the impact of health care for this condition. We invite them to consider the contents of this book and decide for themselves the merits and demerits of using quality of life measures in research and clinical settings. Even those who remain unconvinced will, we hope, recognise the imperative behind our own and other researchers' efforts to promote the issue of quality of life as an integral aspect of the management of epilepsy. Quality of life research places the perspective of persons with epilepsy centre-stage. By doing so, it enables them to have a genuine role in the decision-making process and challenges the sometimes unfounded assumptions made by health care providers about what does and does not constitute a good outcome of care.

References

Adamolekun, B. (1999) Living with epilepsy in the developing countries. *Epilepsia*, **40**(Suppl.2), S213. Keynote presentation given at the 23rd International Epilepsy Congress, Prague, Sept 1999.

Aldenkamp, A.P. (1995) The impact of epilepsy on cognitive development and learning behaviour. In: Aldenkamp, A.P., Dreiffus, F.E., Renier, W.O., Suurmeijer, Th.P.B.M. (eds.) *Epilepsy in Children and Adolescents*. Boca Raton: CRC Press, 225–238.

Arnston, P., Drodge, D., Norton, R., Murray, E. (1986) The perceived psychosocial consequences of having epilepsy. In: Whitman, S., Hermann, B. (eds.) *Psychopathology in Epilepsy: Social Dimensions*. Oxford: Oxford University Press, 143–161.

Baker, G.A., Jacoby, A., Buck, D., Stalgis, C., Monnet, D. (1997) Quality of life of people with epilepsy: a European study. *Epilepsia*; **38**, 353–362.

Bharucha, N.E., Shorvon, S.D. (1997) Epidemiology in developing countries. In: Engel, J Jr., Pedley, T.A. (eds.) *Epilepsy: A Comprehensive Textbook*. Philadelphia: Lippincott-Raven, 105–118.

Brazier, J., Deverill, M., Green, C., Harper, R., Booth, A. (1999) A review of the use of health status measures in economic evaluation. *Health Technology Assessment*; Vol. 3 No. 9.

Buck, D., Baker, G.A., Jacoby, A., Chadwick, D. (1997) Patients' experiences of injury as a result of epilepsy. *Epilepsia*; **38**, 439–444.

Bury, M. (1982) Chronic illness as biographical disruption. *Sociology of Health and Illness*; **4**(2), 167–182.

Bury, M. (1988) Meanings at risk: the experience of arthritis. In: Anderson, R. and Bury, M. (eds.) Living with chronic illness: The experience of patients and their families. London: Unwin Hyman.

Canger, R., Cornaggia, C. (1985) Public attitudes towards epilepsy in Italy: results of a survey and comparison with USA and West German data. *Epilepsia*; **26**, 221–226.

Caveness, W.F., Gallup, G.H. (1980) A survey of public attitudes towards epilepsy in 1979 with an indication of trends over the past thirty years. *Epilepsia*; **21**, 509–518.

Chadwick, D. (1994) Standard approach to antiepileptic drug treatment in the United Kingdom. *Epilepsia*; **35**(Suppl. 4), S3-S10.

Chadwick, D. (1995) Do anticonvulsants alter the natural course of epilepsy? Case for early treatment is not established. *British Medical Journal*; **310**, 176–178.

Collings, J. (1990) Psychosocial well-being and epilepsy: an empirical study. *Epilepsia*; **31**, 418–426.

Conrad, P. (1990) Qualitative research on chronic illness: a commentary on method and conceptual development. *Social Science and Medicine*; **30**, 1257–1263.

CSAG (Clinical Standards Advisory Group) (2000) *Epilepsy: a report by the Clinical Standards Advisory Group*. London: HMSO.

Dell, J.L. (1986) Social dimensions of epilepsy: stigma and response. In: Whitman, S., Hermann, B. (eds.) *Psychopathology in Epilepsy: Social Dimensions*. Oxford: Oxford University Press, 185–210.

Engel, J., van Ness, P.C., Rasmussen, T.B., Ojemann, L.M. (1993) Outcome with respect to epileptic seizures. In: Engel, J. (ed.) *Surgical treatment of the epilepsies*. New York: Raven Press, 609–621.

Falk, G. and Gorman, J. (1972) The epileptic: a study in status-role relations. Australian *Journal of Social Issues*; **7**, 56–66.

Fenwick, P. (1987) Epilepsy and psychiatric disorders. In: Hopkins, A. (ed.) *Epilepsy*. London: Chapman & Hall.

Friedson, E. (1970) *Profession of Medicine: A Study of the Sociology of Applied Knowledge*. New York: Russell Sage Foundation.

Harrison, R., West, P. (1977) Images of a grand mal. *New Society*; **40**, 762–782.

Hauser, W.A., Hesdorffer, D.C. (1990) *Epilepsy: Frequency, Causes and Consequences*. Maryland, US: Epilepsy Foundation of America.

ILAE (1989) Commission on Classification and Terminology of the International League against Epilepsy. Proposal for revised classification of epilepsies and epileptic syndromes. *Epilepsia*; **30**, 389–399.

Jacoby, A. (1994) Felt versus enacted stigma: a concept revisited. *Social Science and Medicine*; **38**, 261–274.

Jacoby, A., Johnson, A.L., Chadwick, D.W. (1992) Psychosocial outcomes of antiepileptic drug discontinuation. *Epilepsia*; **33**, 1123–1131.

Jacoby, A., Baker, G.A., Chadwick, D.W., Johnson, A.L. (1993) The impact of counselling with a practical statistical model on patients' decision-making about treatment for epilepsy. *Epilepsy Research*; **16**, 207–214.

Jacoby, A., Baker, G.A., Steen, N., Potts, P., Chadwick, D.W. (1996) The clinical course of epilepsy and its psychosocial correlates: findings from a UK community study. *Epilepsia*; **37**, 148–161.

Jensen, R. and Dam, M. (1992) Public attitudes towards epilepsy in Denmark. *Epilepsia*; **33**, 459–463.

Lechtenberg, R. (1984) *Epilepsy and the Family*. Cambridge, Massachusetts: Harvard University Press.

Levine, M.N. (1988) Quality of life in Stage II breast cancer: an instrument for clinical trials. *Journal of Clinical Oncology*; **6**, 1798–1810.

Matthews, W.S., Barabas, G. (1986) Perceptions of control among children with epilepsy. In: Whitman, S., Hermann, B.P. (eds.) *Psychopathology in Epilepsy: Social Dimensions*. New York: Oxford University Press, 162–184.

Reynolds, E.H. (1995) Do anticonvulsants alter the natural course of epilepsy? Treatment should be started as early as possible. *British Medical Journal*; **310**, 176–178.

Sander, J.W.A.S. (1993) Some aspects of prognosis in the epilepsies: a review. *Epilepsia*; **34**, 1007–1016.

Scambler, G. (1983) PhD Thesis: *Being Epileptic: Sociology of a Stigmatising Condition*. London: University of London.

Scambler, G. (1984) Perceiving and coping with stigmatising illness. In: Fitzpatrick, R., Hinton, J., Newman, S., Scambler, G., Thompson, J. (eds.) *The Experience of Illness*. London: Tavistock.

Scambler, G. (1989) *Epilepsy*. London: Tavistock.

Schneider, J.W. and Conrad, P. (1981) Medical and sociological typologies: the case of epilepsy. *Social Science and Medicine*; **15A**, 211–219.

Schneider, J.W. and Conrad, P. (1983) *Having Epilepsy: The Experience and Control of Illness*. Philadelphia: Temple University Press.

Scott, D.F. (1993) *The history of epileptic therapy: an account of how medication was developed*. Carnforth, Lancs: Pantheon.

Shorvon, S.D. (1987) The treatment of epilepsy by drugs. In: Hopkins, A. (ed.) *Epilepsy*. London: Chapman and Hall.

Taylor, D.C. (1989) Psychosocial components of childhood epilepsy. In: Hermann, B.P., Seidenberg, M. (eds.) *Childhood Epilepsies: Neuropsychological, Psychosocial and Intervention Aspects*. Chichester: John Wiley and Sons, 119–142.

Turk, D.C. (1979) Factors influencing the adaptive process with chronic illness. In: Sarason, A., Spielberger, C.D. (eds.) *Stress and Anxiety*. Washington DC. Halsted Press.

Vinson, T. (1975) Towards demythologising epilepsy. *Medical Journal of Australia*; **2**, 663–666.

Wenger, N.K. (1988) QOL: *Why the burgeoning interest in clinical and research cardiology communities?* Second Workshop on QOL and cardiovascular disease. Co-sponsored by National Health, Lifestyle and Behaviour Institute and Bowman Gray School of Medicine.

West, P. (1979) PhD Thesis: *Investigation into the social construction and consequences of the label 'epilepsy'*. University of Bristol.

West, P. (1986) The Social Meaning of Epilepsy: Stigma as a Potential Explanation for Psychopathology in Children. In: Whitman, S., Hermann, B.P. (eds.) *Psychopathology in epilepsy: social dimensions*. New York: Oxford University Press, 245–266.

Westbrook, L.E., Bauman, L.J., Shinnar, S. (1992) Applying stigma theory to epilepsy: a test of a conceptual model. *Journal of Pediatric Psychology*; **15**, 633–649.

Wilson, S.J., Saling, M.M., Kincade, P., Bladin, P.F. (1998) Patient expectations of temporal lobe surgery. *Epilepsia*; **39**, 167–174.

CLINICAL MANAGEMENT OF EPILEPSY

Chapter 2

MANAGEMENT OF EPILEPSY: FROM DIAGNOSIS TO INTRACTABILITY

John Paul Leach, Veronica Leach, and David Chadwick

Epilepsy encompasses a spectrum of disorders which together constitute one of the most common neurological diseases seen in man: at its most benign it may manifest as a few self-limiting episodes, while at its worst it can lead to frequent, disruptive, disabling seizures which may be refractory to drug treatment. Many pathologies underlie these bursts of abnormal neuronal activity which result essentially from an imbalance between neuronal excitation and inhibition, either locally or generally throughout the brain. With the lifetime prevalence of seizures and epilepsy exceeding 5% of any given population (Shorvon, 1990), epilepsy may be seen not as a rare curse befalling the individual, but as the price that man and other vertebrates pay for maintaining a plastic and adaptable central nervous system.

SEIZURES: A DEFINITION

A seizure can be defined as an episode of neuronal hyperactivity. The clinical effects of such hyperactivity depend on the functions that the neurones normally serve; seizure activity in neurones responsible for processing sensation will cause sensory symptoms such as tingling or burning, while similar activity in motor neurones will cause twitching or shaking. Spread of such activity will lead to spread of symptoms, culminating in some cases in generalised tonic-clonic convulsions. Clinically, seizures can take a variety of forms, most (but not all) of which, will lead at some stage to a loss of awareness of the environment.

DIAGNOSIS OF EPILEPSY

The diagnostic criteria for epilepsy have remained unchanged for many years, and require that there have been at least two seizures which are unrelated to any other illness or metabolic upset (Chadwick, 1990). In many cases, the picture is straightforward, allowing the diagnosis of epilepsy to be made by the first doctor who is consulted about the attacks. Often, however, caution has to be exercised in ensuring that the diagnostic label is not applied hastily, especially in view of the social implications of a diagnosis of epilepsy (see chapters 3 and 6).

As with other medical conditions, an adequate history is often the most important diagnostic tool (Chadwick, 1990). Where awareness is lost or impaired during attacks, such a history will be required from a third party witness such as a friend or relative. At the first visit to the epilepsy clinic, patients should bring such an eye witness along so that details of the attack's prodrome, duration, and main clinical features are available to the doctor at an early stage. The most useful information available from patients themselves usually concerns the nature of any aura, or the post-ictal symptoms.

The definition of a seizure given above is necessarily vague, since the manifestations of seizures are so very variable. There are a few classification systems currently in use, the most comprehensive of which is the classification by the Commission of the International League Against Epilepsy (ILAE, 1989; Table 1). In everyday use, however, many clinicians still use one of the simplest, the classification of the ILAE Commission (1981; Table 2), which divides seizures into those originating from a localised abnormality in the cortex (partial or localisation-related seizures), and those arising from some innate, perhaps genetic abnormality in neuronal function (primary or idiopathic generalised seizures). The distinction between seizure types becomes important in planning the investigation and treatment of each patient: an adequate classification of seizures and syndromes will lead, where applicable, to consideration of any other pathology underlying the ictal events, which may themselves also require treatment other than antiepileptic drugs (for example — treatment of cerebral tumours or vascular malformations, etc.).

Occasionally, particularly where there is no good eye-witness history, where attacks occur infrequently, or where investigations are all normal, the diagnosis may remain obscure or uncertain. In such cases, there is no case for a 'trial of treatment' with antiepileptic drugs. The diagnosis of epilepsy should not be one of exclusion and, given the social, occupational, leisure, family and driving implications, it should not be entered into lightly.

INVESTIGATION OF EPILEPSY

While clinical history is of the utmost importance in the diagnosis of epilepsy, there are occasions when further investigations become imperative. Most patients will have an electroencephalogram (EEG) done at some stage to help characterise their epilepsy, but it should be borne in mind that, contrary to many doctors' expectations, the EEG is

TABLE 1 ILAE 1989 CLASSIFICATION OF EPILEPSY

1	LOCALISATION-RELATED EPILEPSIES AND SYNDROMES
1.1	*IDIOPATHIC (WITH AGE-RELATED ONSET)*
	• BENIGN CHILDHOOD EPILEPSY WITH CENTROTEMPORAL SPIKES
	• CHILDHOOD EPILEPSY WITH OCCIPITAL PAROXYSMS
	• PRIMARY READING EPILEPSY
1.2	*SYMPTOMATIC*
	• TEMPORAL LOBE EPILEPSIES
	• FRONTAL LOBE EPILEPSIES
	• PARIETAL LOBE EPILEPSIES
	• OCCIPITAL LOBE EPILEPSIES
	• CHRONIC PROGRESSIVE EPILEPSIA PARIALIS CONTINUA OF CHILDHOOD (KOJEWNIKOW'S SYNDROME)
	• SYNDROMES CHARACTERISED BY SEIZURES WITH SPECIFIC MODES OF PRECIPITATION (E.G. REFLEX EPILEPSIES)
1.3	*CRYPTOGENIC*
	• AS IN 1.2, BUT LACK OF AETIOLOGICAL EVIDENCE
2	GENERALISED EPILEPSIES AND SYNDROMES
2.1	*IDIOPATHIC (WITH AGE-RELATED ONSET — LISTED IN ORDER OF AGE OF ONSET)*
	• BENIGN NEONATAL FAMILIAL CONVULSIONS
	• BENIGN NEONATAL CONVULSIONS
	• BENIGN MYOCLONIC EPILEPSY IN INFANCY
	• CHILDHOOD ABSENCE EPILEPSY
	• JUVENILE ABSENCE EPILEPSY
	• JUVENILE MYOCLONIC EPILEPSY
	• EPILEPSY WITH GRAND MAL SEIZURE ON AWAKENING
	• OTHER GENERALISED EPILEPSIES
	• EPILEPSIES PRECIPITATED BY SPECIFIC MODES OF ACTIVATION
2.2	*CRYPTOGENIC OR SYMPTOMATIC (IN ORDER OF AGE OF ONSET)*
	• WEST SYNDROME (INFANTILE SPASMS)
	• LENNOX-GASTAUT SYNDROME
	• EPILEPSY WITH MYOCLONIC ASTATIC SEIZURES
	• EPILEPSY WITH MYOCLONIC ABSENCES
2.3	*SYMPTOMATIC*
	2.3.1 NON SPECIFIC AETIOLOGY
	• EARLY MYOCLONIC ENCEPHALOPATHY
	• EARLY INFANTILE EPILEPTIC ENCEPHALOPATHY WITH SUPPRESSION BURST
	• OTHER SYMPTOMATIC GENERALISED EPILEPSIES NOT DEFINED ABOVE
	2.3.2 SPECIFIC SYNDROMES
	• SEIZURES AS PRESENTATION OF OTHER DISEASES
3	EPILEPSIES AND SYNDROMES UNDETERMINED TO BE FOCAL OR GENERALISED
3.1	*WITH BOTH FOCAL AND GENERALISED SEIZURES*
	• NEONATAL SEIZURES
	• SEVERE MYOCLONIC EPILEPSY IN INFANCY
	• EPILEPSY WITH CONTINUOUS SPIKE-WAVES DURING SW SLEEP
	• ACQUIRED EPILEPTIC APHASIA
	• OTHER UNDETERMINED EPILEPSIES NOT MENTIONED ABOVE
3.2	*WITHOUT EQUIVOCAL FEATURES OF GENERALISATION OR FOCAL SEIZURE*
4	SPECIAL SYNDROMES
4.1	*SITUATION-RELATED SEIZURES*
	• FEBRILE CONVULSIONS
	• ISOLATED SEIZURES OR ISOLATED STATUS EPILEPTICUS
	• SEIZURE ONLY IN THE PRESENCE OF AN ACUTE METABOLIC OR TOXIC EVENT

TABLE 2 1981 ILAE SEIZURE CLASSIFICATION (SAMPLE)

I. PARTIAL EPILEPSIES	II. PRIMARY GENERALISED EPILEPSIES	III. UNCLASSIFIABLE EPILEPSIES
SIMPLE PARTIAL COMPLEX PARTIAL SECONDARY GENERALISED	TYPICAL ABSENCE SEIZURES ATYPICAL ABSENCES TONIC SEIZURES CLONIC SEIZURES MYOCLONIC SEIZURES TONIC-CLONIC UNCLASSIFIED	

more useful in classifying epilepsies than in differentiating them from other causes of episodic symptoms. There is evidence that EEGs soon after the first presentation of epilepsy are helpful in classification of seizures (King *et al.*, 1998). While the interictal EEG can help place the site of the abnormality underlying seizures, a normal EEG does not exclude epilepsy. Conversely, other than epilepsy, there are many conditions, not all of them pathological, which may cause minor EEG changes, so an 'abnormal' EEG does not immediately signal the presence of epilepsy.

Seizures are intermittent, and it is no surprise that some patients with epilepsy will not demonstrate any abnormality on EEG, since it only provides a 'snapshot' of around 30 minutes of cerebral activity. The sensitivity of EEG can be enhanced significantly either by depriving the patient of sleep, or by carrying out long-term monitoring. This can be done with ambulatory systems, where several channels of cerebral activity are recorded for 24 hours at a time. Any potentially ictal symptoms can be flagged up by the patients and the relevant co-incident EEG tracings analysed later by the neurophysiologists.

The increasingly widespread use of video-telemetry has been of great help in the management of some patients. Using this system, the video and EEG features of attacks can be recorded. Both telemetry and ambulatory EEG are more expensive and require more input than 'normal' EEG, but in certain circumstances, both are of undoubted benefit, not only in diagnosing and classifying epilepsy, but also in differentiating epileptic from non-epileptic attacks. (Non-epileptic attacks are attacks which, though they resemble seizures, are not associated with abnormal neuronal excitation.)

Patients presenting later than 20 years of age, or those whose history is suggestive of a focal lesion, will have some form of radiological imaging (usually a CT (computerised tomography) scan) carried out to assess the gross cerebral anatomy (Chadwick, 1990). In their series of 154 patients presenting with partial epilepsy, King *et al.* (1998) showed 17% to have epileptogenic lesions on CT scanning. The yield was predictably higher with MRI (magnetic resonance imaging): nine of 28 patients had a surgically remediable lesion which was apparent on MRI but missed on CT. It should be pointed out that no patients with generalised epilepsy had a lesion on cerebral imaging, so it is not useful to provide imaging for patients in whom such a diagnosis is likely.

Occasionally metabolic disorders may need to be excluded as a cause of recurrent seizures, but this is rare in adult patients. In adults, other causes of loss of consciousness may need to be investigated by, for example, further cardiovascular investigation using ECG, echocardiography or 24 hour ECG.

TREATMENT OF EPILEPSY

In the UK at least, patients who have had a single seizure are not routinely treated with anticonvulsant drugs although, legally, they are still affected by some of the rules and restrictions regarding driving, employment and leisure. In most patients coming to the clinic, two or more unprovoked seizures will have occurred within an interval short enough to merit treatment. Problems do, however, arise in defining a short interval. Most clinicians would take this to mean a period less than 6 months to 1 year, but it may vary from patient to patient, occasionally depending on seizure type or on the patient's ambitions in relation to driving or other pursuits. In a few (rare) cases, the frequency and severity of seizures will be so low that treatment will not be necessary (Chadwick, 1998). Such patients may still remain under follow-up to allow easy access to medical facilities in the event of any deterioration. Even where seizures occur within a sufficiently short timespan, the identification of specific precipitating factors may make counselling and avoidance of risk factors more important than drug therapy. This may apply, for example, in childhood febrile convulsions, or alcohol-withdrawal seizures in adults (Chadwick, 1998). Less commonly, seizures may be precipitated in photosensitive subjects by television, visual display units or other photic stimuli. Avoidance of these may be enough to treat the condition.

Prior to starting antiepileptic drug (AED) treatment in those patients who require pharmacological redress, it is important that the patient understands the implications both of the diagnosis and its treatment. The choice of drug therapy will depend on seizure type, concomitant drug therapy, history of adverse events to other drugs, and gender (Brodie and Dichter, 1996; Dichter and Brodie, 1996).

PROGNOSIS OF EPILEPSY

Prognosis of the Single Seizure

When dealing with patients who have had a single seizure, giving a statistical measure of the likelihood of recurrence has always been difficult, since study methods have varied widely both in terms of speed of review after referral, and duration of follow up. Published recurrence rates have varied greatly (Chadwick, 1992) from 27 to 71%, but as a rule it is probably true that the recurrence rate in the adult patient who has had an isolated seizure with no further events in the first month is probably less than 50%. There has been work done which suggests that the risk of seizure recurrence is increased in the presence of neurological deficit, in those with partial seizures, those at the extremes of age and those with no precipitating factors (Hart *et al.*, 1990). Other studies have highlighted the adverse effect of peri-ictal neurological deficit, family history of epilepsy, generalised EEG abnormalities, and the absence of any acute insult (such as head injury or cerebrovascular accident) (Hauser *et al.*, 1990).

The generally low rate of recurrence justifies the tendency, in the UK at least, to investigate but not necessarily to treat the patient who has experienced only a single seizure. This practice varies elsewhere, particularly in the USA, where medical therapy is more likely to be started at an earlier stage (Hauser *et al.*, 1990).

Prognosis of treated epilepsy

Once the diagnosis has been made, particularly at an early stage, there are still good grounds for optimism. Most patients with epilepsy of recent onset will achieve a long-lasting remission soon after the start of therapy, with minimal side effects. One community-based study (Annegers *et al.*, 1979) showed that 61% of patients were in 5-year remission ten years after presentation, rising to 70% after 20 years. The rates have remained essentially unchanged throughout this century, despite the introduction of modern AEDs (Chadwick, 1992). Given that epilepsy may be seen not as a disease entity but as a lowering of the physiological seizure threshold, we can surmise that for many patients, the lowering of the threshold may only be clinically important for a relatively short time.

For such patients, circumstances may allow for drug withdrawal after two or more years of seizure freedom. Studies are underway to determine what factors can help predict when withdrawal of treatment is likely to succeed. There are algorithms available that can provide information on percentage risks of seizure recurrence depending on a number of factors (SIGN Guidelines, 1997). The factors important in these include the presence of EEG abnormalities, the occurrence of seizures while on medication, and the clinical classification of seizure type. This ability to provide patients and their families with information about the relative risks in withdrawing treatment can be of real help in aiding decision-making.

Other studies have looked at outcome related to the primary diagnosis. As a general rule, those patients with an idiopathic generalised seizure disorder will respond very well to treatment (Jeavons *et al.*, 1977). It would appear that over 80% of those with a clinical and electroencephalographic picture of an idiopathic generalised seizure disorder will be rendered seizure-free on treatment with sodium valproate. Although there is as yet little direct comparative work, lamotrigine may prove to be a reasonable alternative. In those patients with a symptomatic or cryptogenic epilepsy, in contrast, the response rates are somewhat less impressive. Patients experiencing partial seizures are less likely to experience remission than those with only tonic-clonic seizures. The worst prognosis would appear to be in those who have both partial and secondary generalised seizures (Chadwick, 1992).

Largely because of their relatively recent introduction, many studies of refractory patients do not take into account the possible contribution of the newer AEDs. Combining older AEDs has traditionally been seen as helping few patients while hindering many by causing a multitude of side effects. The truth is probably less dramatic, especially with the newer AEDs (Leach and Brodie, 1995); the careful use of combination treatment may be the only option for patients refractory to monotherapy. In essence, as treatments fail to induce freedom from seizures, a law of diminishing returns applies. At the more severe end of the spectrum, it has been estimated that some 20% of patients developing epilepsy have a chronic disorder which cannot be controlled by drugs (Chadwick, 1998). The effect of the newer AEDs in reducing this figure can only be guessed at, but for the most refractory group of patients a different strategy should be employed. Where the likelihood of seizure freedom is low, it may be more prudent not to pursue freedom from seizures, but instead to achieve a balance between reducing seizures and inducing side effects, with the minimum number of AEDs. This acknowledges the fact that drug-related adverse events, especially with AED polypharmacy, can in themselves be disabling and worrying.

Some patients may continue to experience seizures but not be disabled by them; they may have very infrequent seizures or seizures that are minor in their symptomatology or confined to sleep. In such patients, assuming that a single drug has been used appropriate to the seizure type and epilepsy syndrome, there is usually little to be gained from alternative drugs or additional drugs (Chadwick, 1998).

DRUG TREATMENT OF EPILEPSY

Antiepileptic drugs possess four distinct types of toxicity: acute dose-related toxicity, acute idiosyncratic toxicity, chronic toxicity and teratogenicity. The older drugs (Table 3) have been used as the mainstay of treatment for many years. Their long- term use is not without problems, however, and in the late eighties a new era of anticonvulsant therapy began (Table 4) using drugs that are generally much more specific in action, have fewer pharmacokinetic interactions, and have fewer adverse events than their older counterparts (Leach and Brodie 1995). Some of the new treatments have been shown to have efficacy that may be comparable with the older AEDs but most, in contrast, have yet to demonstrate this property, particularly with respect to gaining freedom from seizures (Walker and Sander 1996).

MONOTHERAPY OR POLYPHARMACY?

For any epilepsy patient, the ideal outcome would be seizure freedom while on no drug therapy. For some patients, as outlined above, particularly those with one of the more benign idiopathic generalised seizure disorders, this may be a realistic and attainable goal. For others, it would hopefully go without saying that they should be controlled on the lowest possible number of drugs at the lowest possible dose.

Patients who continue to be have seizures despite treatment with optimal dosage of a single drug demand further careful consideration. One recent retrospective study (Smith *et al.*, 1999) looked at 92 patients who had been referred to an epilepsy clinic with seizures deemed refractory to treatment. After review, twelve patients (13%) were not thought to have epilepsy, having already endured the significant lifestyle restrictions appropriate for a diagnosis of epilepsy. A further 18% were rendered seizure-free on manipulation of their drug treatment. A

TABLE 3 THE ESTABLISHED ANTIEPILEPTIC DRUGS

DRUG	YEAR INTRODUCED	MODES OF ACTION[1]	ADVERSE EVENTS			
			ACUTE DOSE RELATED	ACUTE IDIOSYNCRATIC	CHRONIC TOXICITY	TERATOGENICITY
BARBITURATES	1912	MANY	+++ DROWSINESS, UNSTEADINESS	+ RASHES	+ TOLERANCE HABITUATION WITHDRAWAL SEIZURES BEHAVIOURAL CHANGE	++
PHENYTOIN	1939	MANY	++ UNSTEADINESS SLURRED SPEECH CHOREA	+ RASHES LYMPHADENOPATHY HEPATITIS	+++ GUM SWELLING ACNE HIRSUTISM, FOLATE DEFICIENCY	++
CARBAMAZEPINE	1967	MULTIPLE	++ DIZZINESS DIPLOPIA UNSTEADINESS, NAUSEA VOMITING	++ RASHES LOW WHITE CELL COUNT	? NONE DEFINITE	++
SODIUM VALPROATE	1971	MULTIPLE	++ TREMOR, IRRITABILITY, RESTLESSNESS, OCCASIONALLY CONFUSION	+++ GASTRIC INTOLERANCE HEPATOTOXICITY (IN CHILDREN)	? WEIGHT GAIN, ALOPECIA	+++

[1] MANY = MUCH MORE THAN 1; MULTIPLE = MORE THAN 1.
+++ = POTENTIALLY SEVERE
++ = OCCASIONALLY PROBLEMATIC
\+ = RARE

TABLE 4 THE NEW ANTIEPILEPTIC DRUGS

DRUG	YEAR OF UK LICENCE	MODE OF ACTION	EFFICACY IN SEIZURE TYPE (MODE OF USE)	ADVERSE EVENTS			
				ACUTE DOSE RELATED	ACUTE IDIOSYNCRATIC	CHRONIC TOXICITY	TERATOGENICITY
VIGABATRIN	1988	GABA-T INHIBITION	PARTIAL (ADD-ON)	• DROWSINESS • FATIGUE • NERVOUSNESS • IRRITABILITY • DEPRESSION • CONFUSION • MILD GASTROINTESTINAL DISTURBANCES	PSYCHOSIS	VISUAL FIELD DEFECTS	+ ANIMAL MODELS
LAMOTRIGINE	1989	SODIUM CHANNEL BLOCKADE	PARTIAL/GENERALISED, (MONOTHERAPY/ADD-ON)	• NAUSEA • VOMITING • HEADACHE • DIPLOPIA • OEDEMA	RASH	—	NONE DESCRIBED AS YET
GABAPENTIN	1993	-UNCERTAIN- ?GABAERGIC EFFECT ?CA CHANNEL BLOCKADE	PARTIAL (ADD-ON)	• DROWSINESS • HEADACHE • TREMOR	BEHAVIOURAL PROBLEMS (CHILDREN)	—	NONE DESCRIBED AS YET
TOPIRAMATE	1995	• GABAERGIC • NA CHANNEL BLOCK • KAINATE RECEPTOR BLOCK	PARTIAL/?GENERALISED (ADD-ON /?MONOTHERAPY)	• IMPAIRED MEMORY • COGNITION • DROWSINESS • PARAESTHESIA	—	RENAL CALCULI WEIGHT LOSS	+ ANIMAL MODELS
TIAGABINE	1998	GABA REUPTAKE BLOCK	PARTIAL (ADD-ON)	• DIZZINESS • ASTHENIA • NERVOUSNESS • TREMOR • DEPRESSED MOOD	—	—	+ ANIMAL MODELS

+ = RARE
– = NO EVIDENCE AS YET

significant number had had their seizures misclassified, and changing to the appropriate treatment allowed seizure control to be achieved.

Where an antiepileptic drug 'correct' for the specific syndrome has been used unsuccessfully, it is reasonable to turn to a second drug, most usually as monotherapy. In some instances a trial of a two-drug combination may be considered. This requires an understanding from the patient that the second drug will be withdrawn in the absence of a satisfactory sustained response. The major factors that influence the actual choice of antiepileptic drug are comparative efficacy and toxicity (Tables 3 and 4). Where efficacy differences are marginal, the importance of comparative drug toxicity becomes a major consideration in the choice of antiepileptic agent. This may in some cases make the newer AEDs a more acceptable choice, but in a refractory population it is unlikely and unreasonable to expect any of the existing new AEDs to be the magic bullet for epilepsy. Realistically once patients are demonstrably refractory to two different monotherapies, it is unlikely (though the possibility should not be dismissed entirely) that they will fully respond to a third or even fourth monotherapy. For this reason AED polypharmacy will be left as a necessary evil in some patients. The range of different neurochemical and neuropharmacological actions possessed by each of the older AEDs would suggest that polypharmacy would not be generally accepted, but there may be some hope in the development of the newer AEDs (Table 4). Despite the limited effort, there have as yet been no convincing trials proving the advantages of any particular combinations or the presence of synergy between antiepileptic drugs (Leach, 1997). Patients with intractable partial seizures despite adequate drug therapy may benefit from surgical treatment.

ROLE OF SURGERY

A detailed description of all available surgical manoeuvres to treat epilepsy is beyond the scope of this chapter, but it is sufficient to say that in the last twenty years, the role of intracranial surgery for epilepsy has grown considerably. Patients who are refractory to antiepileptic drugs can be considered for surgery if their seizure types fall within certain categories, i.e. if their seizure origin is from an easily resectable area of the brain, most commonly one or other (but not both!) temporal lobes (Polkey and Binnie, 1992). Other operations are available which may help to limit seizure spread. By doing this, some of the more debilitating effects of generalising seizures (such as falls) may be inhibited.

MONITORING TREATMENT

At least in theory, monitoring treatment compliance is relatively easy. On direct questioning, most patients will admit if they have not been adhering to their treatment regime. Measurement of serum concentrations of the relevant drug may confirm the clinician's suspicion that the prescribed dose is being taken infrequently or not at all. The value of routine measurements of serum concentrations of all AEDs is less clear-cut, particularly since the concentration: response relationship is not well defined for most AEDs. As far as the novel AEDs are concerned, there is no value in measuring serum levels unless compliance is an issue. Even then, such assays may only be available at some specialist centres.

Measuring the response to treatment would at first sight seem to be much easier than checking compliance. As an ideal, all patients diagnosed as having epilepsy should be encouraged to keep a diary of their seizures in between clinic visits. This will hardly be necessary where seizures are infrequent, but it can be of help in providing objective information of moderate change in someone with frequent seizures. As well as documenting a change in seizure frequency, these diaries can, with appropriate instruction, be of use in determining whether the seizure type has been affected by any drug therapy.

Patients often look at seizure diaries as a very coarse tool, and this may be true, especially where seizures may not always be witnessed, and the seizure counts may be falsely low. It is useful to explain to patients that although they may be to an extent inaccurate, they are at least *consistently* inaccurate. While such records may not be entirely free of bias, they are much better than a subjective snap judgement by the patient and their family when they are in clinic, and in the long term they can be of great value.

OPTIMISING PATIENT MANAGEMENT

Optimising the management of patients with chronic refractory epilepsy takes more from a doctor than a knowledge of seizures and AEDs. Patients require help to foresee problems associated with their disease and its resultant treatment; they also need an accurate assessment of their progress.

In this respect, realism is essential. The patient who becomes disillusioned will be even less likely to comply with their treatment regime or attend for clinic visits. Patients are more likely to accept drug regimes and lifestyle restrictions if they feel they are aiming for an attainable, realistic goal. Affirmation and support from a dedicated epilepsy specialist nurse can be invaluable in maintaining contact with the epilepsy unit between visits.

Part of the positive aspect of care provision should involve giving each individual patient as much reasonable information about the implications of all possible management options, and letting them decide which of the treatment strategies they prefer. The doctor's role in such situations is as a provider of information, even though more often than not, the patient will be happy to follow the doctor's instincts as to what will work. Sadly, this concept of 'patient empowerment' is not always widely held to be of importance within the medical community.

Above all, it should be remembered that decisions regarding epilepsy treatment are rarely an emergency. Epilepsy is by nature an unpredictable condition, and any changes in seizure frequency should not be used as an excuse to make rapid or ill-considered change to therapy regimes. The only emergency in the management of epilepsy is in dealing with seizures that fall under the rubric of *Status Epilepticus*, and in these cases there is a need for urgent admission to hospital to allow intravenous therapy to be administered. Otherwise, treatment changes should be made only once full clinical information is available to both doctor and patient.

CONCLUSION

The difficulties experienced by patients with epilepsy vary widely from patient to patient, and the management of epilepsy therefore requires a coherent flexible team approach. This helps to deal with difficulties as they arise. The problems caused by individual seizures are markedly different from those caused by the diagnosis of epilepsy; some patients may be more debilitated by any resultant unemployment or the loss of their driving licence than the seizures themselves. Other patients, in contrast, may have their lives inhibited by a dread of seizures that is nurtured by themselves or their family.

It is probably fair to say that while doctors are skilled at minimising the incidence and effect of seizures, it is the other members of the team (nurses, specialist nurses, social workers and clinical psychologists) who have the most important roles to play in reducing the negative effects of epilepsy on the patients and their families. The challenge of such teamwork is part of the attraction of working in a modern epilepsy clinic.

References

Annegers, J.F., Hauser, W.A., Elverback, L.R. (1979) Remission of seizures and relapse in patients with epilepsy. *Epilepsia* **20**, 729–737.

Brodie, M.J., Dichter, M. (1996) Anticonvulsant drugs. *New England Journal of Medicine* **334**, 168–175

Chadwick, D.W. (1990) Diagnosis of epilepsy. *Lancet* **336**, 291–295

Chadwick, D.W. (1992) Seizures and Epilepsy. In: Laidlaw J., Richens, A., Chadwick, D.W. (eds.) *A Textbook of Epilepsy*. London: Churchill Livingstone, 165–204.

Chadwick, D.W. (1998) Rational Drug Therapy for Epilepsy. In: Chadwick D.W., Porter R.J. (eds.) *The Epilepsies 2*. Boston: Butterworth Heinemann, 247–266.

Dichter, M.A., Brodie, M.J. (1996) The Antiepileptic Drugs-2. *New England Journal of Medicine* **334**, 1583–1590

Hart, Y.M., Sander, J.W.A.S., Johnson, A.L., Shorvon, S.D. (1990) National general practice survey of epilepsy: recurrence after a first seizure. *Lancet* **336**, 1271–1274.

Hauser, W.A., Rich, S., Annegers, J.F., Andersen, V.E. (1990) Seizure recurrence after a first unprovoked seizure: an extended follow-up. *Neurology* **40**, 1163–1170.

ILAE Commission on Classification and Terminology (International League Against Epilepsy) (1981) Proposal for revised clinical and electroencephalographic classification of epileptic seizures. *Epilepsia* **22**, 489–501

ILAE Commission on Classification and Terminology (International League Against Epilepsy) (1989) Proposal for revised clinical and electroencephalographic classification of epileptic seizures. *Epilepsia* **30**, 389–399

Jeavons, P.M., Clark, J.E., Maheshwari, M.C. (1977) Treatment of generalised epilepsies of childhood and adolescence with sodium valproate. *Developmental Medicine and Child Neurology* **19**(1), 9–25

King, M.A., Newton, M.R., Jackson, G.D., Fitt, G.J., Mitchell, L.A., Silvapulle, M.J., Berkovic, S.F. (1998) Epileptology of the first seizure presentation: a clinical electroencephalographic, and magnetic resonance imaging study of 300 consecutive patients. *Lancet* **352**, 1007–1011

Leach, J.P. (1997) Polypharmacy with anticonvulsants: focus on synergism. *CNS Drugs* **8**, 366–375

Leach, J.P., Brodie, M.J. (1995) New Antiepileptic Drugs — an explosion of activity. *Seizure* **4**, 5–17

Polkey, C.E., Binnie, C.D. (1992) Neurosurgical treatment of epilepsy. In: Laidlaw J., Richens A., Chadwick D.W. (eds.) *A Textbook of Epilepsy* (4th Edition). London: Churchill Livingstone, 561–611.

Shorvon, S.D. (1990) Epidemiology, classification, natural history and genetics of epilepsy. *Lancet* **336**, 93–96

SIGN (Scottish Intercollegiate Guidelines Network) (1997) *Diagnosis and Management of Epilepsy in Adults: a national clinical guideline*. Edinburgh: SIGN Secretariat.

Smith, D., Defalla, B.A., Chadwick, D.W. (1999) The misdiagnosis of epilepsy and the management of refractory epilepsy in a specialist clinic. *Quarterly Journal of Medicine* **92**, 15–23.

Walker, M.C., Sander, J.W.A.S. (1996) The impact of new antiepileptic drugs on the prognosis of epilepsy: seizure freedom should be the ultimate goal. *Neurology* **46**, 912–914.

Chapter 3

MANAGING COGNITIVE AND BEHAVIOURAL CONSEQUENCES OF EPILEPSY

Albert P. Aldenkamp and Marc Hendriks

Understanding the cognitive and behavioural consequences of epilepsy is an integral part of its clinical management. When reviewing this important topic, it should be noted that the majority of studies in this field are clinical observations that do not allow general inferences. Moreover, research is complicated by methodological pitfalls such as sample selection bias, absence of adequate control groups, controversies as to measures of psychopathology, the possible influence of various confounding variables such as the use of antiepileptic medication, and the effects of economic and social stress associated with chronic disorders in general (Hermann and Whitman, 1984). Nonetheless, the enormous body of research that has been carried out over a period of more than a century provides ample evidence to illustrate that people with epilepsy, as a group, have more cognitive, behavioural and emotional problems than control populations of healthy subjects. In some individuals such problems may be more debilitating than the seizures themselves.

The topics reviewed here represent problem areas on which considerable debate has focused. They can be viewed from the perspectives both of the *indirect effects of having epilepsy* and of the *effects that are directly related* to it. The indirect effects of this, or indeed any other chronic condition, may be severe enough to explain anything from mild depression to paranoid delusions as an understandable psychological reaction to the stress induced by living with a chronic disorder. More specifically for epilepsy, it would be surprising if factors such as the unpredictable and traumatic nature of the seizures, the ignorance and stigma still associated with epilepsy, or the limitations of activities and aspirations resulting from having epilepsy did not have a considerable influence on a person's psychological status. However, the cognitive and behavioural correlates of epilepsy represent more than an understandable reaction to the emotional trauma of physical, social, or cognitive disability; direct neurophysiological-neurochemical mechanisms, particularly those reflecting limbic system dysfunction, may be involved as well. Because the temporal lobe, and the limbic structures contained within it, are known to be important in the mediation of emotional and social behaviour, one might expect that people with epilepsies originating in the temporal lobe are at special risk of developing emotional and social difficulties, psychiatric disorders, and personality problems. Indeed, a high incidence of emotional disorders in people with temporal lobe epilepsy has been reported since the 1950s (Gibbs and Stamps, 1953), suggesting that psychological factors are less important determinants of these disorders than the location of the epileptogenic focus within temporal structures. Both types of effects, direct and indirect, will be considered in this chapter.

A related distinction that is often used in the literature does not focus on the condition itself (i.e. epilepsy), but on its major symptoms, the seizures. This highlights a difference between the *ictal/peri-ictal effects* (effects observed as direct aftermaths of the ictus or seizure) and the *inter-ictal consequences* (effects observed in the periods between the seizures). We should keep in mind that these various sets of factors are not independent of one another. For example, limbic system dysfunction may indeed be an important inter-ictal factor predisposing people with epilepsy to emotional and behavioural disorders, but in individual cases the form and severity of such disorders is likely to depend on an interaction with other factors that only relate indirectly to the epilepsy, including past experience and current psychological and social status (Hermann *et al.,* 1982).

Using the distinctions between direct and indirect effects of epilepsy and between ictal and interictal consequences of seizures, we will discuss the range of cognitive and behavioural consequences of epilepsy. By and large, the separate topics follow the development of an individual from childhood to adult life.

DEVELOPMENTAL PROBLEMS

Although some of the epilepsy syndromes may also cause developmental problems (Arzimanoglou and Aicardi, 1992), there is no evidence for a *direct* relationship between most of the epilepsies and social-emotional development. Nonetheless, epilepsy with onset in early childhood may have a large *indirect* effect on development through its adverse impact on parental and peer group attitudes and the learning of social skills. Restrictions on the child's activities and lifestyle due to epilepsy may interfere with personality maturation and contribute to psychosocial difficulties later in life (Fenton, 1981). Parents may worry about the seizures, about the side effects of antiepileptic medication, or about possible future social handicaps (Ward and Bower, 1978; Suurmeijer *et al.*, 1978; West, 1979). Parents tend to have lower expectations of their children with epilepsy relative to their healthy children (Suurmeijer *et al.*, 1978; Long and Moore, 1979). Because of such special concerns and expectations, parents may behave differently toward their children with epilepsy. There appears to be considerable variation among parents and other members of the family in their reactions to a child with epilepsy, which may range from over-protection to rejection and scapegoating. Various developmental problems may occur due to such reactions, including low self-esteem, lack of social skills (Fenton, 1981), feelings of guilt, or the adoption of the 'sick role' (Lechtenberg, 1984). These may all have significant effects in adult life. The importance of parental expectations is emphasized in studies on so-called 'outgrown epilepsies', in which children are studied after they are considered to be cured of their epilepsy. Most of the studies report that although the children tend to adapt to the new situation, their parents still remain worried and new behaviour patterns of the child are not immediately evaluated positively by the parents (Aldenkamp *et al.*, 1994; 1998).

LEARNING AND EDUCATIONAL PROBLEMS

There is only one peri-ictal phenomenon showing a *direct* relation between ictal discharge and learning or educational impairment: the so-called *'transitory cognitive impairment'*. This concept followed from early observations (Gibbs *et al.*, 1936) that, although epileptic discharge will mostly result in overt clinical symptoms such as automatisms, movements or impaired consciousness (the seizures), epileptic EEG-discharge was also found to occur without observable clinical symptoms. This 'subclinical' ('masked', or 'larval') epilepsy can occur even in persons not known to suffer from epilepsy. Schwab (1939) disclosed the possibility of EEG-discharge, not accompanied by seizures, but by transitory changes in higher cortical functions. In fact 'transitory cognitive impairment' was found to be a seizure with impairment of cognitive function as its only symptom. It is often considered a subclinical form of the absence seizure but is also described in partial epilepsies (Binnie, 1987). Transitory cognitive impairment has been studied extensively over a long period (Prechtl *et al.*, 1965; Aarts *et al.*, 1984) and the concept has proven its value for explaining impairment of complex behaviour patterns, such as episodic learning difficulties and fluctuations during intelligence testing (Aldenkamp *et al.*, 1996).

Because of the significant impact of transitory cognitive impairment, some authors (Binnie, 1987; Stores, 1987) recommend the combination of EEG recording with psychological testing in any patient who shows inconsistent behaviour.

As with developmental processes, the *indirect* effects of epilepsy may nonetheless have a far greater impact on learning. Children with epilepsy as a group are certainly at increased risk of developing learning problems. However, 'learning/educational problems' has been used as a rather ill-defined category and there is no uniformity in assessment methods. Consequently, prevalence estimates of learning/educational problems in children with epilepsy vary widely, percentages mentioned in the literature ranging from five to 50% (Thompson, 1987). Approximately one third receive some form of special educational support (Thompson, 1987; Aldenkamp, 1995). Academic underachievement in children with epilepsy relative to their own abilities has been noted by several authors (Seidenberg *et al.,* 1986; Aldenkamp *et al.,* 1990). Of course, parental attitudes and behaviour may be expected to influence the child's learning behaviour and educational achievement (Suurmeijer *et al.,* 1978), but specific cognitive deficits may also be responsible for learning problems and underachievement. Slowing on tasks involving complex information processing, quick decision making, and attention and concentration difficulties all are well established phenomena in epilepsy (Aldenkamp *et al.,* 1992). These may be examples of direct effects of epilepsy, caused by factors such as the localization of the epileptogenic focus, the seizure activity, and the central nervous system side effects of antiepileptic medication (Vermeulen *et al.,* 1994). Disappointing school achievement, regardless of its origin, may have a considerable impact on the self-perception of the child with epilepsy, and may lead to reduced employment choices and earning potential as an adult.

AFFECTIVE DISORDERS

The four types of affective disorders that are often suggested to be a consequence of epilepsy: depression, anxiety, aggressive behaviour and sexual dysfunction, are discussed below.

Depression and Anxiety

The major *inter-ictal* affective disorders in epilepsy are depression and anxiety, though their exact prevalence is not known and relevant studies are too few to establish an association with specific factors (Hermann and Whitman, 1984). Psychosocially oriented explanations have emphasized the various psychological and social stress factors associated with having seizures, thus the indirect effects of epilepsy. Seizures are essentially unpredictable traumatic events over which the individual has little or no control. The nature of epilepsy may thus be conducive to 'learned helplessness' (Seligman, 1975); and it has been suggested that this may be one way of understanding some of the inter-ictal behavioural concomitants of epilepsy, particularly the apparent high rates of depression and anxiety (Hermann, 1979). Medical misinformation, fear of seizures and fear of death from seizures is widespread among patients and this may affect behaviour in adverse ways. Patients have many concerns about what they think are the potentially destructive effects of epilepsy, such as progressive brain damage, mental deterioration, mental illness and loss of intelligence. A common approach to dealing with such fears and concerns is social and emotional withdrawal. Depression and anxiety in epilepsy may in part be due to such mechanisms.

An example of the direct effect of epilepsy is peri-ictal depression, manifested in feelings of sadness, futility and the like, and unmotivated by the context, which may occur as an aura, during the seizure, or as a sequel to the seizure. Peri-ictal depression is fairly uncommon, occurring in about 1% of the patients with epilepsy, and it is associated with temporal-limbic discharges (Robertson, 1988). The duration of the depression may be brief, lasting for minutes, but unlike other ictal emotions, the mood may persist for days after the seizure. Naturally, the sequelae of such effects may lead to serious emotional complications (Robertson, 1992).

Fear is much more common as part of a seizure and is experienced as a *peri-ictal* phenomenon in about three percent of patients with epilepsy. It may also be produced by experimental electrical stimulation of limbic structures, especially the amygdala. Peri-ictal fear typically occurs with temporal lobe seizures, about 20% of subjects with such seizures reporting episodes of peri-ictal fear, which differs from the normal state in that it arises suddenly, out of context and is undirected. Its duration varies from seconds to minutes, and its intensity ranges from mild anxiety to overwhelming terror.

Aggression

Despite anecdotal reports in the medico-legal literature suggesting that violent events might occur as a *peri-ictal* phenomenon, and thus as a direct effect of epilepsy, the weight of evidence does not support such allegations (Treiman and Delgado-Escueta, 1983; Treiman, 1986). It is extremely unusual for people with epilepsy to behave aggressively during a seizure. Aggressive behaviour sometimes occurs as an aftermath of a seizure, because the person is restrained in an attempt to protect him or her from injury. Aggressive behaviour during seizures, if it occurs at all, is typically simple, stereotyped, unsustained, unplanned, and never supported by a consecutive series of purposeful acts. It is not premeditated and does not occur in response to pre-ictal provocation (Strauss, 1989). It is unlikely therefore that a co-ordinated act of violence or aggression against others could occur as part of a seizure. Interictal aggression, that may be indirectly related to epilepsy, has been studied in hospital-based surveys that have failed to reveal increased aggression in people with epilepsy in general, and temporal lobe epilepsy in particular.

Sexual Behaviour

Few methodologically sound studies have been carried out on sexual function in people with epilepsy. However, the existing data suggest that sexual dysfunction is not uncommon. Hyposexuality, usually in the form of a global loss of performance as well as interest in sex, is the most prominent problem, and appears to be specifically associated with temporal lobe epilepsy. However, presence of temporal lobe epilepsy is presumably only one of several factors that may contribute to sexual dysfunction. The individual's overall mental health is an important consideration; depressed or anxious people often have little interest in sex. The chronic use of antiepileptic drugs may also produce alterations in sex hormone levels and thus affect sexual functioning. Adolescents with epilepsy may have limited opportunities for social and so sexual contacts because of their isolated position in peer groups (Hermann and Whitman, 1984; Strauss, 1989). Thus, a large number of *indirect* relationships exist between epilepsy and the reported problems of sexual behaviour.

PSYCHIATRIC IMPAIRMENT

There is little doubt that overall rates of psychopathology of any type are elevated in people with epilepsy relative to healthy controls. This increased tendency toward psychopathology appears to be due to the problems associated with having *any* chronic disorder, rather than with epilepsy itself. Comparisons with patients with other chronic conditions generally fail to reveal increased overall psychopathology rates in epilepsy. For example, it is frequently reported that personality traits such as excessive religiosity, mental slowness, viscosity, hyposexuality, circumstantiality, irritability, impulsivity and mood fluctuations are associated with epilepsy. However, such traits have never been demonstrated to be more common in people with epilepsy than in those with other chronic brain-related disorders (Hermann and Whitman, 1984; Strauss, 1989).

There is evidence, however, that psychopathology, when present in epilepsy, is more likely to manifest itself as psychosis, particularly schizophrenia-like and paranoid states, than in chronically ill controls (Whitman *et al.,* 1984). This finding might account for the observed over-representation of patients with epilepsy in psychiatric hospitals and the increased rates of previous psychiatric hospitalizations in epilepsy, as patients with psychotic disorders are more likely to receive treatment in inpatient psychiatric settings (Hermann and Whitman, 1984). As yet, there are no population-based studies on the prevalence of psychosis in epilepsy that might resolve the question as to whether or not the combination of epilepsy and psychosis is coincidental. Despite such uncertainties, various explanations for a causal link between epilepsy and psychosis have been advanced (Toone, 1981). It is theorized that the repeated intrusions into consciousness of bizarre and alien seizure-related experiences and affects could have deleterious effects on the patient's mental health, and prepare the ground for a later psychotic development (Pond, 1957). There are some data supporting this hypothesis. For example, patients with complex auras manifest more psychopathology than those with simple auras (Standage and Fenton, 1975); and patients with auras consisting of illusions, hallucinations, and complex automatisms are at increased risk of psychosis, relative to other types of auras (Jensen and Larsen, 1979).

PSEUDO-EPILEPTIC PSYCHOGENIC SEIZURES

A common psychosocial problem in epilepsy is the combination of pseudo-epileptic psychogenic seizures and epileptic seizures (Aldenkamp and Mulder, 1997). Pseudo-epileptic psychogenic seizures were found, for example, in 7–10% of patients referred to specialized epilepsy centres in The Netherlands (Aldenkamp and Mulder, 1997). In theory, the distinction between epileptic and pseudo-epileptic psychogenic seizures is evident. Epileptic seizures are the manifestation of a sudden abnormal change in brain function, accompanied by excessive electrical discharge of brain cells. Pseudo-epileptic psychogenic seizures are not accompanied by abnormal paroxysmal discharges, but are symptoms of emotional disturbances (Williams *et al.*, 1978). However, EEG recording of epileptic seizures is not always possible. Where pseudo-epileptic and epileptic seizures co-exist in the same patient, this may lead to serious diagnostic problems, as interictal EEG-registration does not rule out the possibility of pseudo-epileptic seizures in a patient with epilepsy. As a result, these patients may be diagnosed as suffering from intractable epilepsies and may be overtreated (Ramani *et al.*, 1980).

The definition of pseudo-epileptic psychogenic seizures is hindered by diversity in often conflicting terminology, such as hysterical seizures, psychogenic seizures and functional seizures. Different models have been proposed to explain pseudo-epileptic psychogenic seizures. In some studies these seizures are seen as a symptom of internalized emotional conflicts or coping ego-mechanisms to avoid unconscious conflicts; in others they are seen as learned behaviour, mostly occurring in situations which overrun the individual's stress capacity; and in some cognitive-behaviouristic theories, as a form of dissociation. This latter model may explain the observation that people with epilepsy are highly hypnotizable (Gross, 1979), since hypnosis is also as a state of dissociation. Using DSM-III criteria, Stewart *et al.* (1982) were able to uncover several forms of psychopathology behind the pseudo-epileptic symptomatology. There was a clear tendency in their study for the combination of borderline and antisocial personality disorders in patients with pseudo-epileptic seizures, but hysteria was not a common diagnosis. The conclusion must be therefore that pseudo-epileptic psychogenic seizures are probably a symptom of various affective and psychiatric factors that may seriously complicate the evaluation of relationships between epileptic conditions and psychosocial reactions.

SOCIOECONOMIC STATUS

This chapter closes with a brief consideration of the 'endpoint' of several critical influences and focuses on the social-economic status of the adult with epilepsy. Being able to obtain and maintain a satisfactory job and income is obviously relevant to an individual's psychosocial functioning, if only because unemployment introduces economic pressure, and may reduce opportunities for social interaction and leisure activities. Unfortunately, unemployment and underemployment of people with epilepsy are much more frequent than in the general population. According to So and Penry (1981), the unemployment rate for people with epilepsy is double the national average in the United States. Many young adults with epilepsy experience problems finding work (Fraser, 1980), and it is by no means uncommon for people to lose their job because of seizures. Not surprisingly, people with epilepsy generally have lower than average income.

The relationship between epilepsy and lower socioeconomic status is, however, complex. Characteristics of the seizures may be such that they limit an individual's employment opportunities. Negative personality or behavioural characteristics may contribute to the difficulties. Cognitive functioning may be a significant factor in determining successful or unsuccessful employment status. Neuropsychological investigations of epilepsy have found, for example, that measures of higher cortical function predict vocational status and adequacy of psychosocial functioning (Dikmen and Morgan, 1980; Dodrill, 1980). However, it should also be remembered that epilepsy continues to be associated with considerable stigma and ignorance, manifesting itself in various forms of social discrimination, such as difficulties in obtaining a driver's licence, discrimination in obtaining employment and difficulty in obtaining all types of insurance. The National Commission for the Control of Epilepsy and its Consequences (1978) has outlined the societal sanctions in detail. Such sanctions are conducive to social exclusion and ostracism and may result in limited opportunities for extended social contact. Public attitudes towards epilepsy and misconceptions about this condition may go a long way to accounting for the difficulties experienced in gaining employment.

SUMMARY

A very heterogeneous group of cognitive and behavioural problems is associated with epilepsy. These include, among others, learning and educational problems, changed affect, personality and behaviour difficulties, and psychiatric disorders. This review has focused on the group where such factors coincide. Fortunately, there is evidence that these problems do not occur in the majority of people with epilepsy. Only in a minority, possibly about 15–25%, do such problems manifest themselves. In this latter group however, multiple problems may arise and the need for psychological as well as medical treatment is evident.

Disentangling the causes of the cognitive and behavioural consequences of epilepsy is complex. It is clear that there are direct neuropsychological and neurochemical mechanisms at work, particularly in temporal lobe epilepsy. These probably interact with indirect factors, not the least of which are the popular misconceptions and prejudices that continue to surround epilepsy. Together, they may result in the existence of a subgroup of people with epilepsy who face severe difficulties and poor outcomes. Several epidemiological studies are currently in progress which, hopefully, will elucidate this topic further in the near future.

MAIN MANAGEMENT ISSUES

Management of the cognitive and behavioural consequences of epilepsy includes several key issues, most of these addressed in later chapters. We do, however, want to emphasize some of these aspects:

- A multidisciplinary approach in clinical practice is required for the subgroup where direct and indirect effects of epilepsy coincide and lead to serious cognitive and other behavioural consequences. As the problems have a combined neurological and psychosocial origin, this may seem self-evident. However, day-to-day practice in many hospitals and centres is different and often shows monodisciplinary treatment. Models of multidisciplinary work such as the case-management model (Strang, 1987) should be implemented in epilepsy care. The role of other members of the multidisciplinary team in these treatment models is outlined in later chapters.
- The same multidisciplinary approach must lead to standards of care that stimulate early recognition of cognitive and psychosocial consequences of epilepsy, proper assessment and the use of methods aimed at prevention, such as family counselling.
- Consensus needs to be established on the issue of when psychotherapy and counselling for behavioural consequences of epilepsy (such as psychiatric disorders) requires epileptological expertise (and thus treatment in specialized centres) and when the patient should be referred to more general institutions of mental health. Frequently such institutions do not feel capable of providing treatment when the patient has epilepsy in addition to the major behavioural symptoms for which he/she is referred.
- Treatment of psychogenic pseudoepileptic seizures is stimulated by uniformity in labelling and classification of such seizures. This classification is now either based on negative medical diagnosis such as the label 'non-epileptic seizure' or focused on the similarity of symptoms with an epileptic seizure (Betts and Boden, 1992a; 1992b).

The classification should, however, focus on the psychogenic mechanisms that presumably generate the seizures.

- There is an increasing need for the implementation of neurorehabilitation programmes in clinical practice. Some of these programmes are directly aimed at the treatment of the cognitive handicap, such as memory training; others are aimed at finding alternative forms of behaviour. However, both types of programmes have benefits for patients as they learn how to cope with the handicap (Aldenkamp and Vermeulen, 1992).

References

Aarts, J.H.P., Binnie, C.D., Smit, A.M., Wilkins, A.J. (1984) Selective cognitive impairment during focal and generalised epileptiform EEG activity. *Brain* **107**, 293–308.

Aldenkamp, A.P. (1995) The impact of epilepsy on cognitive development and learning behaviour. In: Aldenkamp A.P., Dreifuss F.E., Renier W.O. *Epilepsy in Children and Adolescents.* Boca Raton, New York: CRC-Press, 225–239.

Aldenkamp, A.P., Mulder O.G. (1997) Behavioural Mechanisms involved in Pseudo-epileptic Seizures: a comparison between patients with epileptic seizures and patients with pseudo-epileptic seizures. *Seizure* **6**, 275–282.

Aldenkamp, A.P., Vermeulen, J. (1992) Neuropsychological rehabilitation of memory function in epilepsy. *Journal of Neuropsychological Rehabilitation* **1**(3), 199–214.

Aldenkamp, A.P., Alpherts, W.C.J., Dekker, M.C.A., Overweg, J. (1990) Neuropsychological aspects of Learning disabilities in Epilepsy. *Epilepsia* **31**(S4), 9–20.

Aldenkamp, A.P., Vermeulen, J., Alpherts, W.C.J., Overweg, J., Van Parijs, J.A.P., Verhoeff, N.P.L.G. (1992) Validity of computerized testing: patient dysfunction and complaints versus measured changes. In: Dodson W.E. and Kinsbourne M. (eds.), *Assessment of cognitive function*, New York: Demos, 51–68.

Aldenkamp, A.P., Blennow, G., Sandstedt, P., Alpherts, W.C.J., Elmqvist, D.D., Heijbel, J., Nilsson, H.L., Nilsson, H., Tonnby, H., Wahlander, L., Wosse, E. (1994) Computerized assessment of Cognitive Function and Quality of Life. In: Dodson W.E. and Trimble M.R. (eds.) *Epilepsy and Quality of Life.* New York: Raven Press, 199–215.

Aldenkamp, A.P., Overweg, J., Gutter, Th., Beun, A.M., Diepman, L., Mulder, O.G. (1996) Effect of epilepsy, seizures and epileptiform EEG discharges on cognitive function. *Acta Neurologica Scandinavica* **93**, 253–259.

Aldenkamp, A.P., Alpherts, W.C.J., Sandstedt, P., Blennow, G., Elmqvist, D., Heijbel, J., Nilsson, H., Tonnby, H., Wahlander, L., Wosse, E. (1998) Antiepileptic drug-related cognitive complaints in seizure-free children before and after drug discontinuation. *Epilepsia* **39**(10), 1070–1074.

Arzimanoglou A., Aicardi, J. (1992) The epilepsy of Sturge-Weber syndrome. *Acta Neurologica Scandinavica* **86**(140), 18–23.

Betts, T., Boden S. (1992a) Diagnosis, Management and Prognosis of a group of 128 patients with non-epileptic attack Disorder. Part I. *Seizure* **1**, 19–26.

Betts, T., Boden S. (1992b) Diagnosis, Management and Prognosis of a group of 128 patients with non-epileptic attack Disorder. Part II. *Seizure* **1**, 27–32.

Binnie C.D. (1987) Seizures, EEG discharges and cognition. In: Trimble M.R., Reynolds E.H. (eds.), *Epilepsy, Behaviour and cognitive function.* New York: John Wiley and Sons, 45–51.

Dikmen, S., Morgan, S.F. (1980) Neuropsychological factors related to employability and occupational status in persons with epilepsy. *Journal of Nervous and Mental Disease* **168**, 236–240.

Dodrill, C.B. (1980) Interrelationships between neuropsychological data and social problems in epilepsy. In: Canger R., Angeleri F., and Penry J.K. (eds.), *Advances in epileptology: XIth Epilepsy International Symposium.* New York: Raven Press, 191–197.

Fenton, G.W. (1981) Personality and behavioral disorders in adults with epilepsy. In: Reynolds E.H., Trimble M.R. (eds.), *Epilepsy and Psychiatry.* Edinburgh: Churchill Livingstone, 77–91.

Fraser, R.T. (1980) Vocational aspects of epilepsy. In: Hermann B.P. (ed.), *A Multidisciplinary Handbook of Epilepsy.* Springfield Ill: Charles C. Thomas, 74–105.

Gibbs, F.A., Stamps, F.W. (1953) *Epilepsy Handbook.* Springfield Ill: Charles C. Thomas.

Gibbs, F.A., Lennox, W.G., Gibbs E.L. (1936) The electroencephalogram in diagnosis and in localisation of epileptic seizures. *Archives of Neurology and Psychiatry* **36**, 1225–1235.

Gross, M. (1979) Hypnosis a diagnostic tool in epilepsy. In: Burrows G.D., Collison D.R., Dennerstein L. (eds.), *Hypnosis*, Biomedical Press, 97–114.

Hermann, B.F. (1979) Psychopathology in epilepsy and learned helplessness. *Medical Hypotheses* **5**, 723–729.

Hermann, B.P., Whitman. S. (1984) Behavioral and personality correlates of epilepsy: A review, methodological critique, and conceptual model. *Psychological Bulletin* **95**, 451–497.

Hermann, B.P., Dikmen, S., Schwarz, M.S., Karnes, W.E. (1982) Psychopathology in TLE patients with ictal fear: A quantitative investigation. *Neurology* **32**, 7–11.

Jensen, I., Larsen, J.K. (1979) Psychoses in drug resistant temporal lobe epilepsy. *Journal of Neurology Neurosurgery and Psychiatry* **42**, 948–954.

Lechtenberg, R. (1984) *Epilepsy and the family*. Boston: Harvard University Press.

Long, C.G., Moore, J.L. (1979) Parental expectations for their epileptic children. *Journal of Child Psychology and Psychiatry* **20**, 299–312.

Pond, D.A. (1957) Psychiatric aspects of epilepsy. *Journal of the Indian Medical Profession* **3**, 1441–1451.

Prechtl, H.F.R., Boeke P.E., Schut, T. (1965) The electroencephalogram and performance in epileptic patients. *Neurology* **11**, 296–302.

Ramani, S.V., Quesney, L.F., Olson, D., Gumnit, R.J. (1980) Diagnosis of hysterical seizures in Epileptic patients. *American Journal of Psychiatry* **137**, 705–709.

Robertson, M.M. (1988) Epilepsy and Mood. In: Trimble M.R., Reynolds E.H. (eds.), *Epilepsy, Behaviour and Cognitive Function*, New York: John Wiley and Sons, 145–157.

Robertson, M.M. (1992) Affect and mood in epilepsy: an overview with a focus on depression. *Acta Neurologica Scandinavica* **86**(140), 127–133.

Schwab R.S. (1939) A method of measuring consciousness in petit mal epilepsy. *Journal of Nervous and Mental Disease* **89**, 690–691.

Seidenberg, M., Beck, N., Geisser, M., Giordani, B., Sackellaras, J.C., Berent, S., Dreiffus, F., Boll, T.J. (1986) Academic achievement of children with epilepsy. *Epilepsia* **29**, 753–759.

Seligman, M.E.P. (1975) *Helplessness*. San Francisco: Freeman.

So, E.L., Penry, J.K. (1981) Epilepsy in adults. *Annals of Neurology* **9**, 3–16.

Standage, K.F., Fenton, G.W. (1975) Psychiatric symptom profiles of patients with epilepsy: A controlled investigation. *Psychological Medicine* **5**, 152–160.

Stewart, R.S., Lovitt, R., Stewart, R.M. (1982) Are hysterical seizures more than hysteria? A research diagnostic criteria, DSM-III, and psychometric analysis. *American Journal of Psychiatry* **139**, 926–929.

Stores G. (1987) Effects on learning of 'subclinical' seizure discharge. In: Aldenkamp A.P., Alpherts W.C.J., Meinardi H., Stores G. (eds.), *Education and Epilepsy*. Lisse/Berwyn: Swets and Zeitlinger, 14–21.

Strang J. (1987) Educational and related treatment considerations concerning the child with epilepsy: a developmental neuropsychological approach. In: Aldenkamp AP, Alpherts WCJ, Meinardi H., Stores, G. (eds.) *Education and Epilepsy*. Berwyn: Swets and Zeitlinger, 118–135.

Strauss, E. (1989) Ictal and interictal manifestations of emotions in epilepsy. In: Boller F., Grafman, J. (eds.), *Handbook of neuropsychology*, Vol. 3, Amsterdam: Elsevier, 315–344.

Suurmeijer, T.P.B.M., Dam, A. van, Blijham, M. (1978) Socialization of the child with epilepsy and school achievement. In: Meinardi H., Rowan J. (eds.), *Advances in Epileptology-1977*. Lisse: Swets and Zeitlinger, 31–39.

Thompson, P.J. (1987) Educational attainment in children and young people with epilepsy. In: Oxley J., Stores G. (eds.), *Epilepsy and Education* London: The Medical Tribune Group, 15–24.

Toone, B.K. (1981) Psychoses of epilepsy. In: Reynolds E.H., Trimble M.R. (eds.), *Epilepsy and Psychiatry*. Edinburgh: Churchill Livingstone, 113–137.

Treimann, D.M. (1986) Epilepsy and violence: medical and legal issues. *Epilepsia* **27**(S2), 77–104.

Treimann, D.M., Delgado-Escueta, A.V. (1983) Violence and epilepsy: A critical review. In: Pedley T.A., Meldrum B.S. (eds.), *Recent Advances in Epilepsy*, Vol. 1, London: Churchill Livingstone, 179–209.

Vermeulen, J., Kortstee, S.W.A.T., Alpherts, W.C.J., Aldenkamp, A.P. (1994) Cognitive performance in learning disabled children with and without epilepsy. *Seizure* **3**, 13–21.

Ward, F., Bower, B.D. (1978) A study of certain social aspects of epilepsy in childhood. *Developmental Medicine and Child Neurology* **39**(S), 1–50.

West, P. (1979) An investigation into the social construction and consequences of the label epilepsy. *Sociological Review* **27**, 719–741.

Whitman, S., Hermann, B.P., Gordon, A. (1984) Psychopathology in epilepsy: How great is the risk? *Biological Psychiatry* **19**, 213–236.

Williams, D.T., Spiegel, H., Mostofsky, D.I. (1978) Neurogenic and hysterical seizures in children and adolescents: differential diagnostic and therapeutic considerations. *American Journal of Psychiatry* **135**, 82–86.

QUALITY OF LIFE ISSUES IN EPILEPSY

Chapter 4

THEORETICAL AND METHODOLOGICAL ISSUES IN MEASURING QUALITY OF LIFE

Ann Jacoby

In the field of epilepsy, the formal assessment of quality of life is a relatively recent science. Increasing emphasis on questions about the effectiveness and cost-effectiveness of treatments for epilepsy, combined with political and philosophical pressures to take note of the patient's perspective in health care, has led to increased demand for tools by which these can be robustly measured. This, in turn, has highlighted a number of theoretical and methodological questions about how quality of life (QoL) should be assessed within the context of this chronic condition. The debate about QoL assessment in epilepsy is part of a much wider debate about QoL assessment in medicine generally, where QoL has been described as 'the new catch phrase' (Slevin, 1992). Despite continuing controversy about whether QoL assessment can best be regarded as sound academic endeavour or mere whim of fashion, it is a topic to which a clear political agenda now attaches and so continues to generate considerable interest in epilepsy, as in other areas of health care provision. In this chapter, the concept of QoL will be reviewed and issues around its assessment will be considered.

HISTORY OF QoL RESEARCH

Though QoL assessment has been described as the 'new paradigm' in medicine (Schipper *et al.*, 1990), the distinction between *quantity* and *quality* of life is one that has absorbed philosophers for centuries. Historically, QoL measurement reflects the shift in medical pre-occupation from the management of acute to chronic disease. It is concerned with evaluating the effectiveness of medicine to control rather than to cure disease, and with issues of morbidity rather than mortality. Clinical interest in QoL issues dates back to the 1940s, during which decade the World Health Organisation published its definition of health as 'a state of complete physical, mental and social well-being'. In the same decade, the Karnovsky Performance Index, frequently cited as the earliest 'quality of life' measure, was published (Karnovsky *et al.*, 1948). Over the next three decades, the idea that non-clinical measures could be relevant indicators of medical outcome gradually gained credibility, the term QoL making its first appearance in *Index Medicus* in the mid-1970s. During the 1980s, a number of authors made the case for QoL measurement in medical settings (McCartney and Larson, 1987; Levine, 1988; Read, 1993). And they apparently did so persuasively — a Medline search of papers with the term 'quality of life' in their title for the years 1966 to 1970 identified only four (Spitzer, 1987); whereas one undertaken in 1995 identified 1000 (Rosenberg, 1995).

The growing support for QoL assessments as important non-clinical outcomes of medical care is clearly evidenced by current requirements of the major UK and international funding bodies that applicants address the issue of QoL in their proposals. Drug licensing agencies are increasingly interested in the role of QoL assessments in the regulatory approval process and the pharmaceutical industry is eager to provide such information (see Chapter 11). Support for QoL assessments has been expressed in the major academic medical journals (Guyatt and Cook, 1994; Lancet Editorial, 1995); and widespread recognition of the need for scientific rigour in QoL assessment is demonstrated by the recent publication of guidelines on the selection, application and reporting of QoL assessments (Staquet *et al.*, 1996; Fayers *et al.*, 1997; Fitzpatrick *et al.*, 1998; Anonymous 1998). An international society for QoL research (ISOQOL), with a dedicated journal, *QoL Research*, was founded in 1994, marking yet another stage in the acceptance of the central role of QoL assessments in the area of health and medical care.

The history of QoL research in epilepsy has been characterised as falling into three 'discernible and overlapping' phases, the most recent of which has borrowed the methods and models of health services research (see Chapter 5). A number of authors (Meador, 1993; Scambler, 1993; Hermann, 1995) have been anxious to emphasise that it is the use of these methods and models that is novel, rather than interest in the impact of epilepsy on QoL. However, we would be doing a disservice to them in leaving unacknowledged the efforts of these 'third phase' researchers in ensuring that QoL assessment is now theoretically driven, methodologically more robust and firmly on the epilepsy outcomes agenda.

Use of the term 'quality of life' is not documented in epilepsy till 1990 (Hermann, 1992), when it made its appearance in the title of the proceedings of a UK Royal Society of Medicine Round Table (Chadwick, 1990). QoL became a main conference topic for the first time in 1991; and results of the first randomised trial of epilepsy treatment to incorporate a comprehensive and systematic QoL assessment were published in 1992 (Jacoby, 1992; Jacoby *et al.*, 1992). Following from these beginnings, the 1990s has seen publication of a significant number of QoL assessment tools for epilepsy, including the Epilepsy Surgery Inventory (Vickrey *et al.*, 1992), the Liverpool QoL Battery (Baker *et al.*, 1993; Baker *et al.*, 1994) and the QoLIE scales (Devinsky *et al.*, 1995); and their application in a range of descriptive studies and clinical trials of treatment for epilepsy. In a recent editorial, Hays (1995) concludes that we have now reached the point in epilepsy where we need to, 'focus efforts on evaluation, fine-tuning and applying the existing arsenal rather than proliferating' new QoL measures. While there will undoubtedly be those who dissent from this position, they will, hopefully, concur with Hays that coordinated and collaborative efforts are likely to be most productive in advancing the QoL cause.

CONCEPTUAL AND DEFINITIONAL ISSUES IN QoL ASSESSMENT

A number of different concepts have driven the development of QoL measures including, among others, the concept of utility, the reintegration concept and gap theory (Box 1; Schipper *et al.*, 1990). The WHO definition of health has been a starting point conceptually for many

The psychological view	QoL reflects the patient-perceived distinction between disease and the *experience* of illness.
The concept of utility	Patients make 'trade-offs' between quantity and *quality* of life.
The community-centred concept	A hierarchy of variables, starting with physical illness and progressing outwards to the patient's social/ community role.
Reintegration to normal living	The ability to do what a person has to or wants to do, following the onset of illness.
The Gap Principle	The gap between a person's expectations and achievements, which may vary over time as health improves or regresses.

Adapted from Schipper *et al.*, (1990)

BOX 1 CONCEPTUAL FORMULATIONS OF QUALITY OF LIFE

descriptive QoL measures which focus on the patient's perception of illness impact and on their experience of illness; whereas individualised approaches to QoL assessment draw heavily on Calman's (1984) Gap Principle — that the more you are able to realise your expectations, the higher your QoL will be. Yet other QoL measures are firmly grounded in the utility approach — that values can be attached to health states and that patients are willing and able to make trade-offs between QoL and survival. The WHO classification of impairment, disability and handicap is intended as a framework within which to consider the different consequences of disease, and has also been suggested as a useful conceptual base for QoL assessment (Fitzpatrick *et al.*, 1998). Schipper *et al.*, (1990) conclude that what has emerged from these various attempts to conceptualise QoL is a functional definition that is measurable and evaluative over time, rests on the patient's own perspective and on the premise that the goal of medicine is to eliminate, or at least reduce, the morbidity and mortality associated with disease.

It has been argued that the problem with the science of QoL assessment is that it has lacked a rigorous theoretical base (Schipper and Clinch, 1988). Conversely, it has been suggested (and the paragraph above might indicate that this is so) that the problem is not a lack of theory, but too much (Fitzpatrick *et al.*, 1998): the different theoretical perspectives of researchers designing the instruments have led to a wide range of definitions, each with their own different emphasis — and this is reflected both in the content of scales and the terms used to describe them. Farquhar (1995) has developed a taxonomy of these differing definitions, which she classifies into global (all-encompassing but telling us little about the possible components of QoL); component (more useful for empirical work, because by identifying a series of QoL components, they make it easier to operationalise the concept); focused (as is the case in *health-related* or *micro-economic* definitions of QoL); and combination (which overlap the first two). She, like a number of other authors, counsels us on the need for a consensus definition, achievable in her view by opening the debate to both lay people and 'experts'. In the meantime, she charges QoL researchers to make explicit the conceptual basis of their measurement attempts.

A number of QoL researchers have proposed possible models of the theoretical links between the sorts of variables that are of primary interest to clinicians and those of more immediate interest to patients. For example, Wilson and Cleary (1995) identify five different levels at which health outcome can be assessed, from biological/physiological

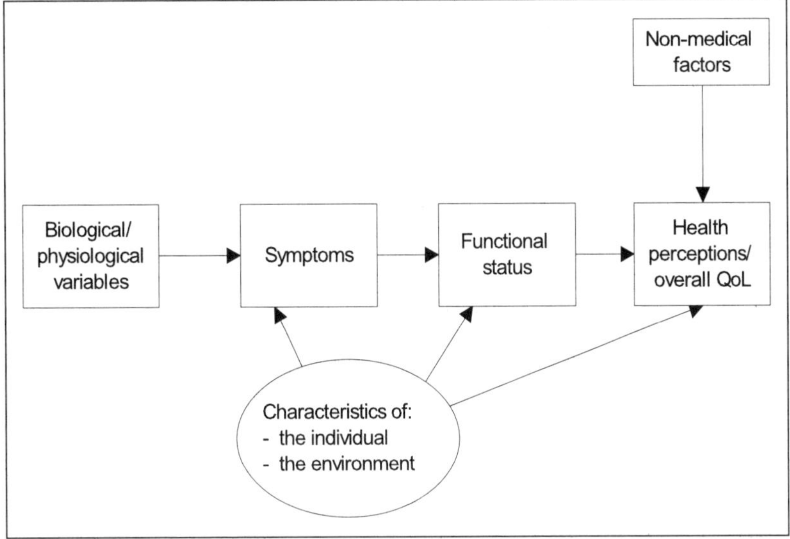

Adapted from Wilson and Cleary (1995)

BOX 2 THEORETICAL LINKS BETWEEN CLINICAL VARIABLES AND HEALTH-RELATED QoL

through to overall QoL; and the mediating role of patient preference and emotional/psychological factors in these (Box 2). They highlight the importance of understanding the complexity of interrelationships between the variables, in making the link between diagnosis and therapy and designing appropriate therapeutic interventions. Likewise, Cramer and Spilker (1998) describe a model of how aspects of a medical treatment at the level of its clinical evaluation (safety and efficacy) are filtered through patients' own beliefs, values and judgements about their health care, to influence their QoL, both within specific domains and globally. In epilepsy, Baker *et al.* (1993) have developed the QoL model originated by Meenan *et al.* (1984), which identifies an operational level at which consideration is given to the effects of their condition on the various aspects of a person's physical, social and psychological functioning; and an operational level, at which measures appropriate to assessing these effects are specified.

Romney and Evans (1996) have taken this theoretical activity one stage further, by adapting and testing a health-related QoL model developed for people with chronic physical or mental illness on a representative sample drawn from the general population. The same five component factors were identified as important across all three groups. Two of the components represented clinical features in the ill groups and features of physical and mental health in the well one; the others represented psychosocial function in all three. Using structural equation modelling to examine the goodness of fit of a series of alternative causal models, the authors were able to show that in people with chronic illness a medical model in which physical and mental health predicted social interrelationships, personal growth and job satisfaction was most appropriate. In contrast, in people who were well, a psychosocial model in which social interrelationships, personal growth and job satisfaction predicted physical and mental health was a better fit. In the context of interventions aimed at improving health outcomes, including QoL, for people who are chronically ill, the important implication of their findings is that symptom reduction will have an important beneficial effect.

A major and fairly fundamental debate is whether, regardless of the theoretical base they adopt, QoL researchers are in fact measuring QoL at all! Hunt (1996) thinks not, suggesting that what QoL researchers in medicine most often do is 'infer quality of life from a variety of indicators' of somewhat questionable validity (Leplege and Hunt, 1997). She argues that future efforts in health and clinical care research should be confined to the measurement of health status and functional capacity which, while acknowledging that patients have their own perspectives on the impact of ill health and treatment, 'implies little or nothing about their quality of life'. Gill and Feinstein (1994) share Hunt's view. After reviewing 75 randomly selected articles with the term 'QoL' in their titles in order to evaluate how well they did, in fact, measure QoL, these authors concluded that what these studies really did was measure different aspects of health status. Because QoL is a highly individual construct, it can only be measured by taking into account patients' own values and preferences; and most of the QoL measures employed in the cited studies made no allowance for this.

In the same edition of JAMA, Guyatt and Cook (1994) responded by pointing out that to argue that individual patients' values should be taken into account in *every* study is too stringent. They maintain that, assuming we can establish that the aspects we ask about are important to patients and that no aspects known to be important to patients are omitted, it is reasonable to conclude *both* that we are measuring the right things and that treatment which improves these things is going to improve QoL. This position is supported by, amongst others, the authors of one of the most frequently used generic health status measures, the MOS Short-Form 36 (Ware and Sherbourne, 1992). Ware and colleagues provide empirical evidence of a positive and substantial relationship between health and quality of life, which suggests that personal evaluations of health status are an extremely good indicator of QoL. Acceptance of the position Guyatt and Cook adopt, does, of course, imply recognition of the importance of actively involving patients in the development of QoL measures — something which has all too often been neglected. There is a clear case here for what has been termed 'discovery research' (Kessler and Mroczek, 1996), both to develop items for inclusion in QoL measures and to examine their comprehensibility to those at whom they are targeted.

The most recent contribution to this debate comes from Smith *et al.* (1999), who used structural equation modelling to examine the relationships between the two constructs, QoL and health status, and three function domains — mental, physical and social — in studies of chronic diseases. Their analysis indicated that QoL and health status are, indeed, distinct constructs; with patients giving greater emphasis to mental health than to physical function when rating QoL and *vice versa* when rating health status. They conclude that many prominent health status measures may be inappropriate for measuring QoL; and that health care evaluations may differ in their conclusions depending on whether QoL or health status measures are chosen to assess treatment outcomes.

QUALITY OF LIFE OR HEALTH-RELATED QUALITY OF LIFE

Another major debate in the science of QoL as applied to medicine revolves around the often interchangeable use of the terms 'QoL' and 'health-related QoL'. This seeming terminological confusion was the subject of debate at an international workshop held in 1991, at which contributors concluded that what QoL concerns is 'the broad range of dimensions of human experience' and not all these dimensions are necessarily health or medical concerns (Patrick and Erickson, 1993). Researchers in this camp argue that we need to focus on dimensions that are — for which reason we should talk about *health-related* QoL (HRQoL), rather than QoL. Needless to say there is an opposing camp, which argues that it is often impossible to separate out health-related and non-health-related aspects of QoL (Hunt, 1997). In the area of epilepsy, Hermann's (1992) distinction between within- and beyond-the-skin variables highlights this impossibility. QoL researchers in the field of health services research increasingly accept that what we are mainly concerned with measuring are those dimensions of QoL which are specific to health and medical care. Most appear fairly comfortable with the definition of QoL in clinical medicine as representing, 'the functional effect of an illness and its consequent therapy upon a patient, as perceived by the patient' (Schipper *et al.*, 1996).

A piece of empirical research that seems to support this emphasis on the health-related aspects of QoL is reported in a recent article by Ann Bowling (1995a). Her work attempted to address the question of whether all the relevant domains are measured in current QoL research. To do so, over 2000 people in Great Britain were interviewed as part of a monthly omnibus survey, about the important things — both positive and negative — in their lives. Informants were asked to identify things that were important, place the items they identified in rank order of importance, rate their current status in relation to each item from as good to as bad as it possibly could be and rate life overall. Informants with limiting long-standing illness or disability were also asked to define and rate the important effects of illness on their lives. Bowling's findings were that the priorities accorded different aspects of life were rather different for those recorded as chronically ill or disabled and those who were not, with the former giving higher priority to health-related aspects (Box 3). Bowling then looked at the coverage of generic HRQoL scales commonly employed in health and health care research and was forced to conclude that not all the domains cited by respondents as important

General population	**Informants with limiting long-standing illness/disability**
Relationships with family (31%)	Ability to get out and about (25%)
Own health (23%)	Availability of/ability to work (14%)
Health of another person (close/dependent other) (20%)	Social life/leisure activities (13%)
Finance/housing/standard of living (10%)	Symptoms (9%)
Relationships with other people (4%)	Other activity restrictions (7%)

*Percentages in brackets are proportions of respondents who ranked each item as first most important.

BOX 3 FIRST MENTIONED 'IMPORTANT THINGS' IN LIFE*

were covered and, conversely, that not all domains covered were identified by respondents as important. Her work also suggests a number of other conclusions, amongst which are the importance of deriving scale items from the populations in which they will be applied; that QoL is multidimensional and questionnaires should independently reflect and measure each relevant dimension; that it may be necessary to weight the different dimensions of QoL; and that generic measures may be best suited to application in general populations and less relevant to people who are ill or have health problems.

MAJOR APPROACHES TO QoL ASSESSMENT

The way in which the researcher conceptualises QoL broadly determines how he or she goes on to measure it (Avis and Smith, 1994). Basically, as highlighted above, there are three broad approaches to QoL measurement: standardised descriptive instruments, both disease-specific and generic; utility (preference-based) measures; and individualised approaches.

The descriptive approach is the one used most often in QoL assessments, perhaps in part because descriptive measures are easiest to apply, many being suitable for patient self-completion. It includes both generic and disease- or condition-specific measures, the advantages and disadvantages of which have been discussed at length in the literature (Patrick and Deyo, 1989; Guyatt and Jaeschke, 1990; Fitzpatrick *et al.*, 1998) and will not be revisited here. However, it is worth noting that evidence about the responsiveness of condition-specific measures compared to generic ones is conflicting (Wiebe *et al.*, 1997; Bessette *et al.*, 1999). A huge number of condition-specific measures is currently available. Bowling (1995b) lists around 30 for cancer, 25 for respiratory conditions, and 20 for cardiovascular conditions. The list for epilepsy is also expanding rapidly, as the review in the next chapter illustrates. Descriptive (or profile) measures provide assessments of several different dimensions of functioning — and this is one of their problems, because it can be difficult to make sense of conflicting outcomes across the different domains. Some researchers have responded to this problem of multiple comparisons by developing summary scales (as in the SF-36, the Epilepsy Surgery Inventory and the QoLIE scales). However, a recently reported study suggests that the solution may not be as simple as this response suggests. Simon *et al.*, (1998) showed that though patients reported modest impairment on the physical function, role physical, pain and general health perceptions subscales of the SF-36 at baseline and moderate improvements at three months follow-up, the physical component summary score indicated neither baseline impairment nor subsequent improvement. In an accompanying editorial, McHorney (1998) makes the point that had Simon and his colleagues used only the summary scales, they would have reached a conclusion that was inconsistent with other evidence. She therefore recommends that summary scales be tested alongside their base profile measures, to elucidate under what circumstances they will produce discrepant results.

The utility approach draws on a specific set of assumptions from economic and decision theory (Fitzpatrick *et al.*, 1998). It elicits the personal preferences of individuals and societal preferences regarding health states. Utilities can be assessed directly by means of an interview using time trade-off, standard gambol and so on; or indirectly, using standardised questionnaires to which previously derived weighted scores are attached. Well-known examples of the latter are the EuroQoL EQ-5D (EuroQol Group, 1990; Dolan *et al.*, 1995) and the Health Utilities Index (Feeny *et al.*, 1995). There can be problems in measuring health states directly, since patients do not always find the tasks they have to perform easy and so interviews can be labour-intensive and time-consuming. That said, a recent cost-utility study of treatment for MS involved a time trade-off exercise with a subset of patients, of whom only a minority reported finding it difficult (Parkin *et al.*, 1998). The object of utility measures is to generate a single index score, thus providing an unambiguous answer as to which of a number of alternative treatments is to be preferred. However, doing so means that there is no disaggregated evidence about individual dimensions of health, with the result that specific advantages or disadvantages may not be detected. There are also questions in the literature about the validity of the methods used to derive values for all possible health states (Brooks and the EuroQoL Group, 1996).

In individualised assessments of QoL, respondents are allowed to focus on those aspects of their life they themselves consider to be most important either in its overall quality (O'Boyle *et al.*, 1992) or as affected by their condition (Ruta *et al.*, 1994), rather than these being predetermined by the investigator. In this sense, individualised approaches have high content validity and could be seen as the 'gold standard' approach to QoL assessment. However, they are labour and time-intensive, and require highly trained interviewers. As a result their use, so far, has been limited. In epilepsy, the main proponents of the patient-generated approach are Kendrick and Trimble (1994) and their colleagues, whose work is described in detail in the next chapter in this volume. Since, in Kendrick's method, informants' responses are probed until at least two constructs have been elicited in each of five QoL areas defined as key by WHO and adopted by the researchers, their approach seems less clearly patient-generated than they suggest. It is nonetheless a very appealing one.

Because of the various unresolved issues relating to each of these three approaches, a common response has been to back all horses and to use a combination. This idea is well-established in relation to the combined use of generic and condition-specific descriptive measures (Cox *et al.*, 1992); it is also not uncommon to use both descriptive and preference-based QoL measures within a single study. Correlations between descriptive and preference-based measures appear weak (McHorney, 1998) but this may be a product of the heterogeneity of the patient groups in whom both have been applied (Bult *et al.*, 1998) and is not necessarily problematic, except where the one type of measure is used to predict responses on the other. The limitations of descriptive measures from a pharmacoeconomic perspective has stimulated research into their transformation to utility measures (Brazier *et al.*, 1998). Recently, Juniper *et al.*, (1992) have offered a possible compromise to the question of individualised versus standardised measures. They allowed patients to identify for themselves up to five items additional to those already included as standard in an asthma QoL questionnaire, and to assess the extent to which they perceived these 'individualised items' as being affected by their condition.

SOFT DATA OR THE MISSING MEASUREMENT?

One of the major criticisms levelled against QoL assessments is that they are subjective and therefore not 'hard' scientific data. This has been vigorously challenged by writers such as Fallowfield (1990) who has described QoL as the vital 'missing measurement in health care'. There is plenty of evidence that the notion of so-called 'hard' data is, in itself, flawed. For example, Feinstein (1977) reviewed the choice of clinical variables used in medical research in the area of cancer and reported 'striking' variability for both intra- and inter-rater reliability among pathologists and radiologists. Focusing on the area of interest for this volume, it is now thought that up to 20% of epilepsy is misdiagnosed, because seizures — the so-called hard evidence of the condition — are not always easy to recognise or identify.

It was because of the pre-occupation with the notion of objectivity that the earliest QoL measures (mainly developed by clinicians) were intended for completion by clinicians rather than patients. However, work by Slevin *et al.*, (1988) and several other authors subsequently showed that not only is there little agreement on QoL between patients and health professionals, neither is there agreement between health professionals themselves. It is also increasingly clear that patients' pre-occupations and the judgements they make about health care often differ significantly from those of clinicians (Wynne, 1989; Guyatt *et al.*, 1993). Such revelations mean that the idea that clinicians are in a good position to complete QoL assessments on behalf of their patients quickly looks less than convincing. However, they also beg the question whether obtaining QoL information from *any* source other than the patient him or herself can be regarded as valid. Since, for patients who are too ill or impaired to complete questionnaires themselves QoL data would otherwise be entirely missing, a considerable body of work has focused on comparing QoL assessments made by patients themselves and their informal caregivers (Sprangers and Aaronson, 1992; Hays *et al.*, 1995; Sneeuw *et al.*, 1997). This shows that agreement is generally good for more observable aspects of QoL, but less good for the less easily observable aspects such as mood or psychological status. It also appears that carers tend to over-estimate effects on some domains and under-estimate others. Hays *et al.* (1995) found only modest correlations between the self-reports of adults with epilepsy and their designated proxies and that the lack of agreement was sufficiently large in some areas as to introduce bias.

A particularly useful piece of research has been reported in relation to proxy assessments in stroke, a condition where the cognitive and communication deficits experienced by some patients means they are often the only possibility. Sneeuw and his colleagues (1997) compared the level of agreement on responses to the Sickness Impact Profile (SIP) between stroke patients and their lay carers. Correlations between patient and proxy ratings on SIP were moderate to high. Differences between patient and proxy ratings were statistically significant for seven of the 11 subscales and the total SIP score, but the magnitude of differences was small, suggesting that only modest bias would be introduced by using proxy information. The differences were also all in same direction, with proxies consistently rating patients as having greater functional limitations than patients themselves. One important finding was that the magnitude of the differences was dependent on the level of the patient's impairment, with bias more pronounced the more impaired the patient. Accepting that there will inevitably be limitations to using proxy data, studies such as theirs at least enable QoL researchers to begin to quantify the degree of bias associated with doing so and make a reasoned decision about whether or not to accept data obtained in this way.

ESTABLISHING THE PSYCHOMETRIC ROBUSTNESS OF QoL MEASURES

Developers of QoL measures need to demonstrate and potential users need to be convinced that they are good science. A recent UK Health Technology Assessment Programme review (Fitzpatrick *et al.*, 1998) highlights eight basic criteria on which QoL measures should be judged (Box 4): appropriateness (to the research question under scrutiny); validity (the ability of the instrument to measure what it purports to measure); reliability (its ability to produce the same results on repeated occasions under similar test conditions); responsiveness (its ability to detect clinically important changes); precision (of the measure's response categories and of its ability to reflect true change); interpretability (the meaningfulness of scores and any changes in scores); acceptability (to patients completing it); and feasibility (with regard to ease of administration).

Judging the appropriateness of a QoL measure depends on the researcher asking him or herself whether it is fit for the purpose for which it is intended. Generally speaking, it is fairly easy to establish validity and reliability, less easy to establish responsiveness. Relatively little work has been done to date about the precision or interpretability of QoL measures, but with regard to the former, it should be recognised that, 'scales with equal reliabilities . . can differ dramatically in their range of precision.' (Kessler and Mroczek, 1996). It has been suggested (Kessler and Mroczek, 1996) that to assure precision, scale developers need to move beyond classical psychometric theory to more recently developed procedures such as item response theory (Streiner and Norman, 1989; Hays, 1998), which takes account of the way in which a person's underlying traits determine his or her responses to questionnaire items.

The problem of interpretability of QoL measures relates to some extent to lack of use (Fitzpatrick *et al.*, 1998). Whereas we know enough about the range of measurement on commonly applied clinical variables to be able to interpret their meaning, their relative infancy means that the same cannot be said to be true of QoL measures. A range

- **Appropriateness:**
  - should be clearly focused on patients' concerns
  - should be relevant to the health problem studied
  - should show evidence of a clear rationale behind selection
- **Validity:**
  - face (what an item appears to measure, based on manifest content)
  - content (how well a measure covers all important domains)
  - construct (does the measure relate to others in previously hypothesised ways)
  - criterion (refers to relationship of the selected measure to another regarded as a 'gold standard' or criterion variable)
  - predictive (whether scores for the selected measure correlate with future values of the criterion variable)
- **Reliability:**
  - internal consistency reliability (examines homogeneity of scale items to ensure that they are measuring a single construct)
  - reproducibility (the degree of agreement between scores at two time-points)
- **Responsiveness:**
  - change scores (significant correlations of change scores on the measure with changes in other available variables)
  - effect size (size of change in group scores on a measure compared with variability of scores; calculated as the difference between mean scores divided by the standard deviation of baseline scores)
  - standardised response mean (differs from effect size in that the denominator is the standard deviation of group change scores)
  - relative efficiency (square of the ratio of the t-statistic for the selected measure relative to another with which it is compared)
  - sensitivity and specificity (transforms change scores into categorical data and tests the sensitivity and specificity of categories against independent evidence)
- **Precision:**
  - of response categories (evidence that precision is increased with seven, over five response categories)
  - of numerical codes assigned to response categories (these are generally unweighted and so make assumptions about the

relationships between the different options which may therefore decrease precision)
- floor and ceiling effects (response categories may not allow respondents in poor health to report further deterioration or those in good health to report further improvement)

- **Interpretability:**
  - by reference to normative data (though in practice, such data only exist for the more widely used QoL measures)
  - by standardising QoL scores (by calculating the study sample mean, then relating individual patient scores to the mean for the whole sample)
  - by calibration (of changes in QoL scores against changes for the same instruments associated with major life events
  - by identifying the range within which a minimal clinically important difference (MCID) falls
- **Acceptability:**
  - of length and completion time required
  - of questionnaire format and readability
  - of cultural applicability
  - as indicated by non-completion item omission rates
- **Feasibility:**
  - of mode of delivery
  - of data processing and analysis

BOX 4 CRITERIA FOR JUDGING QoL MEASURES

of possible options for interpreting scores on QoL measures has been suggested, though it is worth noting that these are as yet unevaluated and no one appears to out-rank any other (Liang, 1995). Keller and Ware (1995) provide us with a useful illustration of how a change in a scale score might be interpreted by different audiences. The score change under scrutiny was one of a 7.6 improvement on the SF-36 physical function scale, observed in older patients undergoing heart value replacement surgery. Statistically, this represented a gain of three-quarters of a standard deviation; clinically, they argue, it meant the surgery was successful; from the health payer perspective, it meant a 3% decrease in the hospitalisation rate; from the perspective of employers, it meant a 8% decrease in job losses; and lastly and arguably most importantly, for patients it meant improved functioning and increased 5-year survival rate (from 87% to 92%).

Not surprisingly, Keller and Ware make a strong plea in support of using standardised generic core measures such as their own, since this will allow a more rapid accumulation of generalisable information. However, as Bowling (1995a) has shown, generic scales may not always be appropriate. One way forward, they suggest, would be the development of disease-specific scoring of generic health profiles. Ware (1998) has also argued the case for developing a common metric against which the various health status and QoL measures could be plotted alongside one another.

Ways in which the acceptability of questionnaires (QoL or otherwise) can be maximised and the relative efficiency of different modes of delivery have been the focus of a considerable body of survey methodological activity and are summarised in another recently commissioned UK Health Technology Assessment Programme review (McColl *et al.*, in press). Suffice it to say that QoL researchers need to pay careful attention to matters of questionnaire length and speed of completion, appearance and layout, readability, question formatting and ordering, question response options and so on, as well as to content and coverage. The use of techniques such as cognitive interviewing are receiving increasing emphasis as an integral part of developing and refining QoL measures and have been shown to contribute to an improved instrument with less response error (Harris-Kojetin *et al.*, 1999).

A recent review of QoL measures for epilepsy illustrates the relative lack of psychometric evidence in their support (Jacoby, 1996), a matter explored fully in the following chapter. Nor is there always detailed information available against which they can be judged in relation to the other criteria specified above. It seems reasonable to suppose that a parallel review in any other clinical area would highlight the similar information gaps.

DO QoL ASSESSMENTS OFFER ADDED VALUE?

It has been suggested that QoL measures could be useful both to clinicians in everyday clinical practice and across a wide range of health care research contexts (Fitzpatrick *et al.*, 1992), though there is some argument as to whether these are all entirely appropriate. In everyday practice, Hopkins (1992) proposes their use: to provide baseline data against which effectiveness of subsequent interventions can be measured; to draw attention to areas of difficulty that the clinician may otherwise overlook; to determine disease severity and so the priority given to treating the patient; to understand the illness experience from the patient's viewpoint; to encourage patients to make treatment choices that fully reflect the values they place upon different dimensions of QoL; and to assess the impact of therapy and allow patients a say in planning their treatment. A number of 'mini' measures — shortened forms of the originals — have been produced to meet the requirements of clinical practice; in epilepsy, for example, the authors of the QoLIE scales suggest their 10-item version for use in this context. Likewise, Ware and colleagues have recently published a yet shorter form of the Short-Form 36, the SF-12 (Ware *et al.*, 1996).

Unfortunately, though the idea that using QoL measures might improve clinical practice is an attractive one (at least from the perspective of this sometime patient!), there is little evidence as yet that they make a great deal of difference. Wagner *et al.*, (1997) looked at the routine use of QoL questionnaires for patients with epilepsy and found that though consultation time was lengthened and doctors felt that such measures provided new information about the patient, they did not alter their management of the patient and patients did not report any increase in satisfaction. It has been suggested that one reason for the apparent lack of impact of QoL and other patient-centred measures on routine clinical care is the lack of clarity about how to present the data to clinicians in a useful and manageable way. One attempt to do so in epilepsy, which makes use of computerised methods, is reported later in this book (see Chapter 11). Another difficulty is that few QoL measures have been documented as having adequate reliability for use at the level of the individual, as opposed to with groups of patients, a point discussed in some detail in the next chapter.

With regard to their value in other health care contexts, Battista and Hodge (1996) think QoL measures can reasonably be applied to public health policy making; whereas Ebrahim (1995) thinks they cannot, because of the various unresolved conceptual and methodological issues. He does concede, however, that they have something to offer in clinical trials of new therapies, by virtue of their ability to detect unexpected outcomes. There is certainly some support for the claim that QoL assessments represent added value from published trials of treatment for epilepsy (see Chapter 12). Despite the expression of some misgivings, it is now generally accepted that trials should incorporate QoL or other patient-centred measures, unless it is clear that they are not relevant outcomes (Fitzpatrick *et al.*, 1998). Interestingly, a review in the British Medical Journal's special edition on 50 years of clinical trials, highlighted how rarely QoL outcomes have so far been reported (Sanders *et al.*, 1998). In the ten years from 1987 to 1997, they were mentioned in only 5% of all published trials identified through the UK Cochrane Collaboration database. This dearth of publications has been attributed to the lengthy life-span of most large multicentre trials (Lancet Editorial, 1995) and so, it is suggested, will naturally be redressed by time. At present, QoL measures are most often used as secondary outcomes in clinical trials, though there are some examples of their use as primary ones, particularly in the field of oncology.

CONCLUSION

In the context of medicine, QoL research, though no longer in its infancy, is still a relatively young science. Yet despite its youthfulness it can reasonably claim to be becoming increasingly sophisticated at both a theoretical and methodological level. Early QoL research in the medical setting was largely empirically driven and less than adequately informed by attention to conceptual and theoretical issues. The criticisms levelled at it have been important in emphasising the need to address such shortcomings robustly; and the suggestion by Avis and Smith (1994) that the term 'quality of life' be applied 'more judiciously' is one that is difficult to disregard. QoL researchers have taken the various challenges seriously, and knowledge is rapidly accumulating not only on how to develop measures that satisfy basic psychometric criteria, but also on the meaning of QoL data from the points of view of its various protagonists, and on the relationships of different QoL measures to one another and to traditional clinical measures. The fact that there is a continuing political agenda for QoL research (Secretary of State for Health, 1997; Tilson and Tierney, 1999), coupled with rapid methodological and technological advances in its implementation, would suggest that it will continue to be seen as central to the assessment of health care outcomes, at least for the foreseeable future.

References

Avis, N.E., Smith, K.W. (1994) Conceptual and methodological issues in selecting and developing quality of life measures. In: Fitzpatrick, R., (ed.) *Advances in medical sociology*. London: JAI Press Inc, 255–280.

Baker, G.A., Smith, D.F., Dewey, M., Jacoby, A., Chadwick, D.W. (1993) The initial development of a health-related quality of life model as an outcome measure in epilepsy. *Epilepsy Research* **16**, 65–81.

Baker, G.A., Jacoby, A., Smith, D., Dewey, M., Johnson, A., Chadwick, D. (1994) Quality of life in epilepsy: the Liverpool initiative. In: Trimble, M.R., Dodson, W.E., (eds.) *Epilepsy and Quality of Life*, New York: Raven Press Ltd, 135–150.

Battista, R.N., Hodge, M.J. (1996) Quality of life research and health technology assessment: a time for synergy. *Quality of Life Research* **5**, 413–418.

Bessette, L., Sangha, O., Kuntz, K.M., Keller, R.B., Lew, R.A., Fossel, A.H., Katz, J.N. (1999) Comparative responsiveness of generic versus disease-specific and weighted versus unweighted health status measure in carpal tunnel syndrome. *Medical Care* **36**(4), 491–502.

Bowling, A. (1995a) What things are important in people's lives? A survey of the public's judgements to inform scales of health related quality of life. *Social Science and Medicine* **41**(10), 1447–1462.

Bowling, A. (1995b) *Measuring disease*. Buckingham: Open University Press.

Brazier, J., Usherwood, T., Harper, R., Thomas, K. (1998) Deriving a preference-based single index from the UK SF-36 Health Survey. *Journal of Clinical Epidemiology* **51**(11), 1115–1128.

Brooks, R.H. and the EuroQoL Group (1996) EuroQoL: the current state of play. *Health Policy* **37**, 53–72.

Bult, J.R., Hunink, M.G., Tsevat, J., Weinstein, M.C. (1998) Heterogeneity in the relationship between the time tradeoff and Short Form-36 for HIV-infected and primary care patients. *Medical Care* **36**(4), 523–532.

Calman, K.C. (1984) Quality of life in cancer patients — a hypothesis. *Journal of Medical Ethics* **10**, 124–127.

Chadwick, D.W. (1990) *Quality of life and quality of care in epilepsy. RSM Round Table Series No. 23*, London: Royal Society of Medicine.

Cox, D.R., Fitzpatrick, R., Fletcher, A.E., Gore, S.M., Spiegelhalter, D.J., Jones, D.R. (1992) Quality of life assessment: can we keep it simple? *Journal of the Royal Statistical Society* **155**(3), 353–393.

Cramer, J., Spilker, B. (1998) *Quality of Life and Pharmacoeconomics: an introduction*, Philadelphia: Lippincott-Raven.

Devinsky, O., Vickrey, B.G., Cramer, J., Perrine, K., Hermann, B.P., Meador, K., Hays, R.D. (1995) Development of the quality of life in epilepsy inventory. *Epilepsia* **36**(1), 1089–1104.

Dolan, P., Gudex, C., Kind, P., Williams, A. (1995) *A social tariff for EUROQOL: results from a UK general population survey*. University of York: Centre for Health Economics.

Ebrahim, S. (1995) Clinical and public health perspectives and applications of health-related quality of life measurement. *Social Science and Medicine* **41**(10), 1383–1394.

EuroQoL Group (1990) EuroQoL — a new facility for the measurement of health-related quality of life. *Health Policy* **16**, 199–208.

Fallowfield, L. (1990) *The Quality of Life: The Missing Measurement in Health Care*, London: Souvenir Press.

Farquhar, M. (1995) Definitions of quality of life: a taxonomy. *Journal of Advanced Nursing* **22**, 502–508.

Fayers, P.M., Hopwood, P., Harvey, A., Girling, D.J., Machin, D., Stephens, R. (1997) Quality of life assessment in clinical trials — guidelines and a checklist for protocol writers: the UK Medical Research Council experience. *European Journal of Cancer* **33**(1), 20–28.

Feeny, D., Furlong, W., Boyle, M., Torrance, G.W. (1995) Multi-attribute health status classification systems: health utilities index. *Pharmacoeconomics* 7, 490–502.

Feinstein, A.R. (1977) Hard science, soft data and the challenges of choosing clinical variables in research. *Clinical Pharmacology and Therapeutics* **22**, 485–498.

Fitzpatrick, R., Fletcher, A., Gore, S., Jones, D., Spiegelhalter, D., Cox, D. (1992) Quality of life measures in health care. I: applications and issues in assessment. *British Medical Journal* **305**, 1074–1077.

Fitzpatrick, R., Davey, C., Buxton, M.J., Jones, D.R. (1998) Evaluating patient-based outcome measures for use in clinical trials. *Health Technology Assessment* 2(14).

Gill, T.M., Feinstein, A.R. (1994) A critical appraisal of the quality of quality-of-life measurements. *Journal of the American Medical Association* **272**(8), 619–626.

Guyatt, G.H., Cook, D.J. (1994) Health status, quality of life, and the individual. *Journal of the American Medical Association* **272**(8), 630–631.

Guyatt, G., Jaeschke, R. (1990) Measurements in clinical trials: choosing the appropriate approach. In: Spilker, B., (ed.) *Quality of life assessments in clinical trials*. New York: Raven Press, 37–46

Guyatt, G., Feeny, D.H., Patrick, D.L. (1993) Measuring health-related quality of life. *Annals of Internal Medicine* **118**, 622–629.

Harris-Kojetin, L.D., Fowler, F.J., Brown, J.A., Schnaier, J.A., Sweeny, S.F. (1999) The use of cognitive testing to develop and evaluate CAHPS^{TM} 1.0 core survey items. *Medical Care* 37(3), MS10-MS21

Hays, R.D. (1995) Directions for future research. *Quality of Life Research* **4**, 179–180.

Hays, R.D. (1998) Item response theory models. In: Staquet, M.J., Hays, R.D. and Fayers, P.M. (eds.) *Quality of Life Assessment in Clinical Trials: Methods and Practice*, Oxford: Oxford University Press, 183–190.

Hays, R.D., Vickrey, B.G., Hermann, B.P., Perrine, K., Cramer, J., Meador, K., Spritzer, K., Devinsky, O. (1995) Agreement between self reports and proxy reports of quality of life in epilepsy patients. *Quality of Life Research* **4**, 159–168.

Hermann, B.P. (1992) Quality of life in epilepsy. *Journal of Epilepsy* **5**, 153–165.

Hermann, B.P. (1995) The evolution of health-related quality of life assessment in epilepsy. *Quality of Life Research* **4**, 87–100.

Hopkins, A. (ed.) (1992) *Measures of the quality of life, and the uses to which such measures may be put*. London: Royal College of Physicians.

Hunt, S.M. (1997) The problem of quality of life. *Quality of Life Research* **6**, 205–212.

Jacoby, A. (1992) Epilepsy and the quality of everyday life: findings from a study of people with well-controlled epilepsy. *Social Science and Medicine* **43**(6), 657–666.

Jacoby, A. (1996) Assessing quality of life in patients with epilepsy. *Pharmacoeconomics* **9**(5), 399–416.

Jacoby, A., Johnson, A.L., Chadwick, D.W. (1992) Psychosocial outcomes of antiepileptic drug discontinuation. *Epilepsia* **33**(6), 1123–1131.

Juniper, E.F., Guyatt, G.H., Epstein, R.S., Ferrie, P.J., Jeneschke, R., Hiller, T.K. (1992) Evaluation of impairment of health-related QoL in asthma: development of questionnaire for use in clinical trials. *Thorax* **47**(2), 76–83.

Karnovsky, D.A., Abelmann, W.H., Craver, L.F. (1948) The use of nitrogen mustards in the palliative treatment of carcinoma. *Cancer* **1**, 634–656.

Keller, S.D., Ware, J.E. (1995) Interpretation strategies for health status scores. *Medical Outcomes Trust Bulletin* 3(5), 2–4.

Kendrick, A.M., Trimble, M.R. (1994) Repertory grid in the assessment of quality of life in patients with epilepsy: The quality of life assessment schedule. In: Trimble, M., Dodson, W., (eds.) *Epilepsy and quality of life*, New York: Raven Press Ltd, 151–164.

Kessler, R.C., Mroczek, D.K. (1996) Some methodological issues in the development of quality of life measures for the evaluation of medical interventions. *Journal of Evaluation in Clinical Practice* 2(3), 181–191.

Lancet Editorial (1995) Quality of life and clinical trials. *The Lancet* **346**, July 1–2.

Leplege, A., Hunt, S. (1997) The problem of quality of life in medicine. *Journal of the American Medical Association* **278**(1), 47–50.

Levine, M.N. (1988) Quality of life in Stage II breast cancer: an instrument for clinical trials. *Journal of Clinical Oncology* **6**, 1798–1810.

Liang, M.H. (1995) Evaluating measurement responsiveness. *Journal of Rheumatology* **22**(1), 1191–1192.

McCartney, C.F., Larson, D.B. (1987) Quality of life in patients with gynaecological cancer. *Cancer* **60**(suppl. 2), 129–2136.

McColl, E., Jacoby, A., Thomas, L., Soutter, J., Bamford, C., Thomas, R., Harvey, E., Garrett, A., Bond, J. (2000) Designing and using patient and staff questionnaires: a review of best practice. *Health Technology Assessment*, in press.

McHorney, C.A. (1998) Methodological inquiries in health status assessment. *Medical Care* **36**(4), 445–448.

Meador, K.J. (1993) Research use of the new Quality-of-life in Epilepsy Inventory. *Epilepsia* **34**, S34-S38

Meenan, R.F., Anderson, J.J., Kazis, L.E. (1984) Outcome assessment in clinical trials. *Arthritis and Rheumatism* **27**, 1344–1352.

O'Boyle, C.A., McGee, H., Hickey, A., O'Malley, K., Joyce, C.R.B. (1992) Individual quality of life in patients undergoing hip replacement. *The Lancet* **339**, 1088–1091.

Parkin, D., McNamee, P., Jacoby, A., Miller, P., Thomas, S., Bates, D. (1998) A cost-utility analysis of interferon beta for multiple sclerosis. *Health Technology Assessment* **2**(4).

Patrick, D.L., Deyo, R.A. (1989) Generic and disease-specific measures in assessing health status and quality of life. *Medical Care* **27**(suppl. 3), S217-S232

Patrick, D.L., Erickson, P. (1993) Assessing health-related quality of life for clinical decision-making. In: Walker, S.R. and Rosser, R.M., (eds.) *Quality of life assessment: Key issues in the 1990s*, Lancaster: Kluwer Academic Publishers.

Read, J.L. (1993) The new era of quality of life assessment. In: Walker, S.R., Rosser, R.M. (eds.) *Quality of life assessment: Key issues in the 1990s.* Lancaster: Kluwer Academic Publishers.

Romney, D.M., Evans, D.R. (1996) Toward a general model of health-related quality of life. *Quality of Life Research* **5**, 235–241.

Rosenberg, R. (1995) Health-related quality of life between naturalism and hermeneutics. *Social Science and Medicine* **41**(10), 1411–1415.

Ruta, D.A., Garratt, A.M., Leng, M., Russell, I.T., Macdonald, L.M. (1994) A new approach to the measurement of quality of life. *Medical Care* **32**(11), 1109–1123.

Sanders, C., Egger, M., Donovan, J., Tallon, D., Frankel, S. (1998) Reporting on quality of life in randomised controlled trials: bibliographic study. *British Medical Journal* **317**, 1191–1194.

Scambler, G. (1993) Epilepsy and quality of life research. *Journal of the Royal Society of Medicine* **86**, 449–450.

Schipper, H., Clinch, J. (1988) Assessment of treatment in cancer. In: Teeling-Smith, G. (ed.) *Measuring health: a practical approach*. Chichester: John Wiley and Sons, 109–139.

Schipper, H., Clinch, J., Powell, V. (1990) Definitions and conceptual issues. In: Spilker, B. (ed.) *Quality of life assessments in clinical trials.* New York: Raven Press, 11–24.

Schipper, H., Clinch, J., Olweny, C.L.M. (1996) Quality of life studies: definitional and conceptual issues. In: Spilker, B., (ed.) *Quality of life and pharmacoeconomics in clinical trials*, 2nd edn. New York: Lippincott Raven, 11–24

Secretary of State for Health (1997) *The new NHS*. London: The Stationery Office.

Simon, G.E., Revicki, D.A., Grothaus, L., Vonkorff, M. (1998) SF-36 summary scores: are physical and mental health truly distinct? *Medical Care* **36**(4), 445–448.

Slevin, M.L. (1992) Current issues in cancer. Quality of life: philosophical question or clinical reality? *British Medical Journal* **305**, 466–469.

Slevin, M.L., Plant, H., Lynch, D., Drinkwater, J., Gregory, W.M. (1988) Who should measure quality of life, the doctor or the patient? *British Journal of Cancer* **57**, 109–112.

Smith, K.W., Avis, N.E., Assmann, S.F. (1999) Distinction between quality of life and health status in quality of life research: a metanalysis. Quality of Life Research 8(5), 447–59.

Sneeuw, K.C.A., Aaronson, N.K., de Haan, R.J., Limburg, M. (1997) Assessing quality of life after stroke: the value and limitation of proxy ratings. *Stroke* **28**(8), 1541–1549.

Spitzer, W.O. (1987) State of science 1986: quality of life and functional status as target variables for research. *Journal of Chronic Diseases* 40(6), 465–471.

Sprangers, M.A.G., Aaronson, N.K. (1992) The role of health care providers and significant others in evaluating the quality of life of patients with chronic disease: a review. *Journal of Clinical Epidemiology* 45(7), 743–760.

Staquet, M., Berzon, R., Osoba, D., Machin, D. (1996) Guidelines for reporting results of quality of life assessments in clinical trials. *Quality of Life Research* 5, 496–502.

Streiner, D.L., Norman, G.R. (1989) *Health measurement scales: a practical guide to their development and use*, Oxford: Oxford Medical Publications.

Tilson, H., Tierney, W.M. (1999) Pharmacoeconomics and Pharmaceutical outcomes research: new trends, new promises, new challenges. *Medical Care* 37(4), AS1-AS3

Vickrey, B.G., Hays, R.D., Graber, J., Rausch, R., Engel, J., Brook, R.H. (1992) A health-related quality of life instrument for patients evaluated for epilepsy surgery. *Medical Care* 30(4), 299–319.

Wagner, A.K., Ehrenberg, B.L., Tran, T.A., Bungay, K.M., Cynn, D.J., Rogers, W.H. (1997) Patient-based health status measurement in clinical practice: a study of its impact on epilepsy patients' care. *Quality of Life Research* 6, 329–341.

Ware, J. (1998) *Interpreting quality of life scores*. Talk given at ISOQOL workshop, 5th Annual Conference of ISOQOL, Baltimore, USA, November 1998.

Ware, J.E., Sherbourne, C.D. (1992) The MOS 36-item Short-Form Health Survey (SF-36). I. Conceptual framework and item selection. *Medical Care* 30(6), 473–483.

Ware, J.E., Kosinski, M., Keller, S.D. (1996) SF-12 An even shorter health survey. *Medical Outcomes Trust Bulletin* 4(1), 2–2.

Wiebe, S., Rose, K., Derry, P., McLachlan, R. (1997) Outcome assessment in epilepsy: comparative responsiveness of quality of life and psychosocial instruments. *Epilepsia* 38(4), 430–438.

Wilson, I.B., Cleary, P.D. (1995) Linking clinical variables with health related quality of life: a conceptual model of patient outcomes. *Journal of the American Medical Association* 273(1), 59–65.

Wynne, A. (1989) Is it any good? The evaluation of therapy by participants in a clinical trial. *Social Science and Medicine* 29(11), 1289–1297.

Chapter 5

A REVIEW OF CURRENTLY AVAILABLE QUALITY OF LIFE MEASURES

Nicole V. Steinbüchel, Sabine Heel and Monika Bullinger

A BRIEF HISTORY

The formal assessment of quality of life in epilepsy has a short history, through it has long been a concern to clinicians in everyday clinical routine. However, the measurement of quality of life has only recently been considered fruitful and feasible. According to Hermann (1995), the assessment of health-related quality of life in epilepsy has evolved through three phases. The first phase emphasised measuring clinical features of epilepsy in terms of cognitive function and intelligence (e.g., Fetterman and Barnes, 1932; Matthews and Klove, 1967; Dikmen *et al.,* 1975; Dikmen and Matthews, 1977; Seidenberg *et al.*, 1981). Behavioural and emotional correlates of epilepsy were also investigated (Guerrant *et al.*, 1962; Hermann and Whitman, 1984; Whitman and Hermann, 1986). In this phase, researchers were concerned with the phenomenology of this chronic neurological condition rather than with patients' ability to adjust to the disease. In the second phase, the need to develop epilepsy-related psychological instruments became apparent. Two different approaches can be distinguished (Hermann, 1995). One approach was to design self-report inventories for patients to assess the psychosocial consequences thought to be particularly associated with epilepsy, as in the 'Washington Psychosocial Seizure Inventory' (WPSI; Dodrill *et al.,* 1980) and the 'Social Effects Scale' (Chaplin *et al.,* 1990). The other approach involved developing scales referring to more specific problems or concerns in epilepsy, like fear of seizures (Mittan and Locke, 1982; Mittan, 1986; Goldstein *et al.,* 1990) or perceived stigma (Ryan *et al.*, 1980). The third phase is characterised by an increased focus on developing disease-specific instruments and on applying concepts from health-care research. This has led to a new generation of instruments focusing on wider quality of life (QoL) issues.

DEFINING QUALITY OF LIFE IN EPILEPSY

The term 'Quality of life in Epilepsy' (EQoL) represents a construct which can be operationalised by relevant dimensions. This immediately presents three questions: 1. Which are the relevant dimensions of EQoL, and how many are there? 2. Which instrumental approach fits the EQoL construct best? and 3. who is the appropriate person to evaluate EQoL? The view that EQoL is a multidimensional construct (Hermann, 1992, 1993; Baker *et al.*, 1993; Cramer, 1993, 1997; and Kendrick, 1997) is supported by empirical investigations (Chaplin *et al.*, 1990, 1992; Gilliam *et al.*, 1997) showing numerous areas of concern in people with epilepsy. To develop a comprehensive instrument for the assessment of all aspects of epilepsy, it is necessary both to define quality of life in epilepsy as comprehensively as possible, and to empirically determine the areas of importance. Hermann (1992) provides an excellent overview of life domains important for assessing EQoL, suggesting fundamental areas such as functional status (self-care, mobility, physical activity), role activities (work, household management), social functioning (personal interactions, intimacy, community interactions), emotional status (anxiety, stress, depression, locus of control, spiritual well-being), as well as cognition, sleep and rest, energy and vitality, health perceptions, and general life satisfaction. The Liverpool Initiative (Baker *et al.*, 1993) suggests a similar approach: EQoL should be assessed across physical (daily functioning), social (work, finance, relations), cognitive and emotional (subsumed under psychological) domains. Devinsky *et al.*, (1995) point out that as it is a subjective concept the patient is the expert on his or her quality of life, and maintains that 'the ways in which the disorder and the seizures impact on a person's life are as individual as fingerprints.' However, proxy reports can and should provide important supplementary information (Hermann, 1993).

MEASUREMENT APPROACHES IN EQoL ASSESSMENT

In this chapter, we will review currently available measures of EQoL. Two methodological approaches to assess quality of life in patients with epilepsy can be distinguished: a quantitative approach, using scales derived from quantitative analyses (global, generic, condition-specific, and utility measures), and a qualitative approach. We will consider both approaches. According to Kirshner and Guyatt (1985), the quantitative approach is represented by three different types of instruments, which can be distinguished according to their application: discriminative, evaluative, or predictive (for further discussion, see: Jaeschke and Guyatt, 1990; Testa and Nackley, 1994; Guyatt *et al.*, 1996). While discriminative instruments are designed to make distinctions among (groups of) individuals with respect to a criterion at a single point in time (cross-sectional), evaluative instruments separate individuals with a major change in the criterion from those with a minor one (longitudinal). In considering the various measures identified by our review, we will comment both on their psychometric properties and on their usefulness as discriminative, evaluative or predictive instruments.

IDENTIFYING EQoL MEASURES

To identify relevant EQoL instruments, evaluation studies, descriptive and clinical investigations, several Medline and PsychLit searches were conducted in 1998, going back to 1966 and using the key words 'Quality of life', 'Life Quality', and 'Social Adjustment' in combination with 'epilepsy'. The final literature search yielded 371 sources. The first study identified as evaluating EQoL dates back to 1979 (National Institutes for Health, 1979). After revision, 174 records with EQoL as key words were included for further analyses. Of these, 37% were related to conceptual and theoretical issues (e.g., QoL and definition, antiepileptic drug treatment, surgery, cost utility, measurement, review of scales), 12% consisted of psychometric and evaluative studies, and 51% were empirical investigations. Of the latter, 18% investigated children, 6% cost utility issues, 4% were studies with generic instruments, 35% with instruments without any published psychometric study, and 37% were studies using epilepsy-specific, validated scales in any context. Most of the latter studies were descriptive or epidemiological investigations (23). Finally, six controlled and four randomised clinical trials included QoL as an outcome criterion (Appendix 1). For review, we selected epilepsy-specific scales which were validated in a psychometric study and used in at least one empirical investigation. The construction principle, the underlying model and content of the scale, psychometric criteria, and, if available, their evaluation in clinical studies are described.

PSYCHOMETRIC CRITERIA FOR SCALE ASSESSMENT

The following psychometric concepts are critical for the evaluation of health-related measures of QoL related to epilepsy: reliability (reproducibility, internal consistency), validity (content, construct), and responsiveness. Some important aspects of each are discussed below.

Reliability

Test-retest reliability, which denotes the association between test scores over time across individuals is commonly validated by the Pearson correlation coefficient. This procedure, however, raises problems (Bland and Altman, 1986; Johnson, 1994; Streiner and Norman, 1995). As an alternative, the intraclass correlation coefficient, based on an analysis of variance, has been suggested (Streiner and Norman, 1995). Only a few investigators in the EQoL field take the problem of the Pearson correlation into account. Because of that, in accordance with Nunally and Bernstein (1994), we chose a Pearson correlation coefficient of $r_{tt} = 0.70$ as an acceptable criterion to prove stability over time for the scales discussed below.

Internal consistency, which refers to the association of items within one scale, defines another aspect of reliability. Cronbach's α — as a function of the number of items and their average intercorrelation — provides one way to assess internal consistency. As a criterion for group comparison, which is the main aim of scale development and the application of EQoL assessment at the moment, a coefficient alpha of 0.80 was chosen in accordance with Nunally (Nunally and Bernstein, 1994; for critical discussion of the concept of Cronbach's α see Clark and Watson, 1995).

Validity

Validating a scale is a continuing process. It involves evaluating what a scale purports to measure. Face validity, content validity, construct validity, and criterion validity represent different approaches, although 'all validity is at its base some form of construct validity' (Guion, 1977). Of special relevance for the quality-of-life field are both content and construct validity (for detailed definitions see Nunally and Bernstein, 1994; Streiner and Norman, 1995).

There are two different ways to prove content validity. It can be achieved by experts' judgements (Johnson, 1994) that the scale covers the aspects which the construct was intended to measure; or by patient validation. Items in scales which claim to validate QoL of patients should be generated from a data pool reflecting patients' concerns. To uphold the content validity of a scale, as comprehensive a data pool as possible, including patients' concerns and experts' judgements, is recommended.

Discriminant and divergent validity are considered part of construct validity since they examine the conceptual boundaries of the QoL construct. To simultaneously examine both convergent and discriminant validity, the multitrait-multimethod matrix is recommended (Campbell and Fiske, 1959). Construct validity can be supported by the known-groups approach, which involves comparison of mean scores on the scale in different groups (for example, groups divided according to seizure frequency). Factor analysis can provide evidence for the proposed dimensionality of the scale, and implicitly for the dimensions of the construct. Independent of the technique, a comprehensive interpretation of the results is most important.

Responsiveness

Evaluative instruments must be responsive, which means they should be sensitive to change due to an intervention on the time-axis. To estimate a responsiveness index (Guyatt *et al.*, 1989) it is necessary to detect treatment effects as well as to avoid large Type II errors (assuming no difference when a true difference due to intervention really exists (Testa and Nackley, 1994)). High floor or ceiling effects compromise an instrument's responsiveness because they prevent evaluation of effects in those patients concentrated at the top or the bottom of the scale. Therefore, the range of an instrument is also of importance. If ceiling/floor effects are high in a scale an interpretation by the investigators should be provided. Finally, one must ask whether a statistically relevant change reflects a substantial change in QoL, or if this change is clinically relevant. Values for clinical relevance exist for measures such as the SF-36 (Ware and Sherbourne, 1992) which forms the generic core of a number of epilepsy-specific instruments. The time window of the scales, the time required to complete them and the response rate are all important as indicators of feasibility. Each instrument presented below will be discussed according to the above mentioned criteria.

QUANTITATIVE MULTIDIMENSIONAL APPROACHES

Single Scales

The Epilepsy Surgery Inventory (ESI)-55: Published in 1992, the ESI-55 was developed to assess the outcome of surgery for epilepsy (Vickrey *et al.*, 1992; Vickrey, 1993). Based on the generic core of the RAND 36-Item Health Survey (SF-36; Ware and Sherbourne, 1992; Hays *et al.*, 1993), Vickrey and co-workers added a 19-item supplement, including 12 epilepsy-specific items addressing role limitations due to memory problems, cognitive function, and epilepsy-specific health perceptions.

In addition, five items referring to the health-perception scale and the role-limitation scale and two items on overall quality of life were included (Table 1). The underlying health-related model of quality of life includes three distinct dimensions (physical, mental, and social), as well as general health. A literature review and expert information were cited to justify the method (Vickrey, 1993).

In its initial assessment, the ESI-55 was completed by 200 patients (response rate: 89%), 53% of whom were female; the mean age was 34 years; 83% had undergone epilepsy surgery, and the rest had been evaluated for (although not undergone) surgery. For most items, a time window of four weeks was chosen. The question concerning a change in health covers a period of one year. The ESI-55 requires about 15 minutes to complete.

Data analysis showed Cronbach's α ranged from 0.68–0.88; nine of the 11 scales equalled or exceeded 0.80. Hypothesised subscales were empirically supported, showing that no item correlated significantly higher with any subscale than with its own. A subsequent study by Langfitt (1995) involving 71 patients confirmed these results. Content validity was established by the judgements of nine professionals and eight patients. Construct validity was supported by three different analyses. First, an exploratory, common-factor analysis was conducted to examine the interrelationships among the scales. Three factors (mental, physical and cognitive/role limitation) were extracted. In a second step, the ESI-55 and an administered mood profile were correlated. Convergent and discriminant validity was established for two subscales (emotional well-being/energy) and discriminant validity was established for the physical function subscale. The authors showed that seizure-free patients scored significantly higher on all 11 subscales than those still experiencing auras or seizures; the health perceptions and energy/fatigue scales discriminated best. This result was reproduced in further studies (Vickrey *et al.,* 1993; Vickrey, 1995a; O'Donoghue *et al.,* 1998). However, only the health-perception scale detected more sensitive differences following seizure classification into three groups (seizure-free, auras only, seizures).

One problem relating to the evaluative aspect of the ESI-55 should be mentioned. In the initial study (Vickrey *et al.*, 1992), as well as in a study by Langfitt (1995), the ESI-55 showed high ceiling effects. The question is whether this has consequences for its responsiveness. Recently, Wiebe *et al.* (1997) compared the responsiveness of the ESI-55, the WPSI (Dodrill *et al.*, 1980), and the Symptom Checklist-90-

TABLE 1 LISTING OF IMPORTANT ASPECTS OF THE ESI-55 (VICKREY *ET AL.*, 1992)

PURPOSE	ITEM GENERATION	SCORING	SUBSCALES ACCORDING TO FACTOR STRUCTURE	NO. OF ITEMS	CRONBACH'S α
OUTCOME MEASURE FOR PATIENTS WITH INTRACTABLE EPILEPSY UNDERGOING EPILEPSY SURGERY	54 ITEMS IN 11 SUBSCALES AND ONE ITEM ON OVERALL CHANGE IN HEALTH GENERIC CORE: SF-36 SUPPLEMENTAL ITEMS DERIVED FROM OTHER MEASURES AND EXPERT OPINION	VARIOUS FORMATS: SINGLE SCALES CONSIST OF ITEMS WITH DIFFERENT RESPONSE FORMATS. EACH SUBSCALE SCORE IS TRANSFORMED ONTO A 0–100-POINT SCALE. AN OVERALL SCORE AND THREE COMPOSITE SCORES (REFLECTING THE UNDERLYING FACTOR MATRIX) CAN BE DERIVED BY WEIGHTING AND SUMMING SUBSCALE SCORES. HIGHER VALUES INDICATE BETTER FUNCTIONING.	GENERAL:		
			HEALTH PERCEPTION	9	0.85
			ENERGY/FATIGUE	4	0.85
			OVERALL QUALITY OF LIFE	2	0.76
			SOCIAL FUNCTION	2	0.68
			MENTAL:		
			EMOTIONAL WELL-BEING	5	0.82
			COGNITIVE FUNCTION	5	0.83
			ROLE LIMITATIONS DUE TO EMOTIONAL PROBLEMS	5	0.86
			ROLE LIMITATIONS DUE TO MEMORY PROBLEMS	5	0.81
			PHYSICAL:		
			ROLE LIMITATIONS DUE TO PHYSICAL PROBLEMS	5	0.85
			PHYSICAL FUNCTION	10	0.88
			PAIN (FREEDOM FROM)	2	0.80

Revised in a prospective cohort of 57 patients, comparing baseline and follow-up after one year. Forty-three patients had undergone epilepsy surgery, and 14 were being treated medically. Assessing differences in change between surgically- and medically-treated patients, the ESI-55 showed greatest responsiveness, in particular on the health perception, energy/fatigue and emotional well-being subscales. In general, the study supports the responsiveness of the ESI-55. However, the superior sensitivity to change was mainly ascribed to the generic SF-36 scales rather than to the epilepsy-specific ones (with the exception of the health-perception subscale). In a prospective, controlled trial by McLachlan *et al.* (1997), health-related quality-of-life outcomes in 51 patients undergoing temporal lobectomy and 21 patients continuing medical management were compared, assessing EQoL before and at 6, 12 and 24 months after treatment. At 24 months, five of the eleven subscales (health perceptions, energy/fatigue, overall quality of life, social function, cognitive function) and the overall score distinguished among patients who had experienced an at least 90% seizure reduction and those who had not.

The Quality-of-Life-in-Epilepsy Scales 89, 31 and 10: The Quality-of-Life-in-Epilepsy Scale (QOLIE-89, Devinsky *et al.*, 1995) was developed to assess quality of life in patients with epilepsy whose seizures are controlled and for those with a low-to-moderate seizure frequency. Following the same construction principle used for the ESI-55, the RAND 36-Item Health Survey was chosen as a generic core, supplemented by 48 epilepsy-specific items, nine additional generic items, and six items concerning attitudes towards epilepsy and self-esteem (Table 2). After field testing, a visual-analogue scale on overall health and one on satisfaction with sexual functioning were added. The final version of the QOLIE-89 contained 86 items in 17 scales and three single items. The WHO definition of health (WHO, 1948) was chosen as the underlying model for scale development (Perrine, 1993).

The initial 99-item version of the QOLIE-89 was completed by 304 patients from 25 epilepsy centres in the United States (response rate 100%). Fifty-seven percent were women; the mean age was 36 years; mean age at seizure onset was 17.9 years. Twenty-one were seizure free, 116 showed a low seizure frequency, 136 had a moderate seizure frequency, and 31 had a high seizure frequency. For most items, a time window of four weeks was chosen. The QOLIE-89 requires about 15 to 25 minutes to complete (Devinsky *et al.*, 1995).

TABLE 2 LISTING OF IMPORTANT ASPECTS OF THE QOLIE-89 (DEVINSKY *ET AL.*, 1995)

PURPOSE	ITEM GENERATION	SCORING	SUBSCALES ACCORDING TO FACTOR STRUCTURE	NO. OF ITEMS	CRONBACH'S α	TEST-RETEST
COMPREHENSIVE SCALE FOR CLINICAL STUDIES; FOR AED RESEARCH, TO DETERMINE OUTCOMES OF SPECIFIC INTERVENTIONS AND TO DEFINE HEALTH-CARE COST ISSUES AND POLICIES	86 ITEMS IN 17 SCALES AND 3 SINGLE ITEMS*; GENERIC CORE: SF-36 SUPPLEMENTAL ITEMS WERE DERIVED FROM LITERATURE REVIEW, EXPERIENCE OF PROFESSIONALS AND INTERVIEWS WITH 30 PATIENTS	ON YES/NO FORMAT, 3-,4-,5- AND 6-POINT FORMAT; THE SINGLE SCALES CONSIST OF ITEMS WITH DIFFERENT RESPONSE FORMAT. SUBSCALE-SCORES ARE TRANSFORMED ONTO A 0–100 POINT-SCALE. AN OVERALL SCORE AND FOUR COMPOSITE SCORES (REFLECTING THE UNDERLYING FACTOR MATRIX) CAN BE DERIVED BY WEIGHTING AND SUMMING SUBSCALE SCORES. A HIGHER SCORE REFLECTS BETTER FUNCTIONING.	EPILEPSY-TARGETED			
			SEIZURE WORRY	5	0.79	0.84
			MEDICATION EFFECTS	3	0.78	0.64
			HEALTH DISCOURAGEMENT	2	0.82	0.73
			WORK/DRIVING/SOCIAL FUNCTION	11	0.86	0.86
			COGNITIVE			
			LANGUAGE	5	0.88	0.72
			ATTENTION/CONCENTRATION	9	0.92	0.86
			MEMORY	6	0.88	0.82
			MENTAL HEALTH			
			OVERALL QUALITY OF LIFE	2	0.79	0.84
			EMOTIONAL WELL-BEING	5	0.83	0.77
			ROLE LIMITATIONS SCALE	5	0.81	0.67
			SOCIAL ISOLATION	2	0.88	0.73
			SOCIAL SUPPORT	4	0.84	0.78
			ENERGY/FATIGUE	4	0.84	0.75
			PHYSICAL HEALTH			
			HEALTH PERCEPTIONS	6	0.78	0.84
			PHYSICAL FUNCTION	10	0.89	0.75
			ROLE LIMITATIONS: PHYSICAL	5	0.81	0.58
			PAIN	2	0.87	0.69
			OVERALL SCORE	86	0.97	0.88

*SINGLE ITEMS: CHANGE IN HEALTH, SEXUAL FUNCTIONING, AND OVERALL HEALTH

Multitrait scaling yielded 86 items placed in 17 scales with reliability estimates (Cronbach's α) ranging from 0.78 to 0.92, with 13 exceeding 0.80. Only the two role-limitation scales (emotional, physical) showed high ceiling effects (> 40%). Test-retest reliability was assessed in 232 stable patients with a time interval between one and 21 days; the two role-limitation scales, pain, and medication effects failed to reach the 0.70 standard. A comparison of scale content with the answers to an open-ended question about additional QoL concerns was thought to contribute to content validity. It showed that most patients' concerns were covered by the QOLIE-89 (Devinsky *et al.*, 1995).

To support construct validity, the authors applied exploratory factor analysis, yielding four factors (epilepsy targeted, cognitive, mental, and physical health). Those four factors were intercorrelated, justifying the aggregation to one overall score. Moreover, correlations among several scales and the QOLIE, as well as group comparisons (according to seizure frequency), were computed. One important finding was that all the QOLIE scales correlated highly with the Profile of Mood States (POMS; McNair, *et al.*, 1982), whereas correlations with neuropsychological tests were low. Moreover, correlations between two toxicity scales and the four QOLIE factor scores, as well as the overall score, were found to be negative. High correlations indicated a relationship between QOLIE and AED toxicity. In addition, for all scales there was a trend for patients with lower seizure frequency to have higher QoL scores, compared with patients with higher seizure frequency. The epilepsy-targeted subscales — seizure worry, health discouragement and work/driving/social function — were most sensitive in discriminating among seizure groups, since seizure-free patients and those with low seizure frequency scored significantly better than those with moderate- and high-frequency seizures. However, sensitivity to group differences does not equate to responsiveness. In principle, it can be assumed that the generic core of the SF-36 will contribute to the responsiveness of the QOLIE-89. This assumption is supported by recent investigations where the ESI-55 (based also on the SF-36) was found to be a responsive scale (Wiebe *et al.*, 1997). However, the ability to discriminate among treatment groups remains to be validated.

Derivatives of QOLIE-89: The QOLIE-10 (Cramer *et al.*, 1996), and QOLIE-31 (Cramer *et al.*, 1998) were derived from the QOLIE-89. Consequently, only one evaluation sample exists. For the QOLIE-10, six items were selected from the epilepsy-targeted scale (seizure worry, medication effects, work/driving/social function), three from the mental-health scale, and one from the cognition scale. The QOLIE-10 requires about 2–5 minutes to complete (Devinsky, 1993). A factor analysis yielded three factors: 'epilepsy effects', 'mental health', and 'role function'. Reliability estimates (Cronbach's α) for the three factors were poor, none exceeding 0.51. Construct validity was assessed by correlating scores on the QOLIE-10 with two toxicity scales, but the results do not, in our opinion, confirm validation. Discriminant validity was supported by significant differences among seizure groups; but the lack of sufficient information about these data precludes further comment.

The items of the QOLIE-31 were empirically selected, choosing those QOLIE-89 subscales that were considered most important in epilepsy patients' reports. The QOLIE-31 takes about 5–15 minutes to complete (Devinsky, 1993). Reliability estimates are more convincing than for QOLIE-10, ranging from 0.77 to 0.85. Item-to-scale correlations showed that all individual items correlated significantly higher with their own scales than with other scales. Factor analysis yielded two factors, one reflecting emotional/psychological issues, the other mental efficiency. Correlations with other scales supported the convergent validity of the energy, emotional, and overall QoL scales. There seemed to be a relationship between one toxicity scale and the QOLIE-31, but not another. Of particular interest is that the seizure-worry and social-functioning scales could distinguish among patients according to their seizure frequency, with inverse correlations between QoL and seizure frequency.

The Subjective-Handicap-of Epilepsy Scale (SHE) Scale: Initially based on the WHO definition of handicap (ICIDH; WHO, 1980), where six dimensions of handicap (mobility, orientation, physical independence, occupation, social integration, and economic self-sufficiency) with nine levels of severity for each area are defined, O'Donoghue and co-workers (1998) developed this instrument to assess the subjective outcome of epilepsy (Table 3). Given the continuing debate about the conceptual boundaries of health-related quality of life, the authors opted to use the central ideas of the handicap concept, assuming that 'most of the consequences of epilepsy operate at the level of handicap' (O'Donoghue *et al.,* 1998).

The scale was completed by two separate sample groups. Group A (response rate 77%) consisted of 287 clinical patients with a median age of 34 years, 54% of whom were female; the median duration of epilepsy was 22 years. Fifty-nine percent had a localisation-related

TABLE 3 LISTING OF IMPORTANT ASPECTS OF THE SHE-SCALE (O'DONOGHUE *ET AL.*, 1998)

PURPOSE	ITEMS	SCORING	SUBSCALES AND SPECIFIC CONSTRUCTS	NO. OF ITEMS	CRONBACH'S α	INTRA-CLASS COEFFICIENT
TO ASSESS THE LONG-TERM IMPACT OF MEDICAL, PSYCHOLOGICAL, AND SURGICAL INTERVENTIONS ON THE HANDICAP ASSOCIATED WITH EPILEPSY	32 ITEMS IN SIX SUBSCALES; ITEMS DERIVED FROM LITERATURE REVIEW, SCALE REVIEW, 100 OPEN INTERVIEWS WITH PATIENTS, AND EXPERT OPINION	IS ON A FIVE-POINT LIKERT SCALE; THE SUBSCALE SCORE, (SUM OF THE ITEM SCORES) IS TRANSFORMED ONTO A 0–100 SCALE. A HIGHER SCORE INDICATES LESS HANDICAP.	WORK AND ACTIVITY DIFFICULTIES IN OBTAINING AND MAINTAINING EMPLOYMENT BEING IN EMPLOYMENT WHICH IS NOT ONE'S FIRST CHOICE PROBLEMS AT WORK DUE TO SEIZURES AND MEDICATION TRAVELLING AND DRIVING ALTERATION IN DAILY ROUTINE DUE TO SEIZURES OR MEDICATION EFFECT OF EPILEPSY ON LEISURE AND RECREATION	8	0.88	0.89
			SOCIAL AND PERSONAL LIFE DIFFICULTIES SECONDARY TO 'REVEALING' EPILEPSY ALTERATION IN THE DEVELOPMENT OF SOCIALISATION DUE TO CHILDHOOD EPILEPSY ALTERATION IN RELATIONSHIP WITH PARTNER AND FRIENDS DUE TO EPILEPSY SOCIAL LIMITATIONS DUE TO TRAVELLING AND ECONOMIC CONSTRAINTS SEXUAL LIFE	4	0.86	0.86
			SELF-PERCEPTION STIGMATISATION FEELING OF NOT BEING IN CONTROL OF ONE'S FUTURE FEAR OF SEIZURES LEADING TO INJURY OR DEATH FEAR OF SEIZURES IN PUBLIC	5	0.87	0.88
			PHYSICAL SEIZURE-RELATED INJURIES AND SYMPTOMS SUBJECTIVE EFFECT OF MEDICATION ON WELL-BEING	4	0.72	0.87
			LIFE-SATISFACTION HAPPINESS WITH ONE'S WORK, LEISURE, AND SOCIAL LIFE	4	0.79	0.86
			SELF-REPORTED CHANGE ACROSS ALL DOMAINS	7	0.88	0.83

epilepsy syndrome with known etiology, 21% were cryptogenic, 14% suffered from idiopathic generalised epilepsy, 2% had generalised cryptogenic/symptomatic seizures, and 4% were unclassified. Group B (response rate 84%) were patients who had undergone epilepsy surgery; the median age of the 105 responders was 31 years; 55% were female; the median duration since operation was 28 months. When the questions required a time window, an interval of six months was chosen. The overall-change scale refers to a time period over one year. The median time required to complete the questionnaire is eight minutes.

As data analysis was very elaborate, we shall only mention a few important issues. Floor and ceiling effects in each scale did not exceed 5% except on the 'social and the personal' scale (18%). All items showed higher within-scale correlations than inter-scale correlations, as an indicator of scale fit. Test-retest reliability analysis, examined at three time intervals (24 hours, 1 week, 4–8 weeks) was performed with intra-class correlation coefficients and confidence intervals and ranged between 0.83 and 0.89, thereby exceeding the 0.80 criterion. Moreover, there was no bias producing a shift in retest scores. Content validity was supported by the scale-construction process. Construct validity was assessed and supported as follows: in Group A, three of the six subscales (work and activity, physical, and self-perception scales) discriminated between patient groups experiencing differing levels of seizure frequency, whereas the life-satisfaction and change scales discriminated between seizure-free patients and patients with continuing seizures. In Group B, a decrease in SHE score was associated with an increase in seizure frequency. All SHE scores were higher for those in employment in both groups. All subjects who thought their job had been affected by epilepsy and all who assumed epilepsy to be the determining factor in their quality of life scored lower. Correlations with the ESI-55 summary scales were between 0.5 and 0.6; subscales with related content suggested a clear relationship. Factor analysis yielded six factors, underlining the subscale structure and accounting for 65% of the variance. Longitudinal studies assessing responsiveness are in progress.

In summary, the SHE scale appears to be highly related to the handicap concept and to be a complexly-designed and validated measure of the long-term consequences of epilepsy. It was developed as a global health-status scale, and it does not directly measure mental health, physical or cognitive disabilities.

Batteries

The Health-Related Quality-of-Life Questionnaire for People with Epilepsy (HRQLQ-E): Following Patrick's recommendation (Patrick and Deyo, 1989; Patrick and Erickson, 1993a), a group of investigators in the United States decided to choose a modular approach, including generic and specific measures of health-related quality of life to assess the impact of epilepsy and the burdens as well as the benefits of its treatment (Wagner *et al.,* 1995). Based on a literature review, clinical experience, and discussions with patients, the authors developed a 171-item questionnaire (Table 4) comprised of the UK version of the RAND 36-item Health Survey (Jenkinson *et al.,* 1993) with some augmentations; additional measures of general health; previously validated measures of epilepsy impact (Jacoby *et al.*, 1993) and seizure severity (Baker *et al.*, 1991); items relating to epilepsy concerns; an epilepsy-specific mastery scale, adapted from Pearlin and Schooler (1978); a checklist assessing symptom occurrence and impact related to the use of AEDs; as well as two open-ended questions.

The questionnaire was completed by 136 ambulatory patients from three clinics (response rate: 91%); 60% were female; mean age: 21.8 years; mean duration of epilepsy: 14 years. Based on the ILAE classification (ILAE Commission, 1981), 79% had partial seizures, and 21%, primarily generalised tonic-clonic seizures. The time required to complete the questionnaire is about 40 minutes.

As data analysis was very comprehensive, only a few important issues will be mentioned here. While showing low floor effects, ceiling effects in seven of the ten SF-36 scales were higher than 20%. In four of the additional general scales, over 20% of the patients scored maximum points, as well as in two of the epilepsy-specific scales. As an indicator of scale fit, correlations between items and their hypothesised subscales upheld the groupings, except for the concentration and the attention scales and the percept subscale of the Liverpool seizure-severity scale.

Content validity was supported by an analysis of the two open-ended questions, which overlapped clearly with the aspects assessed. Criterion validity was assessed with regard to time since last seizure and self-reported symptom status. There was a general trend for patients with seizures to have lower scale scores than those who were seizure free on all of the scales, the SF-36 Role Physical Scale being the most sensitive to these distinctions. The six epilepsy-specific scales were among the best ten discriminative scales. In contrast, the generic HRQoL scales were

TABLE 4 LISTING OF IMPORTANT ASPECTS OF THE HRQLQ-E BATTERY (WAGNER *ET AL.*, 1995)

PURPOSE	ITEM GENERATION	SCORING	DOMAINS AND SUBSCALES	NO. OF ITEMS	CRONBACH'S α	TEST-RETEST
TO ASSESS	171 ITEMS IN 31	ON LIKERT-RESPONSE	GENERAL HRQoL-SF-36 SCALES			
HRQoL	SCALES.	FORMAT; SYMPTOM	PHYSICAL FUNCTIONING	10	0.92	0.77
BURDEN OF	IMPORTANT DOMAINS	CHECKLIST: YES/NO	ROLE PHYSICAL	4	0.87	0.72
EPILEPSY, AS	WERE IDENTIFIED	RAW SCORES ARE	BODILY PAIN	2	0.79	0.74
WELL AS THE	BASED ON CLINICAL	TRANSFORMED ONTO	GENERAL HEALTH PERCEPTION	5	0.85	0.85
BURDEN AND	EXPERIENCE,	A 0–100 SCALE	VITALITY	4	0.87	0.71
BENEFITS OF	INFORMAL	(EXCEPT SEIZURE	SOCIAL FUNCTIONING	2	0.78	0.71
AEDS	DISCUSSIONS WITH	SEVERITY AND	ROLE EMOTIONAL	3	0.87	0.65
	PATIENTS, AND A	IMPACT OF EPILEPSY	MENTAL HEALTH (MHI-5)	5	0.81	0.80
	REVIEW OF THE	SCALE).	AUGMENTED ROLE PHYSICAL	5	0.85	0.75
	PSYCHOSOCIAL AND	ZERO INDICATES THE	AUGMENTED ROLE EMOTIONAL	4	0.85	0.66
	CLINICAL LITERATURE,	LEAST FAVOURABLE	GENERAL HRQoL-ADDITIONAL SCALES			
	INCLUDING	HEALTH-STATUS.	ANXIETY	4	0.82	0.81
	INFORMATION ABOUT		DEPRESSION	4	0.80	0.80
	AED DEVELOPMENT.		BEHAVIOURAL/EMOTIONAL CONTROL	5	0.76	0.78
			POSITIVE WELL-BEING	6	0.82	0.78
			EMOTIONAL TIES	4	0.74	0.76
			CURRENT HEALTH	4	0.83	0.82
			MOS COGNITION†	6	0.92	0.69
			CONFUSION	2	0.81	0.62
			THINKING	2	0.70	0.74
			CONCENTRATION	2	0.81	0.63
			ATTENTION	2	0.51	0.55
			PSYCHOMOTOR FUNCTION	3	0.80	0.66
			EPILEPSY-SPECIFIC HRQoL SCALES			
			MASTERY	6	0.70	0.74
			IMPACT OF EPILEPSY	8	0.89	0.82
			EXPERIENCE	13	0.86	0.84
			WORRY	9	0.83	0.74
			AGITATION	2	0.79	0.73
			DISTRESS	2	0.82	0.70
			SEIZURE SEVERITY SCALE			
			PERCEPT	8	0.43	0.76
			ICTAL	12	0.88	0.88
			SYMPTOMS	16		
			OPEN-ENDED QUESTIONS	2		

† MEDICAL OUTCOMES STUDY (MOS; STEWART *ET AL.*, 1992A; STEWART *ET AL.*, 1992B)

TABLE 5 SUMMARY OF INVESTIGATED SCALES OF THE LIVERPOOL HRQoL BATTERY

NOVEL SCALES	ADAPTED SCALES
SEIZURE SEVERITY SCALE	MASTERY SCALE
IMPACT OF EPILEPSY SCALE	SELF-ESTEEM SCALE
LIFE FULFILMENT SCALE	AFFECT BALANCE SCALE
ADVERSE DRUG EVENTS PROFILE	HOSPITAL ANXIETY AND DEPRESSION SCALE (HAD)
	STIGMA SCALE

best at differentiating between groups of patients according to the Symptom-Checklist. The most valid scales seemed to be the SF-36 Social Functioning Scale, the Role-Emotional Scale, the Mental-Health Scale and the MOS Cognition Scale (Medical Outcome Study; Stewart *et al.*, 1992). A principal components analysis of the SF-36 confirmed a two-factor structure in agreement with previous research (McHorney *et al.*, 1993; Ware *et al.*, 1995). In summary, this evaluation study provides important, although not longitudinal, information about the validity of several scales. It offers a comprehensive approach to the assessment of EQoL, with close similarities between it and the QOLIE-89, but has yet to be used in any evaluative studies.

The Liverpool HRQoL Battery: HRQLQ-E drew heavily on another battery measure, the Liverpool HRQoL Battery. Based on an epilepsy-specific QoL model (Baker *et al.*, 1993; Baker, 1998) adapted from Meenan *et al.* (1984), the Liverpool Battery was developed to assess the effects of epilepsy on a patient's physical, social, and psychological ability to function. It combined newly developed scales and items with existing measures (Table 5).

Coverage of the battery was informed by a series of in-depth interviews with people with epilepsy of varying severity (Jacoby, 1996) and discussion with expert neurologists. Depending on the particular research question, the Liverpool Battery allows differing combinations of the various instruments (Jacoby, 1996; Baker, 1998). This might be a problem, as it prevents cross-study comparison. We shall comment on a version which suggests inclusion of the following:

1. *Seizure Severity Scale*

There is evidence that seizure severity in patients with poorly controlled epilepsy may have a greater impact on psychosocial well-being than seizure frequency (Arntson *et al.*, 1986; Smith *et al.*, 1991). Baker and co-workers (1991; 1998) developed an instrument based on the patient's perception of seizure severity, assuming it to be determined by two factors: the severity of the ictal and the postictal phase, and the patient's perception of control of their seizures (Table 6).

Ninety-seven patients from an epilepsy clinic in the UK, of whom 51% were female, and with a mean age of 32 years, completed the scale. Twenty percent had simple partial seizures, 60% had complex partial seizures with or without generalised seizures, and 20% had primary generalised seizures. Thirty-two reported the ability to differentiate between two types of seizures (minor/major) they experienced and therefore were asked to complete the scale separately for each seizure type (Baker *et al.*, 1998). The time window — referring to seizures patients had experienced — was four weeks.

Cronbach's α for the percept subscale applied to major seizures was 0.68 and for the corresponding ictal/postictal subscale 0.72. Applied to minor seizures, the percept subscale showed an internal consistency of 0.86 and the ictal/postictal subscale one of 0.78. Test-Retest scores exceeded 0.70 for all subscales. Criterion validity seemed to be supported by significant differences in the mean scores of the two subscales, indicating the scale could distinguish between patients with major and with minor seizures.

As a contribution to construct validity, the initial validation study (Baker *et al.*, 1991) suggested that the original 10-item version of the ictal/postictal scale could distinguish among seizure types based on the ILAE classification (except for primary and secondary generalised, tonic-clonic seizures), while the percept scale showed no significant differences. The lack of discriminant validity of the percept scale may be due to the heterogeneity of the contents (Wagner *et al.*, 1995). The ictal/postictal scale also demonstrated its responsiveness in a double-blind crossover trial comparing lamotrigine to placebo (Smith *et al.*, 1993a). The reported responsiveness, however, reflects sensitivity to group differences (lamotrigine vs. placebo means on this scale) rather than change in scores (longitudinal change in lamotrigine scores relative to longitudinal change in placebo scores), limiting interpretability. The scale has recently been revised to include 12 items relating to the ictal/post-ictal subscale and eight to the percept subscale (Baker *et al.*, 1998). A clinically meaningful change in scores has yet to be published.

2. *The Impact of Epilepsy Scale*

This scale was developed by Jacoby *et al.* (1993) to describe the perceived impact of epilepsy on the quality of a patient's life (Table 7). The scale was initially completed by 75 patients from a UK hospital;

TABLE 6 LISTING OF IMPORTANT ASPECTS OF THE REVISED LIVERPOOL SEIZURE SEVERITY SCALE (BAKER *ET AL.*, 1998)

PURPOSE	ITEM GENERATION	SCORING	SCALES	NO. OF ITEMS	CRONBACH'S α	TEST-RETEST
TO ASSESS SEIZURE SEVERITY FROM A PATIENT-BASED VIEWPOINT	20 ITEMS IN TWO SUBSCALES ITEMS DEVISED BY TWO EXPERTS	IS ON FOUR- AND FIVE-POINT LIKERT FORMAT; THE HIGHER THE SCORE, THE MORE SEVERE THE SEIZURES.	MAJOR PERCEPT SUBSCALE MAJOR ICTAL/POSTICTAL SUBSCALE MINOR PERCEPT SUBSCALE MINOR ICTAL/POSTICTAL SUBSCALE	8 12 8 12	0.68 0.72 0.86 0.78	0.96 0.93 0.72 0.78

TABLE 7 LISTING OF IMPORTANT ASPECTS OF THE IMPACT OF EPILEPSY SCALE (JACOBY *ET AL.*, 1993)

PURPOSE	ITEM GENERATION	SCORING	ITEMS BUILDING THE SCALE	CRONBACH'S $\alpha^{\dagger}$
TO PROVIDE A BRIEF AND SIMPLE SCALE TO MEASURE THE IMPACT OF EPILEPSY ON A NUMBER OF DIFFERENT ASPECTS OF DAILY LIFE	EIGHT ITEMS IN ONE SCALE IDENTIFIED THROUGH GROUP DISCUSSIONS AND IN-DEPTH INTERVIEWS WITH PATIENTS	IS ON FOUR-POINT LIKERT FORMAT; A TOTAL SCORE IS CALCULATED BY SUMMING ALL ITEM SCORES; THE HIGHER THE SCORE, THE GREATER THE IMPACT OF THE EPILEPSY.	IMPACT OF EPILEPSY RELATIONSHIP WITH SPOUSE/PARTNER RELATIONSHIP WITH OTHER CLOSE FAMILY MEMBERS SOCIAL LIFE/SOCIAL ACTIVITIES HEALTH (WORK)† RELATIONSHIP WITH FRIENDS FEELINGS ABOUT SELF PLANS AND AMBITIONS FOR THE FUTURE	0.82

† CRONBACH'S α, IF ITEM WORK WAS EXCLUDED

43% were female, the mean age was 33 years; the mean age of onset was 15 years. Thirteen patients had simple partial seizures, 26 had complex partial seizures with or without secondary generalised seizures, and 36 had primary generalised tonic-clonic seizures.

Cronbach's α was found to be 0.82 when one of the original 'work' items was deleted. Principal-component factor analysis yielded one underlying factor which accounted for 54% of the variance. Correlations among seven measures of psychological well-being (part of the Liverpool Battery) and the total score of the new scale were shown to be significant. A predictive model, including 13 explanatory variables, accounted for 70% of the variance in the impact score. Individual examination proved a strong relationship to self esteem, life fulfilment, perceived quality of life, seizure type, frequency of minor seizures, and marital status. A more detailed interpretation by the authors of correlations and the regression analysis would contribute to construct validity and add helpful information to understand more about the conceptual boundaries of the impact of epilepsy on patients' lives. Evidence of the discriminant validity of the Impact of Epilepsy Scale is provided by several studies by its authors. It has been shown to distinguish clearly between groups of patients who are seizure-free, experiencing infrequent seizures and experiencing frequent seizures (Jacoby *et al.*, 1996) and between groups of patients experiencing different seizure types (Baker *et al.*, 1997). The Impact Scale was also sensitive when comparing seizure-free patients with patients unsuitable for surgery, and those having more than ten seizures per year post-operatively (Kellet *et al.*, 1997).

3. *Life Fulfilment Scale*

Based on a concept developed by Krupinsky (1980), the Liverpool group developed a scale to assess the discrepancy between actual and ideal circumstances of patients with epilepsy (Table 8; Baker *et al.*, 1994a). Patients first rate how important 12 specified areas are for them (perceived importance) and then how satisfied they are with their actual circumstances (expressed satisfaction). The actual score is calculated by multiplying the perceived importance in one area by the level of expressed satisfaction with that area. The ideal score is calculated by multiplying the importance score by four (maximum possible score for satisfaction). The difference between the actual and the ideal score is an indicator of the discrepancy in any one area; consequently, the sum of the differences is a measure of discrepancies in life fulfilment.

TABLE 8 LISTING OF IMPORTANT ASPECTS OF THE LIFE-FULFILMENT SCALE (BAKER *ET AL.*, 1994A)

PURPOSE	ITEM GENERATION	SCORING	SUBSCALES ACCORDING TO FACTOR STRUCTURE	CRONBACH'S α
TO GRASP THE DISCREPANCY BETWEEN PATIENTS' ACTUAL AND DESIRED ASPECTS OF QUALITY OF LIFE	12 ITEMS IN TWO SUBSCALES IDENTIFIED ON THE BASIS OF PREVIOUS RESEARCH, CLINICAL EXPERIENCE, AND THROUGH INTERVIEWS WITH EPILEPSY PATIENTS	IS ON FOUR-POINT LIKERT FORMAT; THE HIGHER THE DIFFERENCE BETWEEN ACTUAL AND IDEAL SCORE, THE HIGHER THE DISCREPANCY IN LIFE FULFILMENT IN AN AREA.	PERSONAL FULFILMENT HAVING A GOOD FAMILY LIFE HAVING CLOSE FRIENDSHIPS HAVING A HAPPY MARRIAGE PARTICIPATING IN ENJOYABLE SPARE-TIME ACTIVITIES ENJOYING A GOOD SOCIAL LIFE BEING IN GOOD HEALTH BEING HAPPY WITH YOURSELF HAVING A SATISFYING JOB	0.68
			MATERIAL FULFILMENT BEING HAPPY WHERE YOU LIVE HAVING HOUSING WHICH MEETS YOUR NEEDS HAVING AN ADEQUATE STANDARD OF LIVING HAVING ENOUGH MONEY TO DO THINGS IMPORTANT TO YOU	0.78

Seventy-five patients from a UK epilepsy clinic, 43% female, with a mean age of 33 years and a mean age at onset of 15 years, completed the questionnaire. Thirteen patients had simple partial seizures, 26 had complex partial seizures, and 36 had primary generalised tonic-clonic seizures.

Factor analysis yielded two factors, termed material and personal fulfilment, accounting for 13% and 29% respectively of the variance, which is only a moderate indication of an underlying subscale structure. Internal consistency of those subscales were Cronbach's $\alpha = 0.68$ for the personal fulfilment and 0.78 for the material fulfilment subscale. The personal fulfilment scale showed absolute correlations between 0.42 and 0.69 with seven other psychological scales and one single item about overall quality of life, suggesting a relationship with similar concepts. There were no significant correlations between the material-fulfilment subscale and the psychological scales, indicating that this subscale was tapping distinct QoL domains. One importance of this scale is that patients can 'impose their own perspectives on the relative importance of particular areas of their lives and their satisfaction with them' (Baker *et al.*, 1994a). It also allows comparisons with other chronic diseases, as it is a generic rather than a condition-specific scale (Baker *et al.*, 1994a).

4. Adverse Drug Events Profile

The Adverse Drug Events Profile is a 21-item checklist providing information about patients' perceptions of central nervous system (CNS) and non-CNS, dose-related side effects of antiepileptic drug treatment (Baker *et al.*, 1997). Two-hundred and fifty patients who participated in the UK Antiepileptic Drug Withdrawal Study were asked to describe common side effects associated with treatment. The most commonly cited effects were used to form the scale (Baker, 1994b). Internal consistency was assessed in 90 patients, showing Cronbach's α to be 0.89. Content validity was supported by the item-generation process. Moreover, and as an indicator for construct validity, 12 of the 21 items discriminated between four different AED treatment groups (Baker *et al.*, 1997).

5. Validated Scales Incorporated in the Liverpool Battery

In considering the previously validated scales included in the Liverpool Battery, we refer to the results of an investigation by that group (Baker *et al.*, 1993), as it represents a central validation process of these scales

TABLE 9 LISTING OF VALIDATED SCALES IN THE LIVERPOOL QoL BATTERY

NAME	NO. OF ITEMS	SCORING	CRONBACH'S α	TEST RETEST
MASTERY	7	FOUR-POINT LIKERT;	0.74	0.76
		HIGHER SCORES =		
		HIGHER MASTERY		
SELF-ESTEEM	10	FOUR-POINT LIKERT;	0.80	—
		HIGHER SCORES =		
		HIGHER SELF-ESTEEM		
AFFECT BALANCE	10	YES/NO RESPONSE;	0.74	—
		POSITIVE SCORES =	FOR POSITIVE ITEMS; 0.60	
		POSITIVE AFFECT	FOR NEGATIVE ITEMS	—
HOSPITAL ANXIETY	14	FOUR-POINT LIKERT;	0.85	—
& DEPRESSION		HIGHER SCORES =	FOR ANXIETY;	
		HIGHER LEVELS	0.73	
		OF ANXIETY/DEPRESSION	FOR DEPRESSION	—
STIGMA	3	YES/NO RESPONSE;	0.72	—
		HIGHER SCORES =		
		GREATER STIGMA		

in patients with epilepsy. The scales comprise the following: Mastery (Pearlin and Schooler, 1978); Self-Esteem (Rosenberg, 1965); Affect-Balance (Bradburn, 1969); Hospital Anxiety and Depression Scale (Zigmond and Snaith, 1983); and Stigma (Hyman, 1971). Eighty-patients completed the questionnaires, 60% of them women, with a mean age of 38 years and mean age of onset of 12 years.

Internal consistency (Cronbach's α) for the various scales is presented in Table 9. In support of construct validity, the mastery scale was sensitive to group differences among patients with epilepsy of differing severity, as defined by time since last seizure (Wagner *et al.*, 1995). Both the Mastery Scale and the Affect-Balance Scale distinguished significantly between two different treatment groups (Smith *et al.*, 1993a) though unfortunately, the same problem of interpretability arises as mentioned above in the discussion of the Seizure Severity Scale. The Self-Esteem Scale could neither distinguish between patient groups according to seizure frequency nor prove its responsiveness in a comparison of Lamotrigine vs. Placebo (Smith *et al.*, 1993a). Investigations by Jacoby (1994) suggest a relatively high relationship between stigmatisation and self-esteem in accordance with Rosenberg's definition. Self-Esteem scores were significantly lower in patients with intractable epilepsy than those in patients whose epilepsy was in remission (Jacoby *et al.*, 1992). Both subscales of the Affect-Balance Scale were shown to distinguish between groups of patients according to the impact of their epilepsy. There was a clear relationship between the

HAD scale and seizure frequency: both subscales were sensitive to group differences according to seizure frequency after epilepsy surgery (Kellet *et al.,* 1997). Jacoby *et al.* (1996) computed correlations among clinical, demographic, and psychosocial variables and some scales of the Liverpool battery, finding the highest correlations between seizure frequency and the two subscales of the HAD scale. Comparing Lamotrigine with placebo, neither HAD subscale was sensitive to group differences or to change (Smith, *et al.,* 1993a; Chadwick, 1994). The Liverpool Battery has been validated in a US American patient group only recently (Rapp *et al.*, 1998).

QUANTITATIVE, UNIDIMENSIONAL (PSYCHOSOCIAL) APPROACHES

Single Scales

The Washington Psychosocial Seizure Inventory/WPSI: The WPSI (Dodrill *et al.*, 1980) is one of the earliest and most widely-used scales in the field of epilepsy. It has served as a major tool to assess the psychosocial consequences of epilepsy for almost 20 years. Preliminary work by a group of behavioural experts suggested seven main areas delineating psychosocial problems: 'Family Background', 'Emotional Adjustment', 'Interpersonal Adjustment', 'ocational Adjustment', 'Financial Status', 'Adjustment to Seizures', and 'Medicine and Medical Management', as well as an evaluation of 'Overall Psychosocial Functioning' (Table 10).

Item development and placement was carried out as follows: items covering each aspect of each area were formulated. After pilot testing, a total of 132 items were subsumed to which responses of 'Yes' and 'No' were obtained. Three supplemental validity scales (lie, rare items, number of items left blank) were used to complete the scale. In addition, a psychosocial rating sheet for use by professionals, to assess the targeted areas of function, was included. The professional ratings determined which items to include in a given scale. A profile sheet was developed onto which the WPSI scores can be plotted for individual patients as well as for groups of patients. The profile sheet divides the range of scores for each scale into four categories which reflect clinical significance. The resulting profile is based on multiple regression, where profile scores directly reflect their relationship with professional ratings of adequacy of adjustment (Dodrill *et al.*, 1980; Dodrill and Batzel, 1994).

The inventory was completed by 127 patients (response rate: 82%), 47% were female, the mean age was 29 years, and the mean age at onset

TABLE 10 LISTING OF IMPORTANT ASPECTS OF THE WASHINGTON PSYCHOSOCIAL SEIZURE INVENTORY (DODRILL *ET AL.*, 1980)

PURPOSE	ITEM GENERATION	SCORING	SCALES	NO. OF ITEMS	CRONBACH'S $\alpha^{\dagger}$	TEST-RETEST
TO EVALUATE PSYCHOLOGICAL AND SOCIAL CONCERNS IN ADULTS WITH EPILEPSY	132 ITEMS THROUGH EXPERT OPINION; THOSE ITEMS WITH HIGH CORRELATIONS BETWEEN THE SUM OF THE PROFESSIONAL RATINGS FOR EACH AREA AND EACH ITEM WERE INCLUDED.	IS ON A YES/NO FORMAT FOR ALL ITEMS	FAMILY BACKGROUND	11	0.82	0.83
			EMOTIONAL ADJUSTMENT	34	0.91	0.84
			INTERPERSONAL ADJUSTMENT	22	0.89	0.80
			VOCATIONAL ADJUSTMENT	13	0.84	0.73
			FINANCIAL STATUS	7	0.80	0.87
			ADJUSTMENT TO SEIZURES	15	0.85	0.70
			MEDICINE AND MEDICAL MANAGEMENT	8	0.62	0.66
			OVERALL PSYCHOSOCIAL FUNCTION	57	0.94	0.85
			NUMBER OF BLANK ITEMS			.28
			LIE	10		.58
			RARE ITEMS	17		.58

† LANGFITT, 1995

was 13.7 years. Thirteen percent suffered from elementary partial seizures, 57% from complex partial seizures, 3% from non-convulsive seizures, 5% from minor motor seizures, 8% from more than one of these seizure types, and 14% from convulsive seizures. The WPSI takes between 15 and 20 minutes to complete.

Test-retest reliability ranged from 0.68 to 0.95. Cronbach's α exceeded 0.80, except for the Medicine and Medical Management subscale (Langfitt, 1995). Correlations between a WPSI scale score and the ratings made by professionals for the total sample, which presumably represented criterion validity coefficients, ranged from 0.58 for 'Medicine and Medical Management' to 0.75 for 'Vocational Adjustment'.

With regard to validity, the results of a study by Langfitt (1995) are of interest. Content agreement (the ability of two raters to agree in the classification of items) as an indicator for face validity was rather low, indicating that the sole use of statistical criteria for item-scale assignment lowers face validity. Most WPSI items were categorised under 'Psychological Functioning', upholding content validity and the more specific intent of the WPSI to focus on psychological and social problems. Via multitrait-multimethod analysis, construct validity was tested for the subscales 'Emotional Adjustment', 'Interpersonal Adjustment', and 'Vocational Adjustment', examining intercorrelations among similar subscales of the ESI-55 and the Sickness Impact Profile (SIP; Bergner *et al.*, 1981). Fewer WPSI scales could be identified which measured domains similar to those indicated by the other measures. Dividing a total of 71 patients into three groups by seizure type yielded less sensitivity to QoL differences in the WPSI than in the SIP and the ESI-55. A recent investigation (Wiebe *et al.*, 1997) compared the responsiveness of WPSI, ESI-55, and the Symptom Checklist-90-Revised (SCL-90-R) in a prospective cohort of surgically or medically treated patients with temporal epilepsy, showing WPSI to be less responsive, especially to small and moderate changes in QoL.

In summary, the focus of the WPSI is, as intended, rather narrow and, consequently, provides a less valid description of the full impact of epilepsy on patients' lives. The dichotomous response format might lower the responsiveness of the questionnaire, as might the fact that some questions refer to non-changing events in the past.

A WPSI version for adolescents, the Adolescent Psychosocial Seizure Inventory (APSI), based on the same construction principle, has also been available since 1991 (Batzel *et al.*, 1991). Dodrill and Batzel (1995) have recently developed a 36-item WPSI QoL-scale, acknowledging the limitations of the WPSI in accurately assessing quality of life. Too little information about the psychometric properties of this scale is available to permit comment at the moment.

Social Effects Scale: The under-representation of questionnaires investigating the social effects of epilepsy across the range of epilepsy severity, motivated Chaplin and co-workers (1990) to develop a scale based on patient-validated content. Patients were drawn from a community-based, prospective cohort study of newly-diagnosed epilepsy patients. Initially, a pool of patient-generated statements was created through a series of in-depth interviews over a period of one year, guided by an interview schedule designed to allow patients to describe spontaneously how epilepsy had effected them. Patients and physicians were then asked to group these statements into distinct areas. The resultant 17 domains were supplemented by four areas derived from comparison with other inventories (Derogatis *et al.*, 1974; Dodrill *et al.*, 1980; Hunt *et al.*, 1986). After data analysis, 14 were selected for the final questionnaire (Table 11).

Test-retest scores ranged from 0.37–0.75. Criterion validity was assessed by Spearman's rank correlations between the results of the questionnaire administered to 20 patients and the independent assessment of the subjects' behaviour provided by medical staff closely associated with those patients. As the correlation between attitude and behaviour is often small, Chaplin and co-authors assumed rather low correlation coefficients as an indicator of criterion validity. Those coefficients ranged between 0.30 and 0.54. The questionnaire is highly content-valid with respect to the generation process. One important aspect of this scale is that it provides systematic presentations of patients' concerns and the impact of epilepsy on quality of life as expressed by patients themselves. Consequently, it can be applied to patients who have well-controlled epilepsy, to those with recently-diagnosed epilepsy, and to those with chronic disease. So far, the Social Effects Scale has been used in only one study and there is no published evidence of its responsiveness.

QUALITATIVE APPROACHES

The Quality of Life Assessment Schedule (QOLAS): Emphasising the requirement that quality-of-life assessment be as subject-driven and individualised as possible, Kendrick (1993; 1997; Kendrick and Trimble, 1994) developed a qualitative method derived from the repertory grid technique (Fransella and Bannister, 1977), which was

TABLE 11 LISTING OF IMPORTANT ASPECTS OF THE SOCIAL EFFECTS SCALE (CHAPLIN *ET AL.*, 1990)

PURPOSE	ITEM GENERATION	SCORING	FINAL AREAS	TEST-RETEST
TO DETERMINE THE NATURE AND EXTENT OF PSYCHOSOCIAL PROBLEMS IN EPILEPSY AND THEIR ASSOCIATIONS IN A WIDE RANGE OF PATIENTS	42 ITEMS IN 14 AREAS AREAS ESTABLISHED THROUGH INTENSIVE IN-DEPTH INTERVIEWS WITH PATIENTS ADDITIONAL AREAS DERIVED FROM A QUESTIONNAIRE -COMPARISON	IS ON A FIVE-POINT LIKERT RESPONSE FORMAT; STATEMENTS WEIGHTED IN ACCORDANCE TO THEIR RELATIVE SIGNIFICANCE	ATTITUDE TOWARDS ACCEPTING THE ATTACKS	0.72
			FEAR OF HAVING EPILEPSY	0.62
			FEAR OF STIGMA IN EMPLOYMENT	0.72
			LACK OF CONFIDENCE ABOUT THE FUTURE	0.37
			LACK OF CONFIDENCE ABOUT TRAVELLING	0.50
			ADVERSE REACTIONS ON SOCIAL LIFE	0.67
			ADVERSE REACTIONS ON LEISURE PURSUITS	0.62
			CHANGE OF OUTLOOK ON LIFE/SELF	0.67
			DIFFICULTY IN COMMUNICATING WITH THE FAMILY	0.51
			PROBLEMS WITH TAKING MEDICATION	0.53
			DISTRUST WITH THE MEDICAL PROFESSION	0.71
			DEPRESSION OR EMOTIONAL REACTIONS	0.73
			FEELING OF INCREASED SOCIAL ISOLATION	0.71
			LETHARGY/LACK OF ENERGY	0.75

later streamlined by Selai and Trimble (1995). The very sophisticated modular approach of QOLAS is the key to understanding the method. In accordance with earlier psychological theory, Kendrick and Trimble (1994) assume human nature to be that of a scientist, who formulates hypotheses and theories related to him/herself and the world based on his/her own personal constructions. QoL is a function of the conceptual distance between one's current life situation and one's expectations (Calman, 1984); it is also a comparative phenomenon, where individuals make comparisons between their current life situation, other times in their lives and the lives of other people.

Since the reduced version will probably be more widely used than the original, we shall present the reduced version, the Quality of Life in Epilepsy Schedule (QOLAS-R), in detail and comment only on the main results of the original. After introduction and rapport building, the 'patient is invited to recount what is important for his/her QoL and the way in which their current health condition is affecting their QoL' (Selai, *personal communication*). Ten constructs are then elicited for the following domains: physical functioning, cognitive abilities, emotional status, social functioning and economic/employment status (two constructs each). The patient has to rate all constructs on a five-point Likert scale according to the severity of the construct at the present time. Afterwards, the same procedure is carried out for the question of how much of a problem the patient would like the construct to be. Each of the present (NOW) and desired (LIKE) scores are summed, providing overall NOW and LIKE scores. The difference between the two is an indicator of the gap between actual and desired circumstances.

Testing the psychometric properties of individualised QoL questionnaires raises several problems, especially those related to test-retest reliability (as quality of life is assumed to be a dynamic concept) and the commonly used techniques applied to assess construct validity by correlating different measures and computing convergent and discriminant validity. Even group comparison, for example according to different seizure frequencies, could be problematic, as there is unlikely to be any general agreement on issues within one group. One decision could be to analyse data of one person qualitatively or related to the time axis. However, relatively high test-retest scores for all five areas (range: 0.53–0.75) in 50 patients with chronic epilepsy and 'some degree of validity for two of the three aggregated scores and for all profile scores' are reported (Kendrick and Trimble, 1994) when correlating them with other measures of psychosocial well-being. All of the scores, with the exception of the Work Scale, successfully discriminated between preoperative and postoperative patients undergoing surgery for the relief of severe facial pain. QOLAS-R also seems to be highly sensitive to change when comparing patients with good medical and surgical outcomes with those either untreated or poor outcomes (Selai, *personal communication*).

Choosing this approach requires time and a basic knowledge of the repertory grid technique. It is still in debate whether this approach is as patient generated as the authors suggest (Jacoby, 1996). However, there seems to be a consistent pattern among QoL studies, indicating that the areas applied (physical functioning, cognitive abilities, emotional status, social functioning, economic/employment status) really are those of concern. Standard psychometric criteria are inappropriate for assessing this method. It remains a promising, highly patient-centred content valid approach, based on a sophisticated model. Unfortunately, it is both time- and labour-intensive and therefore less readily applicable to clinical trials.

CONCLUSION

In this chapter we have presented an overview of instruments assessing QoL in epilepsy, or the psychosocial impact of this condition. The scales differ in several aspects: in the underlying model of EQoL and, consequently, in the areas of concern; in the chosen technique; in the evaluation samples and applicability; and in the psychometric properties. These differences lead to two questions: which scale to use for which purpose; and which types of investigations are relevant for EQoL research in the future.

It is evident that the research question determines the choice of a QoL instrument. A measure is best suited when the sample on which it is evaluated and the sample to which it is subsequently applied are similar and when the concept of QoL behind the measure is as comprehensive as the research question requires. A QoL measure also has to fulfil the psychometric criteria of reliability, validity, and responsiveness. Even if all the measures presented above have been proved reliable, the investigation of construct validity of some has to be questioned. The problem of content validity was emphasised recently by Gilliam *et al.*, (1997). In a study including 81 US adults with moderately-severe epilepsy, these authors identified 24 areas, when asking patients to list in order of importance their concerns about living with epilepsy. The resulting concerns were compared with two established EQoL measures, the QOLIE-89 and, implicitly, the ESI-55 (as it contains similar domains), as well as the Impact of Epilepsy and the Life Fulfilment Scales from the Liverpool QoL Battery. In the Life Fulfilment and Impact of Epilepsy Scales, more than half of the listed concerns are not covered (though it should be said that many are covered by other scales in the battery), whereas in the QOLIE-89, primary concerns were evaluated (although nine of the concerns which were listed by less than 20% of patients were not included). It is important to note that one of the most frequently listed domains, 'independence', is not included in any of currently available measures.

Another question is whether a QoL profile or overall QoL score is most useful. To detect treatment effects, a comparison of profiles might be more informative than a single score; for cost-utility studies an overall score is more appropriate. The ESI-55, the QoLIE, the SHE-scale and the HRQLQ-E fulfil both requirements. Finally, and of relevance to practitioners, is the question of individual assessment. None of the scales except the QOLAS was developed to evaluate the QoL of a single patient and they thus fail to meet psychometric criteria for single assessment. Future research has to show which instrument best offers insight into patients' self-perceived health status in the physician-patient interaction, as shown for the QOLIE-31 only recently (Grudzinsky *et al.*, 1998).

The second question concerns necessary investigations in the near future. Since only little is known about the similarities, differences, and qualities of existing scales, further comparative studies like those of Langfitt (1995) or Wiebe *et al.* (1997) are needed. Second, rather little is known about such things as patient subgroup differences according to type of epilepsy, or, for example, to cognitive deficits. International studies will help to compare patterns of problems and gain information about the EQoL construct and special weighting required. More controlled clinical trials are needed to further examine the responsiveness of the scales. Related to this demand, the question arises whether there are any variables or components of the EQoL construct that are more sensitive than others to change due to an intervention. Answers to this question will help detect useful primary endpoints for different types of interventions. From a scientific point of view, it is imperative to formulate and test hypotheses related to the concept of EQoL to obtain insight into its structure and determinants.

In general, it is obvious that a prolific pool of data and instruments exists in the EQoL research field at present, which could be used in the clinical context. Only a systematic synopsis — requiring co-operation — will provide insight. Otherwise, data will only proliferate.

APPENDIX 1 CLINICAL TRIALS INCLUDING QoL AS AN OUTCOME CRITERION

TYPE OF STUDY	INTERVENTION	QoLIE INSTRUMENT	AUTHOR AND YEAR OF PUBLICATION	RESULTS
CONTROLLED CLINICAL TRIAL				
OUTCOME EVALUATION STUDY OF GABAPENTIN	AED	QOLIE-10	BRUNI, 1998	FURTHER SUPPORT OF THE BENEFICIAL EFFECTS OF GABAPENTIN IN SEIZURE CONTROL AS WELL AS TOLERABILITY; POSITIVE EFFECTS DURING THE TREATMENT WITH GABAPENTIN IN ALL SCORES, SIGNIFICANT IMPROVEMENT IN FIVE OF THE TEN QUESTIONS, AND IN THE COMPOSITE SCORE, COMBINING ALL TEN QUESTIONS
OUTCOME EVALUATION OF SURGERY COMPARED WITH MEDICALLY TREATED PATIENTS	SURGERY	ESI-55	MCLACHLAN *ET AL.*, 1997	TEMPORAL LOBECTOMY SEEMS TO BE A MORE EFFECTIVE TREATMENT TO PROMOTE IMPROVEMENT IN HRQoL THAN A CONTINUED MEDICAL MANAGEMENT AMONG PATIENTS WITH INTRACTABLE TEMPORAL LOBE EPILEPSY ALTHOUGH SEIZURE CONTROL IS IMMEDIATE FOLLOWING SURGERY, IMPROVEMENTS IN HRQoL TAKE TIME TO EVOLVE AND FOLLOW-UP ASSESSMENTS AT LESS THAN 2 YEARS MAY NOT DEMONSTRATE IMPROVEMENTS IN VARIOUS DOMAINS OF HRQoL AFTER SURGERY THE YOUNGER THE PATIENT AT THE TIME OF SURGERY, THE BETTER THE HRQoL OUTCOME
OUTCOME EVALUATION OF SURGERY COMPARED WITH MEDICALLY TREATED PATIENTS	SURGERY	ESI-55, WPSI, SCL-90-R	WIEBE *ET AL.*, 1997	FOCUS ON PSYCHOMETRIC ASPECTS: THE ESI-55 CONTAINED THE MOST RESPONSIVE SCALES; THE LARGEST NUMBER OF SCALES WITH LOW RESPONSIVENESS BELONGED TO THE WPSI; SENSITIVITY TO BETWEEN-TREATMENT DIFFERENCES IN CHANGE WERE HIGHEST FOR THE ESI-55 AND THE SCL-90-R; MOST EFFICIENT SUBSCALES OF THE ESI-55 IN DETECTING DIFFERENCES BETWEEN TREATMENT GROUPS WERE THE EMOTIONAL-WELL-BEING AND HEALTH-PERCEPTION SCALES
OUTCOME EVALUATION OF THE INFLUENCE OF PREOPERATIVE NEUROTICISM ON QoLIE	SURGERY	ESI-55, WPSI, MMPI-2	ROSE *ET-AL.*, 1996	PREOPERATIVE: GREATER NEUROTICISM WAS ASSOCIATED WITH LOWER HRQoL POSTOPERATIVE: PREOPERATIVE NEUROTICISM HAD AN IMPORTANT INFLUENCE ON POSTOPERATIVE HRQoL THAT WAS INDEPENDENT OF POSTOPERATIVE SEIZURE OUTCOME
OUTCOME EVALUATION OF SURGERY COMPARED WITH NON-SURGERY PATIENTS	SURGERY	ESI-55, KAS	VICKREY *ET AL.*, 1995B	SURGERY VS. NON-SURGERY PATIENTS DIFFERED AT BASELINE ONLY IN MEDIAN MONTHLY SEIZURE FREQUENCY; AT FOLLOW-UP, SURGERY PATIENTS HAD GREATER DECLINE IN AVERAGE MONTHLY SEIZURE FREQUENCY AND TOOK FEWER AEDS; QoL SCORES WERE HIGHER WITH SURGERY ON 5 OF 11 SCALES THAT WERE ADMINISTERED ONLY AT FOLLOW-UP; NO SIGNIFICANT DIFFERENCES IN EMPLOYMENT STATUS OR PROSPECTIVELY ASSESSED QoL
EVALUATION OF THE EFFECTS OF COMPLETE SEIZURE-RELIEF ON PSYCHOSOCIAL FUNCTIONING	SURGERY	WPSI	SEIDMAN-RIPLEY *ET AL.*, 1993	SUBJECTS FOR WHOM SURGERY PROVIDED COMPLETE SEIZURE RELIEF SHOWED DRAMATIC DECREASE DURING THE FOLLOW-UP PERIOD IN SIX OF THE SEVEN SCALES (EXCEPT FAMILY BACKGROUND); A FOLLOW-UP-BASELINE COMPARISON IN THOSE PATIENTS WITHOUT COMPLETE SEIZURE RELIEF SHOWED MODEST INCREASES IN ALL BUT TWO (FINANCIAL STATUS, ADJUSTMENT TO SEIZURES) OF THE EIGHT SCALES

TYPE OF STUDY	INTERVENTION	QOLIE INSTRUMENT	AUTHORS AND YEAR OF PUBLICATION	RESULTS
RANDOMISED CLINICAL TRIALS				
MONOTHERAPY STUDY EVALUATING THE EFFECTS OF TIAGABINE	AED	WPSI SEVERAL NEUROPSYCH-OLOGICAL TESTS	DODRILL *ET AL.*, 1998	PATIENTS RECEIVING TGB MONOTHERAPY IMPROVED PARTICULARLY IN THE AREAS OF ADJUSTMENT; A LOW DOSE OF TGB WAS MORE LIKELY TO BE ASSOCIATED WITH IMPROVEMENT IN ADJUSTMENT; IN THE AREA OF COGNITIVE ABILITIES PATIENTS WITH HIGH-DOSE TGB PERFORMED BEST; PATIENTS WITHOUT MONOTHERAPY DID NOT PERFORM AS WELL ON MEASURES OF ADJUSTMENT
DOUBLE-BLIND, ADD-ON, PLACEBO CONTROLLED TRIAL OF TIAGABINE	AED	WPSI	DODRILL *ET AL.*, 1997	NO SIGNIFICANT CHANGE IN ANY SCORE OF WPSI, POMS, AND MOOD RATING SCALE IN ANY TREATMENT GROUP TIAGABINE PROVIDED SIGNIFICANT RELIEF FROM SEIZURES IN PATIENTS WITH SEIZURES DIFFICULT TO CONTROL; ONLY FEW ADVERSE COGNITIVE EFFECTS
DOUBLE-BLIND, PLACEBO CONTROLLED TRIAL OF VIGABATRIN	AED	WPSI	DODRILL *ET AL.*, 1995	NO SIGNIFICANT CHANGE IN ANY SCORE OF WPSI, POMS, AND MOOD RATING SCALE IN ANY TREATMENT GROUP VIGABATRIN PROVIDED SIGNIFICANT RELIEF FROM SEIZURES IN PATIENTS WITH SEIZURES DIFFICULT TO CONTROL; ONLY FEW ADVERSE COGNITIVE EFFECTS
DOUBLE-BLIND, PLACEBO CONTROLLED TRIAL OF LAMOTRIGINE	AED	LIVERPOOL BATTERY	SMITH *ET AL.*, 1993A	LAMOTRIGINE WAS EFFECTIVE IN REDUCING SEIZURE FREQUENCY, AND HAD ADDITIONAL FAVOURABLE EFFECTS ON SEIZURE SEVERITY, MOOD, AND PERCEIVED INTERNAL CONTROL (COMPARING PLACEBO WITH LAMOTRIGINE PROVED THAT HAPPINESS AND MASTERY SCORES WERE SIGNIFICANTLY HIGHER IN THOSE TREATED WITH LAMOTRIGINE), MOREOVER, CORRELATIONS AND MULTIPLE-REGRESSION ANALYSIS INDICATED THAT THE EFFECTS ON SEIZURE FREQUENCY, SEIZURE SEVERITY, AND PSYCHOSOCIAL VARIABLES APPEAR TO BE INDEPENDENT OF EACH OTHER

References

Arntson, P., Drodge, D., Norton, R., Murray, E. (1986) The perceived psychosocial consequences of having epilepsy. In: Whitmann, S., Hermann B. (eds.) *Psychopathology in Epilepsy: Social Dimensions.* New York: Oxford University Press, 143–161.

Baker, G.A. (1995) Health-related quality-of-life issues: Optimising patients outcomes. *Neurology* **45**(Suppl.2), S29–S34.

Baker, G.A. (1998) Quality of life and epilepsy: The Liverpool experience. *Clinical Therapeutics* **20**(Suppl. A), A2–A12.

Baker, G.A., Smith, D.F., Dewey, M., Morrow, J., Crawford, P.M., Chadwick, D.W. (1991) The development of a seizure severity scale as an outcome measure in epilepsy. *Epilepsy Research* 8:245–251.

Baker, G.A., Smith, D.F., Dewey, M., Jacoby, A., Chadwick, D.W. (1993) The initial development of a health-related quality of life model as an outcome measure in epilepsy. *Epilepsy Research* **16**: 65–81.

Baker, G.A., Jacoby, A., Smith, D.F., Dewey, M.E., Chadwick, D.W. (1994a) Development of a novel scale to assess life fulfilment as part of the further refinement of a Quality-of-Life model in epilepsy. *Epilepsia* **35**(3), 591–596.

Baker, G.A., Frances, P., Middleton, E. (1994b) Initial development, reliability and validity of a patient-based adverse drug events scale. *Epilepsia* **35** (Suppl. 7), 80.

Baker, G.A., Jacoby, A., Smith, D., Dewey, M., Johnson, A., Chadwick, D. (1994) Quality of life in epilepsy: the Liverpool Initiative. In: Trimble, M.R., Dodson, W.E. (eds.) *Epilepsy and Quality of Life.* New York: Raven Press, 135–150.

Baker, G.A., Jacoby, A., Buck, D., Stalgis, C., Monnet, D. (1997) Quality of Life of People with Epilepsy: A European Study. *Epilepsia* **38**(3), 353–362.

Baker, G.A., Smith, D.F., Jacoby, A., Hayes, J.A., Chadwick, D.W. (1998) Liverpool Seizure Severity Scale revisited. *Seizure* 7, 201–205.

Batzel, L.W., Dodrill, C.B., Dubinsky, B.L., Ziegler, R.G., Connolly, J.E., Freeman, R.D., Farwell, J.R., Vining, E.P. (1991) An objective method for the assessment of psychosocial problems in adolescents with epilepsy. *Epilepsia* **32**(2), 202–211.

Bergner, M., Bobbitt, R.A., Carter, W.B. (1981) The Sickness Impact Profile: Development and final revision of a health status measure. *Medical Care* **19**, 787–805.

Bland, J.M., Altman, D.G. (1986) Statistical methods for assessing agreement between two methods of clinical measurement. *Lancet* **1**, 307–310.

Boyle, G.J. (1991) Does item homogeneity indicate internal consistency or item redundancy in psychometric scales. *Personality and Individual Differences* **3**, 291–294.

Bradburn, N.M. (1965) *The structure of psychological well-being.* Chicago: Aldine.

Bruni, J. (1998) Outcome evaluation of gabapentin as add-on therapy for partial seizures. 'NEON' Study Investigators Group. Neurotonin Evaluation of Outcomes in Neurological Practice. *Canadian Journal of Neurological Sciences* **25**(2), 134–140.

Calman K.E. (1984) Quality of life in cancer patients — an hypothesis. Journal of Medical Ethics **10**, 124–127.

Campbell, D.T., Fiske, D.W. (1959) Convergent and discriminant validation by the multitrait-multimethod matrix. *Psychological Bulletin* **56**, 81–105.

Chaplin, J.E., Yepez, R., Shorvon, S., Floyd, M. (1990) A quantitative approach to measuring the social effects of epilepsy. *Neuroepidemiology* **9**, 151–158.

Chaplin, J.E., Yepez Lasso, R., Shorvon, S.D., Floyd, M. (1992) National general practice study of epilepsy: the social and psychological effects of a recent diagnosis of epilepsy. *British Medical Journal* **304**, 1416–1418.

Clark, L.A., Watson, D. (1995) Constructing validity: Basic issues in objective scale development. *Psychological Assessment* 7(3), 309–319.

Cramer, J.A. (1993) A clinimetric approach to assessing quality of life in epilepsy. *Epilepsia* **34**(Suppl. 4), S8-S13.

Cramer, J.A. (1997) Quality of life as an outcome measure for epilepsy clinical trials. *Pharmacy World and Science* **19**(5), 227–230.

Cramer, J.A., Perrine, K., Devinsky, O., Meador, K. (1996) A brief questionnaire to screen for quality of life in epilepsy: the QOLIE-10. *Epilepsia* **37**(6), 577–582.

Cramer, J.A., Perrine, K., Devinksy, O., Byrant-Comstock, L., Meador, K., Hermann, B.P. (1998) Development and cross-cultural translation of the 31-item quality of life in epilepsy inventory. *Epilepsia* **39**(1) 81–88.

Derogatis, L.R., Lipman, R.S., Rickels, K., Uhlenhuth, E., Coui, L. (1974) The Hopkins symptom checklist (HSCL): a self-report symptom inventory. *Behavioural Science* **19**, 1–15.

Devinsky, O. (1993) Clinical use of the quality of life in epilepsy inventory. *Epilepsia* **34** (Suppl. 4), S39-S44.

Devinsky, O., Cramer, J.A. (1993) Introduction: quality of life in epilepsy. *Epilepsia* **34** (Suppl. 4), S1-S3.

Devinsky, O., Penry, J.K. (1993) Quality of life in epilepsy: the clinician's view. *Epilepsia* **34** (Suppl. 4), S4-S7.

Devinsky, O., Vickrey, B.G., Cramer, J., Perrine, K., Hermann, B., Meador, K., Hays, R.D. (1995) Development of the quality of life in epilepsy inventory. *Epilepsia* **36**(11), 1089–1104.

Dikmen, S., Matthews, C.G., Harley, J.P. (1975) The effect of early versus late onset of major motor epilepsy upon cognitive-intellectual performance. *Epilepsia* **16**, 73–81.

Dikmen, S., Matthews, C.G. (1977) Effect of major motor seizure frequency upon cognitive-intellectual functions in adults. *Epilepsia* **18**, 21–29.

Dodrill, C.B., Batzel, L.W. (1994) The Washington Psychosocial Seizure Inventory and Quality of Life in Epilepsy. In: Trimble M.R., Dodson W.E. (eds.) *Epilepsy and Quality of Life*. New York: Raven Press, 109–133.

Dodrill, C.B., Batzel, L.W. (1995) The Washington Psychosocial Seizure Inventory: new developments in the light of the quality of life concept. *Epilepsia* **36** (Suppl. 3), S220.

Dodrill, C.B., Batzel, L.W., Queisser, H.R., Temkin, N.R. (1980) An objective method for the assessment of psychological and social problems among epileptics. *Epilepsia* **21**, 123–135.

Dodrill, C.B., Arnett, J.L., Sommerville, K.W. (1995) Effects of differing dosages of vigabatrin (sabril) on cognitive abilities and quality of life in epilepsy. *Epilepsia* **36** (2), 164–173.

Dodrill, C.B., Arnett, J.L., Sommerville, K.W. (1997) Cognitive and quality of life effects of differing dosages of tiagabine in epilepsy. *Neurology* **48**, 1025–1031.

Dodrill, C.B., Arnett, J.L., Shu, V., Pixton, G.C., Lenz, G.T., Sommerville, K.W. (1998) Effects of tiagabine monotherapy on abilities, adjustment and mood. Epilepsia **39**(1), 33–42.

Fetterman, J.L., Barnes, M.R. (1932) Serial studies of the intelligence of patients with epilepsy. *Archives of Neurology and Psychiatry* **28**, 370–385.

Fransella, F., Bannister, D. (1977) *A manual for repertory grid technique*. London: Academic Press.

Gilliam, F., Kuzniecky, R., Faught, E., Black, L., Carpenter, G., Schrodf, R. (1997) Patient-validated content of epilepsy-specific quality-of-life measurement. *Epilepsia* **38** (2), 233–236.

Goldstein, J., Seidenberg, M., Peterson, R. (1990) Fear of seizures and behavioural functioning in adults with epilepsy. *Journal of Epilepsy* **3**, 101–106.

Grudzinski, A.N., Hakim, Z., Coons, S.J., Labiner, D.N. (1998) Use of the QOLIE-31 in routine clinical practice. *Journal of Epilepsy* **11**, 34–47.

Guerrant, J., Anderson, W.W., Fischer, A. (1962) *Personality in epilepsy*. Springfield: Charles C. Thomas.

Guion, R.M. (1977) Content validity: Three years of talk — what's the action. *Public Personnel Management* **6**, 407–14.

Guyatt, G.H., Jaeschke, R., Feeny, D.H. (1996) Measurements in clinical trials: choosing the right approach. In: Spilker, B. (ed.) *Quality of life and pharmacoeconomics in clinical trials*. Philadelphia New York:Lippinicott-Raven, 41–48.

Hays, R.D., Sherbourne, C.D., Mazel, R.M. (1993) The RAND 36-item health survey 1.0. *Health Economics* **2**, 217–227.

Hermann, B.P. (1992) Quality of life in epilepsy. *Journal of Epilepsy* 5, 153–165.

Hermann, B.P. (1993) Developing a model of quality of life in epilepsy: the contribution of Neuropsychology. *Epilepsia* **34** (Suppl. 4), S14-S21.

Hermann, B.P. (1995) The evolution of health-related quality of life assessment in epilepsy. *Quality of Life Research* **4**, 87–100.

Hermann, B.P., Whitman, S. (1984) Behavioural and personality correlates of epilepsy: a review, methodological critique, and conceptual model. *Psychological Bulletin* **95** (3), 451–497.

Hunt, S.M., McEwen, J., McKenna, S.P. (1986) *Measuring health status.* London: Croom Helm.

Hyman, M.D. (1971) The stigma of stroke. *Geriatrics* 5, 132–141.

ILAE Commission on Classification and Terminology (International League against Epilepsy) (1981) Proposal for revised clinical and electroencephalographic classification of epileptic seizures. *Epilepsia* **22**, 489–501.

Jacoby, A. (1994) Felt versus enacted stigma: a concept revisited. *Social Science and Medicine* **38**(2), 269–274.

Jacoby, A. (1996) Assessing quality of life in patients with epilepsy. *Pharmaco Economics* **9**(5), 399–416.

Jacoby, A., Johnson, A., Chadwick, D. (1992) Psychosocial outcomes of antiepileptic drug discontinuation. *Epilepsia* **33** (6), 1123–1131.

Jacoby, A., Baker, G.A., Smith, D., Dewey, N., Chadwick, D.W. (1993) Measuring the impact of epilepsy: the development of a novel scale. *Epilepsy Research* **16**, 83–88.

Jacoby, A., Baker, G.A., Steen, N., Potts, P., Chadwick, D. (1996) The clinical course of epilepsy and its psychosocial correlates: Findings from a UK community study. *Epilepsia* **37** (2), 148–161.

Jaeschke, R., Guyatt, G.H. (1990) How to develop and validate a new quality of life instrument. In: Spilker, B. (ed.) *Quality of life assessments in clinical trials.* New York: Raven Press, 47–57.

Jenkinson, C., Wright, L., Coulter, A. (1993) *Quality of life in health care: A review of measures, and population norms for the UK SF-36.* Oxford: Horgan Print Partnership.

Johnson, A.L. (1994) Some statistical issues in quality of life measurement. In: Trimble, M.R., Dodson, W.E. (eds.) *Epilepsy and Quality of Life.* New York: Raven Press, 65–84.

Kellet, M.W., Smith, D.F., Baker, G.A., Chadwick, D.W. (1997) Quality of life after surgery. *Journal of Neurology, Neurosurgery and Psychiatry* **63**(1), 52–58.

Kendrick, A.M. (1993) *Repertory grid technique in the assessment of quality of life in patients with epilepsy.* PhD thesis. University of London.

Kendrick, A.M. (1997) Quality of life. In: Cull, C., Goldstein, L.H. (eds.) *The clinical psychologist's handbook of epilepsy: assessment and management.* London and New York: Routledge, 130–148.

Kendrick, A.M., Trimble, M.R. (1994) Repertory grid in the assessment of quality of life in patients with epilepsy: the quality of life assessment schedule. In: Trimble, M.R., Dodson, W.E. (eds.) *Epilepsy and Quality of Life.* New York: Raven Press, 151–164.

Kirshner, B., Guyatt, G. (1985) A methodologic framework for assessing health indices. *Journal of Chronic Diseases* **38**, 27–36.

Krupinsky, J. (1980) Health and Quality of Life. *Social Science and Medicine* **14** A, 203–211.

Langfitt, J.T. (1995) Comparison of the psychometric characteristics of three quality of life measures in intractable epilepsy. *Quality of Life Research* **4**, 101–114.

Matthews, C.G., Klove, H. (1967) Differential psychological performances in major motor, psychomotor, and mixed seizure classifications of known and unknown etiology. *Epilepsia* **8**, 117–128.

McHorney, C.A., Ware, J.E., Raczek, A.E. (1993) The MOS 36-Item Short-Form Health Status Survey (SF-36): II. Psychometric and clinical tests of validity in measuring physical and mental health constructs. *Medical Care* **31**, 247–263.

McLachlan, R.S., Rose, K.J., Derry, P.A., Bounar, C., Blume, W.T., Girvin, J.P. (1997) Health-related quality of life and seizure control in temporal lobe epilepsy; *Annals of Neurology* **41** (4), 482–489.

McNair, D., Lorr, M., Droppleman, L. (1992) POMS:Profile of Mood States. San Diego, CA: EDITS — Educational and Industrial Testing Service.

Meenan, R.F., Andersen, J.J., Kazis, L.E., Egger, M.J., Altz-Smith, M., Samuelson, C.O. Jr., Willcens, R.F., Solsky, M.A., Hayes, S.P., Bloeka, K.L. (1984) Outcome assessment in clinical trials. Evidence for the sensitivity of a health status measure. *Arthritis and Rheumatism.* **27**, 1344–1352.

Mittan, R.J. (1986) Fear of seizures. In: Whitman S., Hermann B.P. (eds.) *Psychopathology in Epilepsy: Social dimensions.* New York: Oxford University Press, 90–121.

Mittan, R.J., Locke, G. (1982) Fear of seizures: epilepsy's forgotten symptom. *Urban Health* **11**, 30–32.

National Institutes of Health (1979) *Plan for nationwide action on epilepsy. Vol. 1.* Bethesda: Department of Health Education & Welfare.

Nunally, J.C., Bernstein, I.H. (1994) *Psychometric Theory.* New York: McGraw Hill, 3rd ed.

O'Donoghue, M.F., Duncan, J.S., Sander, J.W. (1998) The subjective handicap of epilepsy: A new approach to measuring treatment outcome. *Brain* **121**, 317–343.

Patrick, D.L., Deyo, R.A. (1989) Generic and disease-specific measures in assessing health care status and quality of life. *Medical Care* **27** (Suppl 3), S217-S232.

Patrick, D.L., Erickson, P. (1993a) Assessing health-related quality of life for clinical decision-making. In: Walker, S.R., Rosser, R.M. (eds.) *Quality of life assessment: key issues in the 1990s.* Lancaster: Kluwer Academic Publishers, 11–63.

Patrick, D.L., Erickson, P. (1993b) *Health Status and Health Policy: Allocating Resources to Health Care.* New York: Oxford University Press.

Pearlin, L.I., Schooler, C. (1978) The structure of coping. *Journal of Health and Social Behaviour* **19**, 2–21.

Perrine, K.P. (1993) A new quality of life inventory for epilepsy patients: interim results. *Epilepsia* **34** (Suppl. 4), S28-S33.

Rapp, S., Shumaker, T., Smith, T., Gibson, P., Berzon, R., Hoffman, R. (1998) Adaptation and evaluation of the Liverpool seizure severity scale and Liverpool quality of life battery for American epilepsy patients. *Quality of Life Research* **7**, 353–363.

Rose, K.J., Derry, P.A., Wiebe, S., McLachlan, R.S. (1996) Determinants of health-related quality of life after temporal lobe epilepsy surgery. *Quality of Life Research* **5** (3), 195–202.

Rosenberg, M. (1965) *Society and the adolescent self-image.* Princeton: Princeton University Press.

Ryan, R., Kempner, K., Emlen, A.C. (1980) The stigma of epilepsy as a self-concept. *Epilepsia* **21**, 433–444.

Seidenberg, M., O'Leary, D.S., Berent, D.S., Bell, T. (1981) Changes in seizure frequency and test-retest scores on the Wechsler Adult Intelligence Scale. *Epilepsia* **22**, 75–83.

Seidman-Ripley, J.G., Bound, V.K., Andermann, F., Olivier, A., Gloor, P., Feindel, W.H. (1993) Psychosocial consequences of postoperative seizure relief. *Epilepsia* **34** (2), 248–254.

Selai, C.E., Trimble, M.R. (1995) Quality of life based on repertory grid technique. *Epilepsia* **36** (Suppl. 3), S220.

Smith, D.F., Baker, G.A., Dewey, M., Jacoby, A., Chadwick, D.W. (1991) Seizure frequency, patient perceived seizure severity and the psychosocial consequences of intractable epilepsy. *Epilepsy Research* **9**, 231–241.

Smith, D., Baker, G.A., Davies, G., Dewey, M., Chadwick, D.W. (1993a) Outcomes of add-on treatment with Lamotrigine in partial epilepsy. *Epilepsia* **34** (2), 312–322.

Smith, D., Chadwick, D., Baker, G.A., Davis, G., Dewey, M. (1993b) Seizure severity and the quality of life. *Epilepsia* **34** (Suppl.5), S31-S35.

Stewart, A.L., Hays, R.D., Ware, J.E. (1992a) Health perceptions, energy/fatigue, and health distress measures. In: Stewart, A.L., Ware, J.E. (eds.) *Measuring Functioning and Well-Being: The Medical Outcomes Study Approach.* Durham, NC: Duke University Press.

Stewart, A.L., Ware, J.E., Sherbourne, C.D., *et al.* (1992b) Psychological distress/well-being and cognitive measures. In: Stewart, A.L., Ware, J.E. (eds.) *Measuring Functioning and Well-Being: The Medical Outcomes Study Approach.* Durham, NC: Duke University Press.

Streiner, D.L., Norman, G.R. (1995) *Health measurement scales: a practical guide to their development and use.* Oxford: Oxford University Press, 2nd ed.

Testa, M.A., Nackley, J.F. (1994) Methods for quality of life studies. *Annual Review of Public Health* **15**, 535–59.

Vickrey, B.G. (1993) A procedure for developing a quality of life measure for epilepsy surgery patients. *Epilepsia* **34** (Suppl. 4), S22-S27.

Vickrey, B.G., Hays, R.D., Graber, J., Rausch, R., Engel, J., Brook, R.H. (1992) A health-related quality of life instrument for patients evaluated for epilepsy surgery. *Medical Care* **20** (4), 299–319.

Vickrey, B.G., Hays, R.D., Engel, J. (1995a) Outcome assessment for epilepsy surgery: the impact of measuring health-related quality of life. *Annals of Neurology* **37**:158–166.

Vickrey, B.G., Hays, R.D., Rausch, R., Engel, G., Visscher, B.R., Ary, C.M., Rogers, W.H., Brook, R.H. (1995b) Outcomes in 248 patients who had diagnostic evaluations for epilepsy surgery. *The Lancet* **346**, 1445–49.

Wagner, A.K., Keller, S.D., Kosinski, M., Baker, G.A., Jacoby, A., Hsu, M.A., Chadwick, D.W., Ware, J.E. (1995) Advances in methods for assessing the impact of epilepsy and antiepileptic drug therapy on patient's health-related quality of life. *Quality of Life Research* **4**, 115–134.

Ware, J.E., Sherbourne, C.D. (1992) A 36-item short form health survey (SF-36): Conceptual framework and item selection. *Medical Care* **30**, 473–483.

Ware, J.E., Kosinsky, M., Bayliss, M.S., McHorney, C.A., Rogers, W.H., Raczek, A. (1995) Comparison of methods for the scoring and statistical analysis of SF-36 Health Survey profiles and summary measures: Results from the Medical Outcomes Study. *Medical Care* 33(4), AS 264–279

Whitman, S., Herman, B. (1986) *Psychopathology in epilepsy*. New York: Oxford University Press.

WHO (World Health Organisation;1948) Constitution of the World Health Organization. *Basic documents*. Geneva: World Health Organisation, 15th ed.

WHO (World Health Organization; 1980) *The international classification of impairments, disabilities and handicaps*. Geneva: World Health Organisation.

Wiebe, S., Rose, K., Derry, P., McLachlan, R. (1997) Outcome assessment in epilepsy: comparative responsiveness of quality of life and psychosocial instruments. *Epilepsia* **38** (4), 430–438.

Zigmond, A.S., Snaith, R.P. (1983) The Hospital Anxiety and Depression Scale. *Acta Psychiatrica Scandinavica* **67**, 361–370.

Chapter 6

IMPACT OF EPILEPSY ON QUALITY OF LIFE: A REVIEW

Malachy Bishop and Bruce Hermann

Epilepsy researchers and clinicians have long been interested in understanding the psychosocial correlates of epilepsy and reducing the negative consequences of epilepsy on cognition, emotional and behavioral status, and social and vocational function. However, while the formal study of quality of life in epilepsy is a relatively recent endeavor (Hermann, 1992; 1995; Perrine *et al.*, 1995), the last decade has seen a burgeoning interest in this topic. This interest is reflected in the increasing number of research studies focusing on quality of life in epilepsy, the continually expanding array of health-related quality of life measures (see, for example, Devinsky *et al.*, 1997; Cramer *et al.*, 1999 and Chapter 5), texts on quality of life in epilepsy (e.g. Chadwick, 1990; Trimble and Dodson, 1994), and formal expressions of continued interest in this line of research by national and international epilepsy organizations. In this chapter we will present a review of the current understanding of the various areas in which epilepsy is thought to affect the quality of life.

QUALITY OF LIFE

For persons with a chronic illness such as epilepsy, where a cure is not attainable and therapy may be prolonged, quality of life (QoL) has come to be seen as an important health care outcome (Jacoby, 1992). Nevertheless, the concept of quality of life remains to some a somewhat vague and poorly defined concept, its measurement imperfect. Quality of life is generally conceptualised as a multidimensional construct. A review of the literature shows that a variety of terms have been equated with QoL, including life-satisfaction, self-esteem, well-being, health, happiness, adjustment, functional status and value of life (Frank-Stromborg, 1988). Quality of life may be described in terms of objective measures, such as physical function, employment, income, socio-economic status and support networks; and in terms of subjective measures, such as self-reported attitudes, perceptions and aspirations (Frank-Stromborg, 1988). Padilla and colleagues (1992) identified the main attributes of QoL as: (a) psychological well-being (life satisfaction, goal achievement, and happiness); (b) physical well-being; (c) social and interpersonal well-being; and (d) financial and material well-being.

In epilepsy research, quality of life and health-status outcomes have been used to assess the efficacy of medical, surgical and rehabilitation interventions; to provide an indicator of the quality of care; to predict health care utilisation and health behaviour; to compare impairment across diseases; and to evaluate the cost-benefit ratio of different treatments (Vickrey *et al.*, 1993). With a few exceptions, quality of life research in the field of epilepsy has focused on the health-related quality of life (HRQoL) model. Although this term too has been multiply defined, definitions of HRQoL generally include the three principal components of physical, mental and social health (Devinsky *et al.*, 1997). Vickrey *et al.* (1993, p. 623) defined HRQoL as encompassing physical, mental and social functioning and well being, 'including how well an individual functions in daily living (role functioning), as well as specific disease manifestations.'

Available evidence suggests that a diagnosis of epilepsy may severely reduce the quality of an individual's life (Jacoby, 1992). Along with the potential physical and cognitive sequelae associated with seizures, epilepsy has been associated with psychological and emotional problems, social isolation, and with problems concerning education, employment, family life and leisure activities (Thompson and Oxley, 1993). It should be recognised at the outset that most knowledge concerning the effects of epilepsy on quality of life has been garnered at specialised centers that tend to see the more severely affected among the population of people with epilepsy. These individuals usually appear to be more adversely affected in a variety of ways than persons with epilepsy in the community identified through epidemiological methods, and who may be more representative of the larger population of people with epilepsy.

QUALITY OF LIFE IN EPILEPSY: CURRENT UNDERSTANDING

A broad framework is necessary to incorporate contemporary HRQoL research findings in epilepsy. Bergner (1985) earlier proposed a comprehensive model for use in QoL research which is comprised of the following factors: symptoms, physical function, social function, sleep and rest, energy and vitality, health perceptions, life satisfaction, role activities, emotional status and cognition. This is an appropriately broad model with which to organise and review current understanding of the effects of epilepsy on life quality (Hermann, 1992; Vickrey *et al.*, 1993). The review below will adapt and expand upon this model as a means of presenting the current findings in each domain. Domains to be discussed include: symptoms, stigma, physical, social, cognitive function, family function, role status, psychological function, energy and vitality and life satisfaction.

Symptoms

Despite the substantial literature addressing the psychosocial consequences of epilepsy, only a modest amount of research has been devoted toward understanding the relationship between seizures, psychosocial problems, and QoL (Smith *et al.*, 1995). Seizures are the major symptom of epilepsy. While sometimes brief, they nevertheless have the potential to be tremendously disruptive. Fear of, or concern about, seizures has been found to affect social, psychological, and vocational function (Baker, 1995).

Seizures are generally the main focus in medical treatment (Devinsky and Penry, 1993), and the degree of reduction in seizure frequency has been the traditional outcome measure reported in the literature regarding outcome of various AED trials, epilepsy surgery, or alternative treatments (Vickrey *et al.*, 1993). This emphasis on seizure frequency and its robust effects can be seen most clearly in the epilepsy surgery literature. In a recent study of 94 patients, Kellett *et al.* (1997) found postoperative quality of life to be 'clearly related to seizure outcome'. Patients who were seizure free were found to exhibit significantly higher overall quality of life compared to patients having ten or more seizures a year post-operatively. In a retrospective study of 153 patients in Sweden, HRQoL, as assessed by the SF-36 was found to be correlated with percentage reduction in seizure frequency (Malmgren *et al.*, 1997). A similar correlation between HRQoL and reduced post-surgery seizure frequency was reported by McLachlan *et al.* (1997).

A relationship between seizure variables and quality of life or health status has been found in numerous descriptive studies also. In their large (n >5000) European based survey, Baker *et al.* (1997) found seizure type and frequency to be clearly associated with SF-36 scores. In this study, people with frequent seizures (at least once a month) had lower (worse) SF-36 scores, indicative of poorer QoL, than people with less frequent seizures or those who were seizure free. Also, people with a single seizure type reported better status on every domain of HRQoL than those with mixed seizure types. Further, in the same study, people with mixed or frequent seizures were more likely than the rest to believe that epilepsy affected the various aspects of their daily lives 'some' or 'a lot'.

In another recent study including 300 patients recruited from UK, Germany and France, seizure type and seizure frequency, as well as country of origin, were found to be significant predictors of scores on the Functional Status Questionnaire (FSQ; Baker *et al.*, 1998). Jacoby *et al.* (1996) found, in their survey of an unselected population in the UK (n = 696), that current seizure frequency was related to perceived impact of epilepsy, perceived stigma, marital and employment status, and anxiety and depression levels. These researchers concluded that 'individuals with frequent seizures have significantly poorer psychosocial profiles than those with infrequent or no seizures' (p. 158).

In light of the consistent findings that seizure status is related to QoL ratings, it is important to note that while seizures are relatively objective events, patients vary in their subjective evaluation of the impact seizures may have on their lives. Some researchers have pointed out that the subjective perspective of seizure-related variables may be as important in terms of quality of life as objective seizure variables (Arnston *et al.*, 1986; Collings, 1990; Vickrey *et al.*, 1993; Smith *et al.*, 1995). Reporting on their study of people with epilepsy in the US, Arnston and associates (1986) concluded that psychosocial indices such as stigma, helplessness, self-esteem and life satisfaction were more closely related to individuals' perceptions of how severely their seizures affected their lives than actual seizure frequency.

It appears that the impact of seizures on quality of life is a highly personal and context dependent situation that may be determined by a number of factors including personal and seizure-related, as well as societal attitudes. It has been suggested, for example, that for patients with refractory epilepsy, seizure severity may be a more important determinant of psychosocial well-being than seizure frequency, whereas for patients with mild seizure disorders, the epilepsy label itself might have greater impact (Smith *et al.*, 1993). Cramer (1993) pointed out that the impact of seizures may be based on their outward appearance, suggesting that a simple partial seizure with, 'an obvious and uncontrollable motor component could be more compromising or bothersome to a patient than a brief alteration in consciousness with aphasia that is unnoticed by others' (p. S9). On a societal level, important distinctions between seizure variables are often neglected in creating and maintaining public policy and public attitudes. For example, Smith *et al.* (1995) reported that in the U.K., a distinction between tonic-clonic and simple-partial seizures is not made in determining eligibility to hold a driving license.

Stigma

As seen in this latter example, epilepsy can be, in addition to being a medical diagnosis, a stigmatising social label (Jacoby, 1992). Although data reveal regional and national differences, stigmatising perceptions, negative attitudes, and misperceptions about persons with epilepsy have been found to exist in samples across the world (Livneh and Antonak, 1997). This stigma of epilepsy consists of deeply discrediting attributes such as propensity to crime and violence, sexual deviance, heritability and mental illness, restrictions or denials of common benefits (such as a drivers' license or life insurance) and limitations on opportunities that lead to independence (such as housing or employment discrimination; Livneh and Antonak, 1997).

In attempting to explain the attribution of discrediting characteristics and rejection of persons with epilepsy, researchers have focused on three areas including (1) parental reactions ranging from overprotectiveness and infantilisation to anger, resentment and rejection; (2) the perceptions and practices of professionals including physicians, teachers and other health and education providers; and (3) the attitudes of the general society including peers and employers (Livneh and Antonak, 1997). Scambler (1984) hypothesised that epilepsy is a stigmatising illness because people with epilepsy threaten the social order, first by failing to conform to cultural norms, and second by causing ambiguity in social interactions. This ambiguity is hypothesised to be related to the unpredictability of epilepsy, the dramatic nature of seizures, and the fear on the part of observers of having to cope with the person's seizures (Scambler, 1984).

It has been suggested that if the person with epilepsy internalises the rejection and societal devaluation he or she may express such negative and non-adaptive reactions as denial, anxiety, depression, low self-esteem and hostility, and such maladaptive behaviours as dependency, rigidity, anger and aggression. In which case, according to Antonak and Livneh (1995), the stigma may become self-perpetuating, as with the stigma cycle associated with race, religion or physical unattractiveness described by Goffman (1963) and Ajzen and Fishbein (1980). Because epilepsy may be felt to be a stigmatising and burdensome diagnosis by some, individuals may attempt to conceal their diagnosis or negotiate a less intimidating one. Possessing a characteristic that is potentially discrediting, people with epilepsy must decide what they will disclose and to whom. Hopkins (1984) suggested that a person with epilepsy 'has to act as his own public relations officer, deciding how much to tell and how much to conceal'. Scambler, in his 1984 study, found that secrecy and concealment was a first-choice strategy for many of the respondents and that disclosures, when they happened, were often not voluntary but provoked by clinical symptoms or manifestations of the respondents' condition.

As may be expected, it appears from research to date that more severe epilepsy, in terms of seizure type and control, has a relationship with the degree to which stigma is felt or perceived. In their survey of over 5000 people with epilepsy, including people selected through their participation in epilepsy support groups or neurology outpatient clinics, Baker *et al.* (1997) used a 3-item scale on which people responded whether they felt that others were uncomfortable with them, treated them as inferior, or preferred to avoid them. More than half the respondents in the study (51%) reported feeling stigmatised by their epilepsy and almost one-fifth (18%) answered yes to all three items. Respondents were more likely to feel stigmatised if they had a combination of seizure types or if they had frequent seizures. Conversely, in her 1992 study of a sample of people whose epilepsy was well controlled (the majority had been seizure-free for at least two years), Jacoby reported that only 14% of respondents reported feelings of stigmatisation, based on the same 3-item scale.

Physical function

Discerning the potential effects of epilepsy on physical function is a complex matter. The additional step of examining these effects in terms of their impact on quality of life is even more complicated and it is an effort that has received little research attention to date. Epilepsy represents a wide spectrum of severity from mild to severe and a number of variables, including seizure type, severity and frequency, as well as non-seizure related variables may affect the person's interaction with the environment and thus their quality of life. Although physical disability may occur in people with epilepsy, major physical limitations are not generally evident unless the seizures are due to underlying co-morbid neurological disease (Fraser *et al.*, 1992; Vickrey *et al.*, 1993).

Related to this topic is the issue of physical harm secondary to seizures. Although seizure-related nonfatal accidents are more common than fatal injuries, data about the incidence and predictors of such accidents are not readily available. Some recent surveys do, however, offer some information on the level of seizure-related injury in the general population, and on some of the factors associated with the likelihood of sustaining an injury because of a seizure. These factors include seizure type, seizure frequency, number of seizures during a lifetime and patients' sex (Spitz, 1992; Nakken and Lossius, 1993; Spitz *et al.*, 1994). Kirby and Sadler (1995) found that out of 146,365 visits to four emergency rooms, 0.4% were precipitated by seizures and 14% of these seizures resulted in injury. Seizure related injuries were sustained by 63 patients and some of the patients incurred multiple injuries as a result of their seizures. Head contusions and lacerations were the most common injuries. Head injuries, along with burn injuries, have been shown in a number of studies to be the most common type of seizure-related injury (e.g., Hauser *et al.*, 1984; Hampton, *et al.*, 1988; Buck *et al.*, 1997). In their recent survey of a large (n = 696) unselected, community-based population of patients with epilepsy, Buck *et al.* (1997) reported that of the patients who had had at least one seizure during the previous year, 24% sustained at least one head injury, 16% sustained a burn or scald, 10% a dental injury, and 6% some other fracture. Seizure type, seizure severity, and seizure frequency were found to be key predictors of having sustained at least one of these four seizure-related injuries.

Other concerns related to physical functioning, such as self-care and physical mobility have not been of substantial interest to epilepsy researchers (Hermann, 1992). However, the amount and type of physical activity and exercise by people with epilepsy has been the subject of an increasing number of studies and available evidence suggests that people with epilepsy are only half as active as comparable age-and sex-matched people, and are at lower levels of physical fitness (Nakken *et al.*, 1990).

Cognitive Function

The impact of epilepsy and its treatment on objectively assessed cognitive function has been a major focus of interest in the epilepsy literature. Most traditional domains of higher cognitive functioning have been investigated including intelligence, language, visuo-perceptual and spatial skills, memory and learning, attention and executive functions, cognitive speed and psychomotor processing and sensori-motor abilities. As a rule, patients with epilepsy exhibit more cognitive difficulty than people in the general population, although there is considerable variability across patient groups. Features of epilepsy that are associated with impaired cognitive and behavioural function include symptomatic aetiology, earlier age of onset and longer duration of epilepsy, higher seizure frequency (and poorer seizure control), seizure type, history of *status epilepticus* episodes, number of lifetime generalized tonic-clonic seizures, antiepileptic medications and other factors (Devinsky, 1995). It is important to point out that the HRQoL literature assesses cognitive function through patient self-report, in contrast to formal objective testing. It is now appreciated that patient self-reports regarding the adequacy of their cognitive status are influenced by mood: patients who are depressed or report increased depressive symptoms are also more likely to complain about the adequacy of their mentation. Perrine *et al.* (1995) examined this issue in the QoLIE-89 normative sample. This database included measures of mood state (POMS) and objective neuropsychological performance, as well as self-reported cognitive status. These authors were able to demonstrate the confounding effects of mood status. However, there did appear to be some relationship between objective test performance and subjective ratings of cognitive efficiency. A more accurate understanding of the relationship between patient self-report of cognitive functioning, actual neurobehavioural status as determined from objective neuropsychological assessment and the moderating effects of mood state remains to be fully clarified.

Social Function

The impact of epilepsy on social functioning can be variable. While some people with epilepsy have few, if any, disruptions of social interaction and functioning, others have severe problems that prevent them from engaging in fully productive lives (Austin and deBoer, 1997). Areas of social function that may be affected by epilepsy and its sequelae are inclusive of the many interpersonal, familial and community connections in which a person is involved. Adults with epilepsy have been found to have a higher prevalence of social problems, including social isolation and problems with adaptation, than people in the general population (Austin and deBoer, 1997). Among the potential reasons suggested for problems in social functioning are the development of a dependency role (e.g., due to parental overprotectiveness); severe and frequent seizures and embarrassment or concerns about participating in activities involving social interaction because of fear of having a seizure; low self-esteem from having a chronic disease that carries a stigma; co-occurring conditions or deficits; and academic underachievement (Vickrey *et al.*, 1993; Austin and deBoer, 1997).

Thompson and Oxley (1988) surveyed 92 patients to examine the psychosocial effects of poorly controlled epilepsy and found that social function was the area of greatest dissatisfaction. Sixty eight percent of the respondents reported no personal friends and 34% stated that they never formed true friendships. Only 8% were married or cohabiting, an additional 8% were involved in a steady relationship, and 57% had never had such a relationship. Collings (1990) found similar social isolation in his survey of 392 people with epilepsy.

Few studies have looked specifically at the effects of social support, perceived social support, or social function on quality of life. In a study of quality of life among 468 people with well controlled seizures, social isolation was associated with higher levels of respondent concern about their epilepsy (Jacoby, 1992). Using the WHO quality of life inventory as an outcome measure, Amir *et al.*, (1999) found social support to be strongly associated with quality of life. They further reported that social support was associated with sense of mastery and ability to cope with the limitations associated with epilepsy. Overall, the effect of social isolation on quality of life has not been well assessed to date. Given, however, the apparently high levels of such isolation among people with epilepsy, and the associations reported here between social support and quality of life, there is clearly a need for research on this factor.

Family Function

In a specific area of social function, family function, epilepsy has been found to have a significant impact both for adults in terms of marriage and family life, and for children with epilepsy and their siblings. There is evidence that people with epilepsy are less likely to marry and have children. This is particularly true if the epilepsy is severe or if it exists in the presence of additional handicaps (Dansky *et al.*, 1980; Jacoby, 1992). Higher rates of divorce than in the general population have been found among parents of children with epilepsy (Sillanpaa, 1973). Also, the siblings of children with epilepsy appear to be at a greater risk of psychiatric disturbance (Hoare and Kerley, 1991).

Families of children with epilepsy have been found to be less cohesive, have lower levels of self-esteem and communication, and have lower levels of social support than families of children with other chronic conditions (Ferrari *et al.*, 1983; Austin, 1988). And, as Betts (1988) has pointed out, there is the possibility that a 'cycle of deprivation' exists in families with a child with epilepsy, as 'the child that has had poor parenting as a result of his or her own epilepsy is likely to make a poor parent in return'.

Role Status

Role status involves functioning in areas such as employment and household management. The problematic employment situation for people with epilepsy has been well researched and an extensive body of literature exists on this topic (see, for example, Fraser, 1980; Thorbecke and Fraser, 1997). In the US labour market, the unemployment rate among people with epilepsy who are maintaining an active job search is reported to be 13–25% (Thorbecke and Fraser, 1997). Individuals who have one or more generalised tonic-clonic seizures or complex partial seizures a year have been found to have an even higher unemployment rate, of 50%, although these data are somewhat dated (Emlen and Ryan, 1979). In two recent studies (Elwes *et al.*, 1991; Jacoby, 1995), higher rates of unemployment were found among persons with active epilepsy compared to people whose epilepsy was in remission or well-controlled.

The Epilepsy Foundation of America (EFA) has been very successful in helping people with epilepsy find employment through its Training and Placement Service (TAPS). 'The most effective training and placement service for people with epilepsy worldwide', there are TAPS programmes in 13 American cities and many more privately funded and TAPS-like models throughout the U.S. (Sumner, 1996; Thorbecke and Fraser, 1997). Further, since 1990 the Americans with Disabilities Act (ADA) has provided some recourse to those with disabilities who are seeking employment. The ADA ensures that if an individual is unable to perform a job due to a disability, but is otherwise qualified, the employer must provide reasonable accommodations by making modifications in the job that enable the person to perform the job. In the case of epilepsy, where the disability is not immediately obvious from outward signs, the question of whether or not to disclose disability status to employers at the time of application often arises, and hence the situation described by Hopkins (1984), wherein the person with epilepsy must act as his or her own public relations manager and make a decision about whether or not to reveal the epilepsy diagnosis.

Scambler and Hopkins (1986) stated that among the respondents in their survey, almost all of those with full-time employment experience after the onset of seizures believed epilepsy to be stigmatising. This was despite the fact that fewer than a quarter could recall an occasion when they suspected they had been victims of 'enacted' stigma (as opposed to 'felt' stigma, or the fear of enacted stigma). In the Jacoby (1995) study of people with well-controlled epilepsy (1992) only 2% of those asked recalled an occasion over the preceding two years when they had been treated unfairly at work because of their epilepsy, and only 3% of those asked said that during the same time that they had failed to get a job they applied for because of it. Nevertheless, nearly a third of patients (32%) felt that their epilepsy made it more difficult for them than for others to get a job. Among those who felt that having epilepsy made getting a job more difficult, 39% felt this was because employers preferred not to employ people with disabilities of any kind; a third felt it was because of fear and lack of understanding about epilepsy on the part of employers; and a fifth attributed these difficulties to the potential dangers of seizures in the workplace. Although no specific question about disclosure was asked, a number of respondents commented that they had not disclosed their epilepsy out of fear of discrimination.

Collings (1990) found full-time employment to be a predictor of psychological well-being, and less adequate financial status has also been found to be a predictor of depression (Hermann *et al.*, 1992). Further elucidation of the relationship between employment status and quality of life is needed. Further, very little is known about the ways in which epilepsy affects the role of household management.

Psychological Function

The emotional and psychological problems associated with epilepsy have been studied to a considerable degree. Commonly expressed emotional and psychological reactions to epilepsy include depression, anxiety, anger, denial, increased suicide risk, decreased self-esteem, lowered perceptions of social support and a sense of loss of control or external locus of control, among many others (Hermann *et al.*, 1992; Cummings, 1994; Blumer and Altshuler, 1997; Livneh and Antonak, 1997). People with epilepsy have been found in a number of studies to have higher rates of suicide than the general population (McNamara, 1995). Mendez and colleagues (1986) reported that 78% of psychiatric hospitalisations of patients with epilepsy were for some form of affective disorder. A comprehensive and critical review of the literature goes far beyond the score of this chapter, and we will touch on only a few selected issues regarding perhaps the most commonly expressed emotional reactions which include anxiety and depression (McNamara, 1995; Livneh and Antonak, 1997).

Anxiety

Given the unpredictable nature of epilepsy, it is logical that anxiety levels among people with epilepsy may be higher than those found in the general population, which is indeed the case. The relationship between the experience of epilepsy and anxiety is, however, not a simple one. Anxiety has a 'complex relationship with epilepsy' which is difficult to disentangle owing to the definitional and methodological uncertainties of the various studies which have considered it (Betts, 1981). The fear of having a seizure may foster anxiety. Anxiety may be an integral part of a person's seizure experience, in that some patients have seizures in which anxiety figures pre-, peri-, or post-ictally (Betts, 1981). The stigmatising potential associated with seizures and epilepsy may also lead to increased anxiety levels (Arnston *et al.*, 1986). Finally, Betts (1981) has proposed that there may be a reciprocal relationship between anxiety and epilepsy in that increased anxiety may cause the person to experience more seizures.

Anxiety has been cited in a number of studies as the problem with epilepsy most commonly elicited from patients themselves (see, for example, Arnston *et al.*, 1986; Collings, 1990). In a recent large-scale survey study, Baker and associates (1997) found that almost half of all respondants said that they worried about their epilepsy a lot or some: only 15% in this study stated that they did not worry at all. In her study of a large sample of people with well-controlled epilepsy, Jacoby (1992) found that 23% worried a lot or some about their epilepsy, and a third reported worrying about it just a little. Jacoby *et al.* (1996) in their survey of a community based sample, found a significant relationship between anxiety levels, as measured by the Hospital Anxiety and Depression Scale, and seizure activity and duration of epilepsy.

Depression

As with anxiety, the relationship between depression and epilepsy is not a simple or well-defined one. It has been suggested that protracted anxiety may be a precursor of depression, and indeed, the two problems are well known to commonly co-exist among persons with epilepsy (Robertson *et al.*, 1987). In the last decade, the relationship has been further complicated by evidence that people with major depression are at a higher risk for the development of epilepsy (Kanner and Nieto, 1999). In her exhaustive review of possible organic contributions to depressive illness in epilepsy, Robertson (1989) noted that although there is substantial evidence that depression is common in persons with epilepsy, there is yet no consensus on the characteristics or causes of this depression. Hermann and associates (1992) proposed a multi-etiological model of social and psychological dysfunction in epilepsy including three categories of risk factors. These were neurobiological factors, such as age at onset, seizure control and seizure type; psychosocial factors including for example, locus of control, fear of seizures and adjustment to epilepsy; and medication factors, such as monotherapy versus polytherapy, and the presence or absence of barbiturate medications. The result of their stepwise multiple regression analysis showed increased depression scores to be associated with an increased number of stressful life events in the previous six months, poor adjustment to seizures, financial stress, and female gender.

It is generally accepted that the increased prevalence of depressive symptoms among persons with epilepsy is due not to a single factor, but to the complex combination of factors involved in having, treating and living with a chronic and unpredictable neurological disorder. Kanner and Nieto (1999) describe a triad of processes proposed as responsible for the increased rates of depression: (1) an intrinsic process directly related to the neurochemical and neurophysiological changes that take place in limbic structures in the course of epilepsy; (2) the iatrogenic potential of many of the antiepileptic drugs; and (3) a reactive process to a chronic disorder that demands multiple adjustments.

While an increased rate of depression is well documented among patients with epilepsy as compared with the general population, the explicit association of depression with quality of life, albeit logical, has not been well documented in the literature. There is some recent evidence that demonstrates that patients with co-morbid DSM-IV minor or major depression have considerably reduced quality of life compared to patients with epilepsy with past but not current, or no history of depression (Wiegartz *et al.*, 1999).

Energy and Vitality

While there has been considerable research on the relationship between sleep and seizures and the effects of sleep on abnormal epileptiform discharges, there has been only a modest amount of research on the sleep quality and sleep hygiene in people with epilepsy. The data that do exist suggest that problems with sleep are not uncommon. However, little is known regarding the effects of sleep quality on HRQoL in epilepsy, a unfortunate state of affairs in that the evidence to date suggests that sleep patterns may be disrupted in people with epilepsy (Vickrey *et al.*, 1993). Further, in a recent qualitative study of what people with epilepsy consider important areas of concern, both sleep disturbance and lack of energy were listed (Chaplin *et al.*, 1990). At the same time, sleep has been omitted from most HRQoL instruments (Hays and Stewart, 1992 in Vickrey *et al.*, 1993).

Life Satisfaction

Hall and Johnston (1994) state that the quality of life construct is so encompassing as to be nebulous, and suggest that life satisfaction should be measured as it is a more circumscribed concept. Although life satisfaction is the term most closely related to QoL, the two are not interchangeable. The biggest distinction between the terms is that life satisfaction is purely subjective and refers to a person's feelings of contentment with his or her life, while QoL has both subjective and objective dimensions (Canam and Acorn, 1999). Global measures of overall life satisfaction and general well being have only recently been investigated among people with epilepsy. In Collings' (1990) study of a large sample of people with epilepsy from Great Britain, Ireland and New Zealand, self-reported overall well-being was investigated. Life satisfaction was found to be most strongly associated with the perceived discrepancy between current self with epilepsy and 'anticipated self without epilepsy'. Less strong associations were found with chronicity of epilepsy and seizure frequency. Further research is necessary in this important area.

CONCLUSION

This has been a necessarily limited and selective review of the relationship between epilepsy and quality of life. Additionally, we have used one model of QoL to organise knowledge about the effects of epilepsy, though any one of a number of other models could have been used for this purpose. The most evident point is that there is a growing body of knowledge regarding patients' perspectives about the nature, course, severity and impact of epilepsy that was not heretofore available. While gaps remain, the information available to date has been invaluable. Compared to the literature that has examined patients with epilepsy with conventional cognitive and behavioural measures for instance, there are points of agreement as well as areas of disagreement which remain to be resolved. However, there is little question that the voice of the patient and family has been heard more clearly than ever before because of the HRQoL movement. How to translate what has been heard into effective treatment and prevention efforts remains an important challenge and logical extension of this literature.

ACKNOWLEDGEMENTS

This work was supported in part by NIH grant NS37738.

We sincerely thank Drs. Gus Baker and Ann Jacoby for their many helpful suggestions regarding earlier versions of this manuscript and for graciously providing us with many helpful published and unpublished materials for incorporation into our chapter.

References

Ajzen, I., Fishbein, M. (1980). *Understanding attitudes and predicting public behavior.* Englewood Cliffs, NJ: Prentice Hall.

Amir, M., Roziner, I., Knoll, A., Neufeld, M.Y (1999). Self-efficacy and social support as mediators in the relation between disease severity and quality of life in patients with epilepsy. *Epilepsia* **40**(2), 216–224.

Arnston, P., Droge, D., Norton, R., Murray, E. (1986). The perceived psychosocial consequences of having epilepsy. In Whitman, S., Hermann, B.P. (eds.), *Psychopathology in epilepsy: Social dimensions.* New York: Oxford University Press, 143–161.

Antonak, R.F., Livheh, H. (1995) Development, psychometric analysis and validation of an error-choice test to measure attitudes towards persons with epilepsy. *Rehabilitation Psychology* **40**(1), 25–39.

Austin, J.K. (1988). Childhood epilepsy: child adaptation and family resources.
Journal of Child and Adolescent Psychiatric Mental Health Nursing **1**(1), 18–24.

Austin, J.K., de Boer, H.M. (1997) Disruptions in social functioning and services facilitating adjustment for the child and adult. In Engel, J. Jr., Pedley, T.A. (eds) *Epilepsy: A Comprehensive Textbook.* Philadelphia: Lippincott-Raven, 2191–2201.

Baker, G.A. (1995). Health-related quality of life issues: Optimizing patient outcomes. *Neurology* **46**(Supp.2), S29–S34.

Baker, G.A., Jacoby, A., Buck, D., Stalgis, C., Monnet, D. (1997). Quality of life of people with epilepsy: A European study. *Epilepsia* **38**(3), 353–62.

Baker, G.A., Gagnon D., McNulty, P. (1998) The relationship between seizure frequency, seizure type and quality of life: findings from three European countries. *Epilepsy Research* **30**, 231–240.

Bergner, M. (1985). Measurement of health status. *Medical Care*, **23**, 696–704.

Betts, T. (1981). Epilepsy: Questions and answers. *Nursing Mirror* **153**(24), vi–ix.

Betts, T. (1988) People with epilepsy as parents. In Hoare, P. (ed). *Epilepsy and the Family: a medical symposium on new approaches to family care.* Manchester: Sanofi UK Ltd.

Blumer, D., Altshuler, L.L. (1997). Affective disorders. In J. Engel Jr., T.A. Pedley (eds.), *Epilepsy: A comprehensive textbook.* Philadelphia: Lippincott-Raven Publishers, 2083–2089.

Buck, D., Baker, G.A., Jacoby, A., Smith, D.F., Chadwick, D.W. (1997). Patients' experiences of injury as a result of epilepsy. *Epilepsia* **38**(4), 439–444.

Canam, C., Acorn, S. (1999). Quality of life for family caregivers of people with chronic health problems. *Rehabilitation Nursing* **24**(5), 192–196.

Chadwick, D. (ed) (1990) *Quality of life and quality of care in epilepsy.* Royal Society of Medicine Round Table Series No. 23. London: RSM.

Chaplin, J.E., Yepez, R., Shorvon, S. Floyd, M. (1990). A quantitative approach to measuring the social effects of epilepsy. *Neuroepidemiology* **9**, 151–158.

Collings, J.A. (1990). Epilepsy and well-being. *Social Science and Medicine* **31**, 165–70.

Cramer, J.A. (1993) A clinimetric approach to assessing quality of life in epilepsy. *Epilepsia* **34**(Supp.4), S8–S13.

Cramer, J.A. (1999) Quality of life assessment in clinical practice. *Neurology* **53**(Suppl.2), S49–S52.

Cummings, J.L. (1994). Depression in neurologic diseases. *Psychiatric Annals* **24**(10), 525–531.

Dansky, L.V., Andermann, E., Andermann, F. (1980) Marriage and fertility in epileptic patients. *Epilepsia* **21**, 261–271.

Devinsky, O. (1995) Cognitive and behavioural effects of antiepileptic drugs. *Epilepsia* **36**(Suppl.2) S46–S65.

Devinsky, O., Penry, J.K. (1993). Quality of life in epilepsy: The clinician's view. *Epilepsia* **34**(Supp.4), S4–S7.

Devinsky, O., Baker, G., Cramer, J. (1997) Quantitative measures of assessment. In J. Engel Jr., T.A. Pedley (eds.), *Epilepsy: A comprehensive textbook.* Philadelphia: Lippincott-Raven Publishers, 2211–2225.

Elwes, R.D.C., Marshall, J., Beatty, A., Newman, P.K. (1991). Epilepsy and employment: A community based survey in an area of high unemployment. *Journal of Neurology, Neurosurgery, and Psychiatry* **54**, 200–203.

Emlen, A.C., Ryan, R. (1979). *Analyzing unemployment rates among men with epilepsy*. Paper presented at the 30th annual Western Institute on Epilepsy, Portland, OR.

Ferrari, M., Matthews W.S., Barabas, G. (1983). The family and the child with epilepsy. *Family Process* **22**(1), 53–59

Frank-Stromborg, M. (1988). *Instruments for clinical nursing research*. Norwalk, CT: Appleton and Lange.

Fraser, R.T. (1980) Vocational aspects of epilepsy. In Hermann, B. (ed) *A Multidisciplinary Handbook of Epilepsy*. Springfield: Charles C. Thomas.

Fraser, R.T., Glazer, E., Simcoe, B.J. (1992) Epilepsy. In M.G. Brodwin, F. Telez, S.K. Brodwin (eds.), *Medical, psychosocial and vocational aspects of disability*. Athens, GA: Elliott and Fitzpatrick, 439–454.

Goffman, E. (1963). *Stigma: Notes on the management of a spoiled identity*. Englewood Cliffs, NJ: Prentice Hall.

Hall, K.M., Johnston, M.V. (1994). Outcome evaluation in TBI rehabilitation. Part 1: Measurement tools for a nationwide measurement system. *Archives of Physical Medicine and Rehabilitation* **75**(12), Spec. No., SC 10–18.

Hampton, K.K., Peatfield, R.C., Pullar, T., Bodansky, H.J., Walton, C., Feely, M. (1988). Burns because of epilepsy. *British Journal of Medicine* **296**, 1659–1660.

Hauser, W.A., Tabaddor, K., Factor, P.R., Finer, C. (1984). Seizures and head injury in an urban community. *Neurology* **34**, 746–751.

Hermann, B.P. (1992). Quality of life in epilepsy. *Journal of Epilepsy* **5**, 153-165.

Hermann, B.P., Whitman, S., Anton, M. (1992). A multietiological model of psychological and social dysfunction in epilepsy. In T.L. Bennett (ed.), *The neuropsychology of epilepsy*. New York: Plenum Press, 39–55.

Hoare. P., Kerley, S. (1991) Psychosocial adjustment of children with chronic epilepay and their families. *Developmental Medicine and Child Neurology* **33**(3), 201–15.

Hopkins, A. (1984) *Epilepsy, The Facts*. Oxford: Oxford University Press.

Jacoby, A. (1992). Epilepsy and the quality of everyday life: Findings from a study of people with well-controlled epilepsy. *Social Science and Medicine* **34**, 657–666.

Jacoby, A. (1995) Impact of epilepsy on employment status: Findings from a UK study of people with well-controlled epilepsy. *Epilepsy Research* **21**, 125–132.

Jacoby, A., Baker, G., Steen, N., Potts, P., Chadwick, D. (1996) The clinical course of epilepsy and its psychosocial correlates. *Epilepsia* **37**(2), 148–161.

Kanner, A.M., Nieto, J.C.R. (1999). Depressive disorders in epilepsy. *Neurology* **53**(Supp.2), S26–S32.

Kellett, M.W., Smith, D.F., Baker, G.A., Chadwick, D.W. (1997) Quality of life after surgery. *Journal of Neurology, Neurosurgery and Psychiatry* **63**(1), 52–58.

Kirby, S., Sadler, R.M. (1995). Injury and death as a result of seizures. *Epilepsia* **36**, 25–28.

Livneh, H., Antonak, R. (1997). *Psychosocial adaptation to chronic illness and disability*. Gaithersburg, MD: Aspen Publishers Inc.

Malmgren, K., Sullivan, M., Ekstedt, G. Kullberg, G. Kumlien, E. (1997). Health-related quality of life after epilepsy surgery: A Swedish multicenter study. *Epilepsia* **38**(7), 830–838.

McLachlan, R.S., Rose, K.J., Derry, P.A., Bonnar, C., Blume, W.T., Girvin, J.P. (1997). Health related quality of life and seizure control in temporal lobe epilepsy. *Annals of Neurology* **41**(4), 482–489.

McNamara, M.E. (1995). Neurological conditions: Depression and stroke, multiple sclerosis, Parkinson's disease, and epilepsy. In A. Stoudemire (ed.) *Psychosocial factors affecting medical conditions*. Washington D.C.: American Psychiatric Press, Inc.

Mendez, M.F., Cummings, J.L., Benson, F. (1986). Depression in epilepsy. *Archives of Neurology* **43**, 766–770.

Nakken, K.O., Bjorholt, P.G., Johannessen, S.I., Loyning, T., Lind, E. (1990). Effect of physical training on aerobic capacity, seizure occurrence, and serum levels of antiepileptic drugs in adults with epilepsy. *Epilepsia* **31**, 88–94.

Nakken, K.O., Lossius, R. (1993). Seizure-related injuries in multihandicapped patients with therapy-resistant epilepsy. *Epilepsia* **34**, 836–840.

Padilla, G.V., Grant, M.M., Ferrell, B. (1992). Nursing research into quality of life. *Quality of Life Research* **1**, 341–348.

Perrine, K., Hermann, B.P., Meador, K.J., Vickrey, B.G., Cramer, J.A., Hays, R.D., Devinsky, O. (1995). The relationship of neuropsychological functioning to quality of life in epilepsy. *Archives of Neurology* **52**, 997–1003.

Robertson, N.M. (1989) The organic contribution to depressive illness in patients with epilepsy. *Journal of Epilepsy* **2**, 189–230.

Robertson, M.M., Trimble, M.R., Townsend, H.R.A. (1987) Phenomenology of depression in epilepsy. *Epilepsia* **28**, 364–372.

Scambler, G. (1984). Perceiving and coping with stigmatizing illness. In R. Fitzpatrick, R. Hinton, S. Newman, G. Scambler (eds.), *The experience of illness*. London: Tavistock.

Scambler, G., Hopkins, A. (1986). Being epileptic: Coming to terms with stigma. *Sociology of Health and Illness* **8**, 26–43.

Sillanpaa, M. (1973). Medico-social prognosis of children with epilepsy: Epidemiological study and analysis of 245 patients. *Acta Paediatrica Scandinavica* Suppl.237, 3–104.

Smith, D.F., Baker, G.A., Dewey, M., Jacoby, A., Chadwick, D.W. (1993) Seizure frequency, patient perceived seizure severity and the psychosocial consequences of intractable epilepsy. *Epilepsy Research* **9**, 231–241.

Smith, D., Baker, G.A., Jacoby, A., Chadwick, D.W. (1995). The contribution of the measurement of seizure severity to quality of life research. *Quality of Life Research* **4**, 143–158.

Spitz, M.C. (1992). Severe burns as a consequence of seizures in patients with epilepsy. *Epilepsia* **33**, 103–107.

Spitz, M.C., Towbin, J.A., Shantz, D., Adler, L.E. (1994). Risk factors for burns as a consequence of seizures in persons with epilepsy. *Epilepsia* **35**, 764–767.

Sumner, G. (1996). An employment perspective from the National Multiple Sclerosis Society. In P.D. Rumrill Jr. (ed.), *Employment issues and multiple sclerosis*. New York: Demos Vermande, 127–132.

Thompson, P.J., Oxley, J. (1988) Socioeconomic accompaniments of severe epilepsy. *Epilepsia* **29**, S9–S18.

Thompson, P., Oxley, J. (1993). Social aspects of epilepsy. In Laidlaw, J., Richens, A., Chadwick, D. (eds.), *A textbook of epilepsy. 4th Ed. London: Churchill Livingstone*, 661–704.

Thorbecke, R., Fraser, R.T. (1997). The range of needs and services in vocational rehabilitation. In J. Engel Jr., T.A. Pedley (eds.). *Epilepsy: A comprehensive textbook*. Philadelphia: Lippincott-Raven Publishers, 2211–2225.

Trimble, M.R., Dodson, W.E. (eds)(1994) *Epilepsy and Quality of Life*. New York: Raven Press.

Vickrey, B.G., Hays, R.D., Hermann, B.P., Bladin, P.F., Batzel, L.W. (1993). Outcomes with respect to quality of life. In J. Engel, Jr. (ed.). *Surgical treatment of the epilepsies*. 2nd Ed., New York: Raven Press, Ltd, 2211–2225.

Wiegartz, P., Seidenberg, M., Woodward, A., Gidal, B., Hermann, B. (1999) Comorbid psychiatric disorder in chronic epilepsy: recognition and aetiology of depression. *Neurology* **53** (Suppl.2) S3–S8.

Chapter 7

QUALITY OF LIFE ISSUES FOR CHILDREN AND ADOLESCENTS WITH EPILEPSY

David W. Dunn and Joan K. Austin

Seizures are a common problem in children, with between 4 and 10% having at least one seizure at some time. By 20 years of age approximately 1% of the population can be expected to have had a diagnosis of epilepsy or repeated seizures (Hauser, 1994). Epilepsy is a pervasive disorder that can disrupt a child's physical, psychosocial and academic functioning. Thus it is essential to consider overall quality of life in the measurement of outcome in children with epilepsy. In this chapter we will review the potential problems associated with epilepsy, concentrating on the psychosocial and academic troubles affecting children and their families.

BEHAVIOURAL CONSEQUENCES OF EPILEPSY IN CHILDHOOD

Common mental health problems reviewed here are behavioural problems, disorders of attention, mood disturbance, anxiety disorders, conduct disorder and aggression, autistic disorder, and psychosis.

Behavioural problems have long been documented in children with epilepsy. They have been found to have higher rates of behavioural problems than children with other chronic conditions. Rutter, Graham, and Yule (1970), in a study on the Isle of Wight, UK, found that 29% of children with uncomplicated seizures and 58% of children with both seizures and obvious CNS damage had behavioural problems. In comparison, the prevalence of behavioural problems in the general childhood population was just under 7%.

When Austin and colleagues (1994) compared rates of behavioural problems between children with epilepsy and children with asthma, higher behavioural problem scores for anxiety, depression and disruptive behaviours were found in those with epilepsy. Compared to controls, McDermott *et al.,* (1995) found children with epilepsy to have higher rates of behavioural problems in several areas, including being headstrong, hyperactive and dependent. Children with epilepsy are also generally found to have poorer self-concepts than children with other chronic physical conditions. Austin (1989) found children with epilepsy to rate themselves lower than children with asthma in all six areas studied (behavioural, intellectual function, physical appearance, self-anxiety, popularity, happiness and satisfaction). Results were similar for comparisons made by Hoare and Mann (1994) between epilepsy and diabetes samples.

Impaired attention is one of the more common problems in children with epilepsy and may affect both the psychosocial and school domains of quality of life. In the study by Holdsworth and Whitmore (1974) evidence of inattention was found in 42% of children with epilepsy who were in regular schools; and Hoare and Kerley (1991) found 59% of children with epilepsy to have poor attention as defined by their parents and 77% to have impaired attention based on reports from their teacher. Mitchell *et al.* (1992) found inattention and slow reaction time in children with seizures both on and off antiepileptic drugs. In children with new-onset seizures, those with prior unrecognised seizures had more attention problems than those without (Dunn *et al.*, 1997).

Mood disturbance or depression has been associated with epilepsy in adults, with prevalence rates ranging from 34% to 78%. Brent *et al.*, (1987) showed an increased risk of depression and attempted suicide in children with seizures treated with phenobarbital. McDermott *et al.*, (1995) noted higher rates of depression in children with epilepsy than in children with cardiac disease. Elevated scores on the Child Depression Inventory (Kovacs, 1980/81) were reported in 26% of children aged 7 to 18 years recruited from an epilepsy clinic (Ettinger *et al.*, 1998). Dunn *et al.*, (1999) reported scores on the Child Depression Inventory and the Anxiety/Depression subscale of the Youth Self-report Form (Achenbach, 1991) that suggested risk for depression in 23% of a sample of adolescents aged 12 to 16 years of age.

Children with epilepsy also are possibly at increased risk for anxiety disorders. Ettinger *et al.*, (1998) found that 16% of children with epilepsy had elevated anxiety scores. This may not be only a reflection of epilepsy, however, because children with other chronic illnesses also have elevated physiological anxiety and worry/oversensitivity scores. Compulsive behaviour has also been seen in association with complex partial seizures (Caplan and Gillberg, 1997).

Data on conduct problems are difficult to find, in part because of the use of differing measures and definitions. McDermott *et al.*, (1995) reported ratings for the descriptor 'antisocial,' which were based on items diagnostic for conduct disorder, and for 'headstrong' that list criteria similar to oppositional defiant disorder. In both categories, children with epilepsy were more likely to have problems than children with cardiac disease or controls (antisocial: seizures 18%, cardiac 12%, controls 9%; headstrong: seizure 28%, cardiac 18%, controls 9%). In the series by Caplan *et al.,* (1997), six of 54 children had oppositional defiant disorder and three conduct disorder. Milrod and Urion (1992) reported an interesting association between firesetting, photoparoxysmal response to photic stimulation, and temporal lobe EEG abnormalities that resolve with antiepileptic medication.

There is an overlap between autistic disorder and epilepsy. Approximately one third of children with autistic disorder develop seizures. Seizures may contribute to the regression seen in some children with autistic disorder. Tuchman and Rapin (1997) found that 30% of children with autistic disorder had a history of regression, typically occurring prior to 3 years of age. Regression occurred equally in autistic children with or without epilepsy. However, in the children without epilepsy, 19% of those with regression had spikes on their EEGs, versus 10% of those with no history of regression. Approximately half the children had centrotemporal discharges. Nass *et al.,* (1998) also reported occipital spikes in a group of children with autistic disorder or autistic regression. These children are similar to those with the Landau-Kleffner syndrome, an acquired aphasia, who have severe regression in language and some behaviours similar to those seen in autistic disorder.

Chronic interictal schizophrenia-like psychosis occurs 6–12 times more often in adults with epilepsy than in the general population, and has been linked to discharges in the mediobasal temporal lobe (Sachdev, 1998). Trimble (1991) has described a time lag of approximately 14 years between the onset of epilepsy and psychosis, one possible explanation for the rarity of reported psychosis in children with epilepsy. Nevertheless, children with seizures may be at risk. Caplan *et al.,* (1997) have found an increase in illogical thinking in children with complex partial seizures. In their sample six of 30 children with complex partial seizures had schizophrenia-like symptoms. The illogical thinking in the children with complex partial seizures was related to the presence of global cognitive dysfunction.

RISK FACTORS FOR BEHAVIOURAL PROBLEMS

Although research has not clearly identified factors that account for these higher rates of behavioural problems in children with epilepsy, it is hypothesised that demographic, neurological, epilepsy/seizure, family, and child factors are involved. These are reviewed briefly below.

Demographic variables identified as being potential risk factors for behavioural problems include low socioeconomic status (Hermann and Whitman, 1986; Hermann *et al.*, 1989; Hoare and Kerley, 1991) and young age (Hoare and Kerley, 1991). Studies focusing on gender have been inconsistent. Austin and colleagues (Austin *et al.*, 1992) found female gender to be associated with more behavioural problems, although girls had fewer problems with peer relationships than boys (Austin *et al.*, 1996). In contrast, other studies have found boys to have more behavioural problems than girls (Aman *et al.*, 1992) or found no differences based on sex (Matthews *et al.*, 1982; Mitchell *et al.*, 1994). Few studies have explored interactions among gender and seizure variables. In one study (Aman *et al.*, 1992) boys with partial seizures had more aggression problems than girls with partial seizures or than boys or girls with generalised seizures. In another study, girls with high seizure severity were found to have the most thought, attention, and social problems (Austin *et al.*, 1996).

There is an increased risk of behavioural problems in children with other neurological problems, especially children with learning disabilities. In a population-based study of psychiatric problems in children with both learning disabilities and epilepsy, Steffenburg *et al.* (1996) found that only six percent had no psychiatric condition; they reported autistic disorder in 27% and an autistic-like condition or Asperger's Syndrome in 14%.

Just as children with CNS dysfunction have more behavioural problems than children with other chronic illnesses, children with epilepsy accompanied by obvious neurologic deficits are at increased risk for behavioural disturbance. In the Isle of Wight study (Rutter *et al.*, 1970), children with seizures and additional CNS dysfunction had twice the rate of psychiatric disorders as children with uncomplicated epilepsy. Hoare (1993) found that having disabilities in addition to epilepsy was consistently associated with a negative impact on quality of life. The studies by Hoare (1984) and Dunn *et al.* (1997) showed that in children with new-onset seizures, behavioural problems were more common prior to starting antiepileptic medication or where seizures recurred. These findings suggest that underlying CNS dysfunction contributes significantly both to seizures and behavioural problems.

Studies comparing the role of seizure type have been less successful in predicting behavioural problems in children with epilepsy. Complex partial seizures have been implicated in behavioural problems of adults with seizures and were a risk factor for illogical thinking in the series by

Caplan *et al.* (1997); several other studies have failed to demonstrate a relationship between complex partial seizures and behavioural difficulties in children.

Other seizure variables have also been studied. Seizure frequency and severity have been shown to be consistent predictors of behavioural problems in children. The degree of seizure control was a better predictor than either psychosocial factors or medication in the study by Hermann *et al.* (1989). Hoare (1984) found that seizure control was negatively associated with behavioural problems; and Austin *et al.* (1992) reported a correlation between behavioural disturbance and seizure frequency. Wildrick *et al.* (1996) described an association between continuing seizures and social difficulties. Seizure severity has also been a predictor of quality of life difficulties. Austin *et al.* (1996) showed an association between seizure severity and both psychosocial and social domains of quality of life. Hoare (1993) found the combination of younger age of onset, longer seizure treatment duration, higher seizure frequency, seizure type (complex partial and mixed) and additional neurological difficulties to have adverse effects on both child and family responses.

It has been difficult to demonstrate a definite relationship between antiepileptic drugs and behavioural problems. The exceptions are an association between hyperactivity and the barbiturates or benzodiazepines, and the occurrence of depression with phenobarbital. In a study that assessed behavioural changes prospectively, Williams *et al.*, (1998) found no changes in behaviour during the first six months of therapy. Most of the children were on either carbamazepine or valproate monotherapy. Nevertheless, there are many anecdotal reports of significant behavioural changes with most of the currently used antiepileptic drugs. Gabapentin has been associated with aggressive, hyperactive behaviour; vigabatrin has led to psychotic reactions, hyperactivity, and aggressiveness; and lamotrigine has adversely affected behaviour in children with learning disabilities. Polypharmacy has been associated with depression and inattention in children in some studies but not others (Bourgeois, 1998).

The few studies of family responses to childhood epilepsy suggest that parent responses might be related to child quality of life outcomes. In an early study, Mulder and Suurmeijer (1977) found a positive relationship between parental control and dependency in children with epilepsy. Lothman, Pianta, and Clarson (1990) studied parenting behaviours through observing mother-child interactions and found that the degree to which mothers praised their children was related to the child's competence and positive affect. In contrast, intrusive or over-controlling parenting behaviours were found to be related to decreased child autonomy and confidence.

The few empirical studies exploring the relationship between family variables and child behavioural problems support a relationship between them. For example, Hoare and Kerley (1991) found family stress, epilepsy variables, medication variables and socioeconomic status to be associated with child behavioural problems. Austin, Risinger, and Beckett (1992) also found family stress, high seizure frequency, and low family resources (extended family social support and family mastery and control) to be associated with increased behavioural problems. Although negative parental perceptions about their child's epilepsy are frequently referred to in the clinical literature as causes of behavioural problems, few empirical studies have been conducted. West (1986) found parents' attempts to conceal their child's epilepsy and the parents' perceived stigma from the illness had a negative impact on the child's sense of identity. A study by Hartlage and Green (1972) found a relationship between parental strictness and positive child socialisation and self-direction.

The learned helplessness model may be particularly useful for understanding the impact of their condition on children with epilepsy. DeVellis and DeVellis (1986) have suggested that the episodic, unpredictable nature of seizures and the lack of control over the illness could lead to learned helplessness and so to depression. In partial support of this model, Matthews and Barabas (1986) were able to show that more children with epilepsy had an unknown or external locus of control than children with diabetes mellitus. Dunn *et al.* (1999) have reported an association between unknown or external locus of control and depression in adolescents with epilepsy. The child's attitudes and coping responses have been shown to be important in determining adaptation to epilepsy; Austin and Huberty (1993) found that children with a positive attitude towards epilepsy were less likely to have behavioural problems, depression or poor self-concept. Austin *et al.* (1991) have also shown that a positive coping response (competence, optimism, compliance and support seeking) was associated with positive self-concept and less emotional disturbance; whereas a negative coping response (irritability, feeling different, social withdrawal) was associated with more behavioural problems. A negative attitude toward illness and a lack of satisfaction with family relationships have been associated with depression in adolescents with epilepsy (Dunn *et al.*, 1999).

ACADEMIC ACHIEVEMENT PROBLEMS

Children with epilepsy have a high prevalence of learning disability including mental handicaps with scores of less than 70 on standard intelligence testing and specific learning disorders with achievement below that expected for age and intellectual capacity. The incidence of mental handicap varies with the seizure type, being as high as 89–90% in children with Lennox Gastaut syndrome and 71–85% in children with infantile spasms (Aicardi, 1994). Children with learning disability are at significant risk for seizures, with epilepsy occurring in half of all children with an IQ of less than 50 and in almost one fourth of children with an IQ between 50 and 70 (Hauser and Hesdorffer, 1990). Even controlling for intellectual ability, children with seizures perform poorly in school. Holdsworth and Whitmore (1974) found that 69% of children with epilepsy who were in regular schools were functioning below average, and 16% were seriously delayed. Rutter *et al.* (1970) reported a 2-year delay in reading in 18% of the children with epilepsy versus seven percent of the control group. Both Seidenberg *et al.* (1986) and Mitchell *et al.* (1991) have described learning disability in children with epilepsy, with rates varying from 10 to 50%, depending upon the assessment employed.

Comparisons of academic achievement among children with different chronic conditions have consistently shown that children with neurological disorders have more difficulties. This is the case even when evaluating only those children with no learning disability. Austin *et al.* (1998) compared 117 children with epilepsy to 108 with asthma and found that academic achievement was lower for the children with epilepsy. Even after controlling for gender and illness severity, children with epilepsy continued to show poorer performance.

Children with seizures have difficulties in multiple areas. Seidenberg *et al.* (1986) reported poorer performance in mathematics (33%) and in word recognition (10%). Mitchell *et al.* (1991) documented under-achievement in mathematics in 31% of children with seizures and in reading in 16%. She also found delays in general information in 50%, reading comprehension in 33%, and spelling in 32%.

Sillanpaa *et al.* (1998), in their long term follow-up of children with seizures as they reached their adult years, found that they had fewer years of education and were more likely to be unemployed than controls. Camfield *et al.* (1993) found that even in children of normal intelligence, 34% had experienced school failure and 20% were unemployed.

RISK FACTORS FOR ACADEMIC ACHIEVEMENT PROBLEMS

Compared to studies looking at behavioural problems, there are fewer studies of factors associated with academic achievement problems in children with epilepsy. Factors that have been studied include demographic, neurological, medication, and child and family factors.

Demographic variables investigated indicate differences based on gender. In general, boys have been found to be at increased risk for academic problems. In children with epilepsy, a similar increase in academic problems for boys has been documented in some studies (Holdsworth and Whitmore, 1974: Stores and Hart, 1976: Austin *et al.*, 1998), though less convincingly in others (Seidenberg *et al.,* 1986). In the study by Austin *et al.* (1998) the boys with the highest seizure severity were the most likely to have academic problems.

Neurological factors are important in the aetiology of cognitive impairment in children with epilepsy. Children with CNS malformations or damage delineated by neuroimaging are at increased risk for both epilepsy and learning disability. This has been shown repeatedly in children with infantile spasms, in whom the prognosis is worse in those children with symptomatic seizures and better in those with cryptogenic seizures (Aicardi, 1994). In children with epilepsy but no evidence of learning disability, it has been harder to show a major effect of neurological variables. Seidenberg *et al.* (1986) found an association between academic problems and longer duration of seizures, multiple seizure types, and more intractable seizures. However, there were no significant associations between seizure variables and learning disability in the studies by Mitchell *et al.* (1991) and Huberty *et al.* (1992).

Of the antiepileptic medications, phenobarbital has consistently been associated with cognitive difficulties. Farwell *et al.* (1990) found that children with febrile seizures on phenobarbital had lower IQ scores than control children with febrile seizures not on medication. Even after the phenobarbital was discontinued, the previously treated children still had lower IQ scores. There have been several reports of an organic brain syndrome in association with valproate. Topiramate has been shown to cause mental slowing and pauses in speech. In general, studies of most of the newer agents have not shown significant cognitive side effects (Bourgeois, 1998). Discontinuation studies have shown improvement in alertness, but have not shown significant improvement in cognitive function (Aldenkamp *et al.*, 1998).

Child and family factors have less frequently been studied. One study compared self-perceptions of children with epilepsy to those of matched samples of children with diabetes and healthy children. In that study, children with epilepsy had significantly poorer self-concepts related to intellectual matters and were twice as likely to report they were worried when they had tests at school than the other two groups. They were also twice as likely to report they became nervous when the teacher called on them (Matthews *et al.*, 1983). Austin and colleagues (1998), in their study of academic achievement in children with epilepsy or asthma, found that a positive attitude towards their condition was associated with academic achievement in children in both samples.

Research identifying relationships between family variables and academic achievement in children with epilepsy is also limited. Green and Hartlage (1971) suggest that parent expectations for academic achievement are reduced in children with epilepsy, and these reduced expectations result in poorer school performance. In an early study, parental attitudes were found to be stronger predictors of academic achievement than seizure type or seizure frequency variables (Hartlage and Green, 1972). More recently, Mitchell and colleagues (1991) also found that underachievement in children with epilepsy was more strongly related to family variables than to seizure variables. In that study, academic achievement was predicted by high parent education, educational materials in the home and family participation in developmentally stimulating activities.

TREATMENT AND INTERVENTIONS FOR PROBLEMS AFFECTING QUALITY OF LIFE

Once seizures have begun, a number of steps can be taken to reduce the risk of behavioural and cognitive problems. Unfortunately, there are limited data to show the effectiveness of specific interventions, but education should be helpful. Both parents and children with new-onset seizures have significant worries and concerns. Shore *et al.* (1998) found that six months after the onset of seizures, one third to one half of the mothers were still very worried, expressing concerns about the causes of the seizures; death, brain damage, or loss of intelligence from seizures; and addiction to medication for seizures. The children were worried about social aspects of epilepsy. They had concerns about talking to others about their seizures and about having seizures in public.

Approximately one out of eight were restricting activities for fear of having another seizure (McNelis *et al.*, 1998). Lewis *et al.* (1990; 1991) have conducted one of the few controlled trials of educational intervention. The intervention was divided into child and family components. The children in the experimental group were involved in four interactive sessions reviewing understanding body messages; controlling seizures with medication; telling others about the seizures; and coping and adaptation. The control group of children received three traditional lectures by a physician followed by questions and answers. The children in the experimental group had more knowledge of epilepsy, felt more competent, were better behaved, and had less need for restrictions. The parents in the experimental group were also involved in four discussion sessions about epilepsy; decision-making; working as a family; and coping and adaptation. The mothers in the experimental group had more knowledge of epilepsy and less maternal anxiety. Though implementation was difficult, a similar approach might be used for small groups within a clinic or private practice, with resultant improvement in psychosocial outcome.

Small group sessions have benefits for children and adults with epilepsy. Williams *et al.* (1979) used a group therapy intervention to reduce emotional stress and found improvement in seizure control in 70% of cases. Normal intelligence, partial seizures, and less abnormal EEGs also predicted a positive response. Oosterhuis (1994) used an 8-session psychoeducational approach and demonstrated a reduction in apparently stress-induced seizures.

For children with epilepsy and academic difficulties, standard programmes could improve outcome, though these children need prompt assessment and appropriate intervention. In Baltimore, the Vocational Educational Programme for Adolescents with Epilepsy identified students with epilepsy and provided assessment and individualised services including counselling, help with placement, vocational training and work experience and epilepsy educational programmes (Freeman *et al.*, 1984). Benefits of the programme were decreased rates of school failure, dropout, and unemployment after school.

Children with major behavioural problems associated with epilepsy may benefit from psychotropic medication (McConnell and Duncan, 1998). Factors to consider in choosing a medication include potential effectiveness, tendency to lower seizure threshold and drug interactions. Stimulant medication is first choice for attention deficit hyperactivity disorder. Methylphenidate has been shown not to increase seizure frequency, worsen EEG or alter antiepileptic drug levels. Tricyclic antidepressants and bupropion are effective in attention deficit hyperactive disorder, but lower seizure threshold. For children with depression, the serotonin reuptake inhibitors may be effective and probably do not lower seizure threshold, but may inhibit the cytochrome system involved in the metabolism of phenytoin, carbamazepine and ethosuximde. Tricyclic antidepressants have been used cautiously, among which clomipramine has been most often associated with worsening of seizures. Of the antipsychotic drugs, clozapine and chlorpromazine both lower seizure threshold. The newer atypical antipsychotic agents, risperidone and olanzapine, have not been reported to adversely affect seizure control.

CONCLUSIONS

Children with epilepsy are at risk of reduced quality of life outcomes in the psychosocial and school domains. Children with additional handicaps are at most risk. It is imperative that children receive assessment of behavioural and academic functioning at initial diagnosis. Quality of life measures should also be a part of the periodic follow-up of all children with epilepsy. Additional research is needed both to prevent and adequately treat those children with epilepsy in whom quality of life is compromised by their condition.

References

Achenbach, T.M. (1991) *Manual for the Youth Self-Report* and *1991 Profile.* Burlington, VT: University of Vermont Department of Psychiatry.

Aicardi, J. (1994) *Epilepsy in Children*, Second Edition, New York: Raven Press.

Aldenkamp, A.P., Alpherts, W.C.J., Sandstedt, P., Blennow, G., Elmquist, D., Heijbel, J., Tonnby, B., Wahlander, L., Wosse, E. (1998) Antiepileptic drug-related cognitive complaints in seizure-free children with epilepsy before and after drug discontinuation. *Epilepsia* **39**, (10) 1070–1074.

Aman, M.G., Werry, J.S., Turbott, S.H. (1992) Behaviour of children with seizures: comparison with norms and effect of seizure type. *The Journal of Nervous* and *Mental Diseases* **180**, 124–129.

Austin, J.K. (1989) Comparison of child adaptation to epilepsy and asthma. *Journal of Child and Adolescent Psychiatry and Mental Health Nursing* **33**, 201–215.

Austin, J.K., Patterson, J.M., Huberty, T.J. (1991) Development of the coping health inventory for children. *Journal of Paediatric Nursing* **6**,166–174.

Austin, J.K., Risinger, M.W., Beckett, L. (1992) Correlates of behavioural problems in children with epilepsy. *Epilepsia* **33**,1115–1122.

Austin, J.K., Huberty, T.J. (1993) Development of the Child Attitude Toward Illness scale. *Journal of Paediatric Psychology* **18**, 467–480.

Austin, J.K., Smith, M.S., Risinger, M.W., McNelis, A.M. (1994) Childhood epilepsy and asthma: comparison of quality of life. *Epilepsia* **35**, 608–615.

Austin, J.K., Huster, G.A., Dunn, D.W., Risinger, M.W. (1996) Adolescents with active or inactive epilepsy or asthma: a comparison of quality of life. *Epilepsia* **37**, 1228–1238.

Austin, J.K., Huberty, T.J., Huster, G.A., Dunn, D.W. (1998) Academic achievement in children with epilepsy or asthma. *Developmental Medicine* and *Child Neurology* **40**, 248–255.

Bourgeois, B.F.D. (1998) Antiepileptic drugs, learning, and behaviour in childhood epilepsy. *Epilepsia* **39**, 913–921.

Brent, D.A., Crumine, P.K., Varma, R.R., Allan, M., Allman, C. (1987) Phenobarbital treatment and major depressive disorder in children with epilepsy. *Paediatrics* **80**, 909–917.

Camfield, C., Camfield, P., Smith, B., Gordon, K., Dooley, J. (1993) Biologic factors as predictors of social outcome of epilepsy in intellectually normal children: a population-based study. *Journal of Paediatrics* **122**, 869–873.

Caplan, R., Arbelle, S., Guthrie, D., Komo, S., Shields, W.D., Hansen, R., Chayasirisobhon, S. (1997) Formal thought disorder and psychopathology in pediatric primary generalised and complex partial epilepsy. *Journal of the American Academy of Child* and *Adolescent Psychiatry* **36**, 1286–1294.

Caplan, R., Gillberg, C. (1997) Child psychiatric disorders. In: Engel, J. Jr., Pedley, T.A. (eds.) *Epilepsy: A Comprehensive Textbook*. Philadelphia: Lippincott-Raven Publishers, 2125–2140.

DeVellis, R.F., DeVellis, B.M. (1986) An evolving psychosocial model of epilepsy. In: Whitman, S., Hermann, B.P. (eds.) *Psychopathology in Epilepsy: Social Dimensions,* New York: Oxford University Press, 122–142.

Dunn, D.W., Austin, J.K., Huster, G.A. (1997) Behavioural problems in children with new-onset epilepsy. *Seizure* **6**, 283–287

Dunn, D.W., Austin, J.K., Huster, G.A. (1999) Symptoms of depression in adolescents with epilepsy. *Journal of the American Academy of Child and Adolescent Psychiatry* **38**, 1132–1138.

Ettinger, A.B., Weisbrot, D.M., Nolan, E.E., Gadow, K.D., Vitale, S.A., Andriola, M.R., Lenn, N.T., Novak, G.P., Hermann, B.P. (1998) Symptoms of depression and anxiety in paediatric epilepsy patients. *Epilepsia* **39**, 595–599.

Farwell, J.R., Lee, Y.J., Hirtz, D.G., Sulzbacher, S.I., Ellenberg, J.H., Nelson, K.B. (1990) Phenobarbital for febrile seizures: effects on intelligence and seizure recurrence. *New England Journal of Medicine* **322**, 364–369.

Freeman, J.M., Jacobs, H., Vining, E., Rabin, C.E. (1984) Epilepsy and the inner city schools: a school-based program that makes a difference. *Epilepsia* **25**, 438–442.

Green, J.B., Hartlage, L.C. (1971) Comparative performance of epileptic and nonepileptic children and adolescents. *Diseases of the Nervous System* **32**, 418–421.

Hartlage, L.C., Green, J.B. (1972) The relation of parental attitudes to academic and social achievement in epileptic children. *Epilepsia* **13**, 21–26.

Hauser, W.A. (1994) The prevalence and incidence of convulsive disorders in children. *Epilepsia* **35**, S1-S6.

Hauser, W.A., Hesdorffer, D.C. (1990) *Epilepsy: Frequency, Causes* and *Consequences*, Maryland: Epilepsy Foundation of America.

Hermann, B.P., Whitman, S. (1986) Psychopathology in epilepsy: A multietiologic model. In: Hermann, B.P., Whitman, S. (eds.) *Psychopathology in epilepsy: Social Dimensions.* New York: Oxford University Press, 5–37.

Hermann, B.P., Whitman, S., Dell, J. (1989) Correlates of behavioural problems and social competence in children with epilepsy, aged 6–11. In: Hermann, B., Seidenberg, M. (eds.)*Childhood Epilepsies: Neuropsychological, Psychosocial* and *Intervention Aspects,* Chichester: John Wiley and Sons Ltd, 143–158.

Hoare, P. (1984) The development of psychiatric disorder among school children with epilepsy. *Developmental Medicine* and *Child Neurology* **26**, 3–13.

Hoare, P., Kerley, S. (1991) Psychosocial adjustment of children with chronic epilepsy and their families. *Developmental Medicine* and *Child Neurology* **33**, 210–215.

Hoare, P. (1993) The quality of life of children with chronic epilepsy and their families. *Seizure* **2**, 269–275.

Hoare, P., Mann, H. (1994) Self-esteem and behavioural adjustment in children with epilepsy and children with diabetes. *Journal of Psychosomatic Research* **38**, 859–869.

Holdsworth, L., Whitmore K. (1974) A study of children with epilepsy attending ordinary schools. *Developmental Medicine* and *Child Neurology* **16**, 746–758.

Huberty, T.J., Austin, J.K., Risinger, M.W., McNelis, A.M. (1992) Relationship of selected seizure variables in children with epilepsy to performance on school-administered achievement tests. *Journal of Epilepsy* **5**, 10–16.

Kovacs, M. (1980/81) Rating scale to assess depression in school-aged children. *Acta Paedopsychiatrica* **46**, 305–315.

Lewis, M.A., Salas, I., de la Sota, A., Chiofalo, N., Leal-Sotelo, M. (1990) A randomized trial of a program to enhance the competencies of children with epilepsy. *Epilepsia* **20**, 299–312.

Lewis, M.A., Hatton, C.L., Salas, I., Leak, B., Chiofalo, N. (1991) Impact of the children's epilepsy program on parents. *Epilepsia* **32**, 365–374.

Lothman, D.J., Pianta, R.C., Clarson, S.M. (1990) Mother-child interaction in children with epilepsy: Relations with child competence. *Journal of Epilepsy* **3**, 157–163.

Matthews, W.S., Barabas, G., Ferrari, M. (1982) Emotional concomitants of childhood epilepsy. *Epilepsia* **23**, 671–681.

Matthews, W.S., Barabas, G., Ferrari, M. (1983) Achievement and school behaviour among children with epilepsy. *Psychology in the Schools* **20**, 10–12.

Matthews, W.S., Barabas, G. (1986) Perceptions of control among children with epilepsy. In: Whitman, S., Hermann, B.P. (eds.) *Psychopathology in Epilepsy: Social Dimensions.* New York: Oxford University Press, 162–182.

McConnell, H., Duncan, D. (1998) Treatment of psychiatric comorbidity in epilepsy. In: McConnell, H.W., Snyder, P.J. (eds.*) Psychiatric Comorbidity in Epilepsy.* American Psychiatric Press Inc, 245–361

McDermott, S., Mani, S., Krishnaswami, S. (1995) A population-based analysis of specific behavioural problems associated with childhood seizures. *Journal of Epilepsy* **8**, 110–118.

McNelis, A., Musick, B., Austin, J., Dunn, D., Creasy, K. (1998) Psychosocial care needs of children with new-onset seizures. *Journal of Neuroscience Nursing* **30**, 161–165.

Milrod, L.M., Urion, D.K. (1992) Juvenile fire setting and the photoparoxysmal response. *Annals of Neurology* **32**, 222–223.

Mitchell, W.G., Chavez, J.M., Lee, H., Guzman, B.L. (1991) Academic underachievement in children with epilepsy. *Journal of Child Neurology* **6**, 65–72.

Mitchell, W.G., Zhou, Y., Chavez, J.M., Guzman, B.L. (1992) Reaction time, attention, and impulsivity in epilepsy. *Paediatric Neurology* **8**, 19–24.

Mitchell, W.G., Scheier, L.M., Baker, S.A. (1994) Psychosocial, behavioural, and medical outcomes in children with epilepsy: A developmental risk factor model using longitudinal data. *Paediatrics* **94**, 471–477.

Mulder, H.C., Suurmeijer, T.P.B.M. (1977) Families with a child with epilepsy: A sociological contribution. *Journal of Biosocial Science* **9**, 13–24.

Nass, R., Gross, A., Devinsky, O. (1998) Autism and autistic epileptiform regression with occipital spikes. *Developmental Medicine* and *Child Neurology* **40**, 453–458.

Oosterhuis, A. (1994) A psycho-educational approach to epilepsy. *Seizure* 3, 23–24.

Rutter, M., Graham, P., Yule, W. (1970) *A Neuropsychiatric Study in Childhood*, Lippincott Publishers.

Sachdev, P. (1998) Schizophrenia-like psychosis and epilepsy: the status of the association. *American Journal of Psychiatry* **155**, 325–336.

Seidenberg, M., Beck, N., Geisser, M., Giordani, B., Sackellares, J.C., Berrent, S., Dreifuss, F.E., Boll, T.J. (1986) Academic achievement of children with epilepsy. *Epilepsia* **27**, 753–759.

Shore, C., Austin, J., Musick, B., Dunn, D., McBride, A., Creasy, K. (1998) Psychosocial care needs of parents of children with new-onset seizures. *Journal of Neuroscience Nursing* **30**, 169–174.

Sillanpaa, M., Jalava, M., Kaleva, O., Shinnar, S. (1998) Long-term prognosis of seizures with onset in childhood. *New England Journal of Medicine* **338**, 1715–1722.

Steffenburg, S., Gillberg, C., Steffenburg, U. (1996) Psychiatric disorders in children and adolescents with mental retardation and active epilepsy. *Archives of Neurology* **53**, 904–912.

Stores, G., Hart, J. (1976) Reading skills of children with generalised or focal epilepsy attending ordinary schools. *Developmental Medicine* and *Child Neurology* **18**, 705–716.

Trimble, M.R. (1991)*The Psychoses of Epilepsy*, New York: Raven Press.

Tuchman, R.F., Rapin, I. (1997) Regression in pervasive developmental disorders: seizures and epileptiform electroencephalogram correlates. *Paediatrics* **99**, 560–566.

West, P. (1986) The social meaning of epilepsy: stigma as a potential explanation for psychopathology in children. In: Whitman, S., Hermann, B.P. (eds.) *Psychopathology in Epilepsy: Social Dimensions.* New York: Oxford University Press, 245–268.

Wildrick, D., Parker-Fisher, S., Morales, A. (1996) Quality of life in children with well-controlled epilepsy. *Journal of Neuroscience Nursing* **28**, 192–198.

Williams, D.T., Gold, A.P., Shrout, P., Shaffer, D., Adams, D. (1979) The impact of psychiatric intervention on patients with uncontrolled seizures. *Journal of Nervous* and *Mental Diseases* **167**, 626–631.

Williams, J., Bates, S., Griebel, M.L., Lange, B., Mancias, P., Pihoker, C.M., Dykman, R. (1998) Does short-term antiepileptic drug treatment in children result in cognitive or behavioural change. *Epilepsia* **39**, 1064–1069.

Chapter 8

QUALITY OF LIFE ISSUES FOR OLDER PEOPLE WITH EPILEPSY

Raymond Tallis

With the falling incidence and prevalence of seizures in children and younger adults, older adults with epilepsy and epileptic fits are emerging as probably the single most important group of people with seizures. It is therefore to be regretted that they are also the least researched. There are several reasons for this: the frequency of seizures occurring for the first time in old age is still underestimated by many practitioners (Craig and Tallis, 1991); it is tempting to believe that information obtained more easily in a younger population can be extrapolated to older people with seizures; and, least acceptably of all, it is often assumed that seizures are less important in older people than in younger people.

EPIDEMIOLOGY

Issues relating to quality of life in older people with seizures justify investigation, if only on account of the very large numbers of older people who have this problem. Hauser and Kurland (1975) reported a rise in the prevalence of epilepsy above the age of 50 and an even steeper rise in incidence — from 12/100,000 in the 40–59 year age group to 82/100,000 in those over 60. The same authors confirmed this rise in more recent studies (Hauser *et al.*, 1991; Hauser *et al.*, 1993).

These findings have also been confirmed by studies based in primary care. The United Kingdom National General Practice Study of Epilepsy and Epileptic Seizures, a prospective community-based study, found that 24% of new cases of definite epilepsy were in subjects over the age of 60 (Sander *et al.*, 1990). A study of a primary care database covering 82 practices and nearly 370,000 subjects, 62,000 of whom were over the age of 60, revealed a continuing rise in the incidence of seizures in old age (Tallis *et al.*, 1991): the incidence for the overall population was 69/100,000 but in the 65–69 age group it was 87, in the 70–79 group it was 147 and in the 80–89 group it was 159/100,000. Over a third of all incident cases placed on antiepileptics (AEDs) were over the age of 60. Analysis of a greatly expanded primary care database of over 2 million subjects has generated very similar findings (Wallace *et al.*, 1998).

It may be confidently anticipated that there will be an increase in the numbers of older people with seizures in the next few decades both in absolute numbers and as a proportion of the overall population of people who have seizures. The sharpest rise in the elderly population will be in the old elderly, especially those over 80, and these carry the highest incidence of epilepsy and epileptic fits. This is not surprising as most elderly onset recurrent seizures are due to cerebrovascular disease which has an exponential relation to age. Moreover, with an increasing number of individuals surviving acute strokes due to better acute care and rehabilitation (Langhorne *et al.*, 1993), we may expect more people to have seizures on the basis of cerebrovascular disease.

It may be argued that numbers alone do not justify studying elderly patients separately. However, there are ways in which one might expect seizures to be different in old age as compared with the general adult population, that are relevant to the issue of quality of life. These differences make it inappropriate to try to extrapolate findings in younger individuals to older adults and justify the independent study of quality of life in old age. The underlying causes will be different, with, as already noted, cerebrovascular disease heading the list. Seizures will more often be secondary to systemic disease than in younger adults. Seizures may also present differently. The lack of eye witnesses in individuals living alone makes diagnosis more difficult, as does the problem of differentiating seizures from the many other causes of 'funny turns' in older people. The chances of over or under diagnosis of seizures would be correspondingly higher and the element of uncertainty will have an impact on the patient's perception of the significance of the events. Epidemiological evidence suggests that the likelihood of recurrence after a single seizure is higher in older people (Sander *et al.*, 1990). There is a clinical impression that the control of seizures seems somewhat easier in older people and this is supported by some of the data from Veteran Administration studies (Ramsey and Rowan, 1994) where more elderly patients achieved good control on lower doses and blood levels of AEDs. Against this is the increased possibility of drug interactions with both pharmacokinetic and pharmacodynamic consequences and also the risk of co-prescription of pro-convulsant drugs.

Other important differences arise from the fact that patients will have different life circumstances (often living alone and being relatively poorly off), have different ideas about the condition, different informational needs, and may have their independence severely affected by the fits in a way less often seen in younger patients.

QUALITY OF LIFE ISSUES

In many ways, epilepsy may be seen as analogous to another major problem in old age, one that has been much more widely researched: falls, dubbed one of the 'giants of geriatric medicine'. Like epileptic fits, falls are episodic events which may have continuing and sometimes permanent consequences. Major fits may be thought of as 'falls plus' — the 'plus' being the added factor of loss or disturbance of consciousness and all that results from that.

One way of thinking about quality of life of elderly people with seizures is to divide the impact into immediate and less immediate effects (see Table 1; Tallis, 1993). First and foremost there is the actual experience of the seizure. Apart from the discomfort and embarrassment of coming round to discover that one is incontinent, dishevelled and, perhaps, surrounded by shocked and anxious friends or strangers, there is the added unpleasantness of an often prolonged confusional state. This may be compounded by the trauma of being brought to hospital (which may or may not be appropriate) and the even greater trauma of being admitted to a hospital ward — an experience that no elderly person should be invited to undergo lightly. Possibly because seizures often occur against a background of cerebrovascular disease, post-ictal states may be prolonged in elderly patients. Although this has not been studied systematically, there are some indications from some series that this is the case. Fourteen per cent of subjects in one series suffered a confusional state lasting 24 hours or more and in some cases it persisted as long as a week (Godfrey *et al.*, 1982).

Todd's phenomena are also more common, in particular post-ictal hemiparesis. This may lead to the misdiagnosis of stroke (Norris and

TABLE 1 IMPACT OF SEIZURES

IMMEDIATE	LESS IMMEDIATE (INCLUDES THE IMPACT OF DIAGNOSIS)
EXPERIENCE OF THE SEIZURE	LOSS OF CONFIDENCE
POST-ICTAL CONFUSION	FEAR OF DEATH
TODD'S PHENOMENA	FEAR OF FURTHER FITS
INJURY	FEAR OF INJURY LOSS OF SELF ESTEEM LOSS OF FUNCTIONAL INDEPENDENCE ALTERED RELATIONSHIPS WITH OTHERS/CARERS ANXIETIES OF OTHERS/CARERS IMPACT OF ANTICONVULSANT THERAPY

FROM TALLIS, 1993.

Hachinski, 1982) and this is also likely to happen where fits occur against a background of known cerebrovascular disease and a recurrent stroke may be incorrectly diagnosed (Fine, 1967).

It is important to look beyond the immediate effects of the fit to the wider and more permanent consequences. The debilitating spiral in patients who have sustained a fall in which loss of confidence leads to limitations on mobility, the restriction of total activities and loss of independence is well-described (Vellas, *et al.,* 1987). Older people who fall have reduced activity, walk less even indoors and find it difficult to move outdoors. Fear of falling is also part of the 'post-fall syndrome' (Murphy and Isaacs, 1982). Individuals develop a tendency to clutch and grab and are unable to walk unsupported due to the anxiety of falling.

Syncope is closer to epilepsy than is a simple fall. However, the psychosocial impact of syncope has not been widely studied (Linzer *et al.*, 1991). What data there are highlight the problems of functional disability affecting employment (39%), driving (64%) and interpersonal relationships in recurrent syncope compared to that seen in emphysema, diabetes and arthritis. Some have even advocated that syncope should be classified as a 'new chronic disease' (Linzer *et al.*, 1991). However, there are no studies of quality of life specifically in older patients

Studies of falls have repeatedly confirmed how a fall may mark a watershed in an older persons' life, after which there is a sharp decline in functional independence. In some instances, this decline will be due to the disease underlying the fall; but in many ways it will be due to loss of confidence. The 3-Fs, (Fear of Further Falls, noted above) that may cause an elderly person to become semi-electively housebound must surely have its analogue in Fear of Further Fits. The experience of a fit may also awaken fear of mortality. This may be greater in elderly people, not only because they may have known of a contemporary who has died after a 'funny turn', perhaps of cardiac origin, but also because they may have memories of their childhood when epilepsy was stigmatised, poorly controlled and its effects often exacerbated by the adverse effects of toxic but useless drugs.

The impact of seizures might also be anticipated to include the effect on the attitude of others, including friends, relatives and carers, to the patient. The tendency to marginalise elderly people may rationalise itself into a desire to protect them from danger. Certainly a fit may trigger anxiety in others, and result in exclusion from normal activity and decision-making processes, less grandparental involvement in child-rearing ('Don't let Grandma hold the baby in case she has a fit and drops it') and more susceptibility to interference in their affairs by others. Although the diagnosis of seizures will not have the effects on employment and education it may have in a younger person, the impact on inter-personal relations may be no less important. Elderly people may be more dependent on motorised transport for mobility. If the individual who has the fit is the only licence holder, a ban on driving may mean that two people are housebound.

There will also be the effect of AEDs. There are reasons for anticipating that this may be more marked in older people. If you are near the threshold of failure of a function, then a minor adverse effect may translate into loss of that function. It might be anticipated that this would particularly apply to adverse neuro-psychiatric effects, but recent studies have not confirmed this (Meador *et al.,* 1990; Craig and Tallis, 1994). Indeed, our own studies did not show a significant adverse effect on cognitive function of either sodium valproate or phenytoin. However, other adverse effects, both neuro psychiatric and non-neuropsychiatric, may be more important in older people. Phenytoin-induced osteomalacia will be more likely in an elderly patient with a diet deficient in vitamin D and a life deficient in sunshine (Harrington and Hodkinson 1987). The impact of subjective feelings of unsteadiness in someone who has already lost confidence may be anticipated to lead towards a vicious spiral of functional and social decline. This will be more likely to happen in a patient who, through concurrent disease and co-prescribed medication may already be nearer to the threshold of failure.

QUALITY OF LIFE IN OLDER PEOPLE WITH SEIZURES: WHAT DO WE KNOW?

Given that there is a case for investigation of the impact of seizures on quality of life for older people, it is to be regretted that so little research has been done in this area and remarkably little is known about how seizures impact on older people. Much of what has been said so far in this chapter is speculative. Speculation is vulnerable to refutation and it is therefore salutary that the one detailed study in the literature does not wholly support the assumptions set out above (Baker *et al.,* 2000).

As part of a large prevalence study of epilepsy conducted in one UK Health Region, the burden of epilepsy in older people was compared with that in younger people. There were few differences between older and younger people with regard to their reported quality of life, although younger people were more likely to report to feeling stigmatised by their condition. Older people with epilepsy diagnosed in later life were more anxious and depressed than those diagnosed earlier and their overall perception of quality of life was more likely to be negative. The authors conclude that the data demonstrate that older people do not necessarily experience poorer quality of life than younger people, but those diagnosed for the first time in later life do appear to have a quality of life which is more impaired.

These data must, however, be regarded as preliminary as there were only a small number of subjects with seizures occurring for the first time in later life (35) and the median age of onset was comparatively young (65 years). Significant age effects may not be expected to be seen before the age of 75. More extensive studies looking at larger numbers of older patients in their 70's and 80's urgently need to be done

SPECIAL PROBLEMS OF QUALITY OF LIFE MEASURES IN OLDER PEOPLE

From what has been said so far, it is clear that quality of life issues in older people are likely to be important and have been seriously under researched. Some of the reasons for this lack of research have already been set out. However, perhaps the most important reason is the complexity of the medical and social problems of many old, and especially very old, people. Although evaluating the impact of a medical condition on quality of life is of interest in itself, most quality of life measures are introduced in the hope that they may enable clinicians to determine the impact of medical treatment and other aspects of management in terms that are relevant to the patient's life. This is a preliminary to comparing the benefits obtained from different drugs or management strategies. The assumption is that quality of life measures enable us to evaluate quality of care for medical problems. There are potential difficulties with this assumption in older people who may have a multiplicity of medical and social problems and rapidly changing social circumstances.

The assumptions behind the widespread use of quality of life measures in evaluating clinical practice are: that quality of life is a sensitive measure of health; and that changes in quality of life may be related to health interventions and the quality of those interventions. Quality of life measures tend to be global and it has been argued elsewhere (Tallis, 1991; Tallis, 1992) that global outcome measures (especially when applied to global packages of care) have held back progress in certain areas of medicine. This is particularly evident in the area of rehabilitation which has been illuminated to only a moderate degree by the tendency to use 'higher level' outcome measures. What matters, in rehabilitation, we are told, is not how rehabilitation improves, say, the strength of the patient, but how the impact of the treatment translates into functional gain and, more importantly, how this translates into a reduction of handicap (nowadays called 'participation') and ultimately quality of life.

Of course the measure of the effectiveness of our treatments should ultimately be understood in terms of what we do for patient happiness. Patients are quite rightly uninterested in whether or not we normalise those kinds of things that doctors traditionally observe or measure — for example, serum potassium. However, this is likely to be less true of conditions such as frequency of fits in which patient and doctor concur in acknowledging their importance. Moreover when we move from the level at which we think we are having our effect (for example, reducing fit frequency by using AEDs), the chain of causation linking our intervention to observed changes becomes more frail and the 'signal to noise ratio' falls off quite rapidly. A wide variety of other factors are brought into play: fluctuating co-morbid illness, other medical and social interventions, other life events and so on. That is why higher level quality of life scales may be less effective in determining the effects of a package of care or even of one element of such a package, such as drug treatment. It is possible therefore that higher level quality of life scales may not give us as much information about the effectiveness of our rather specific interventions as we might hope. Holistic care is good of course, but medical science should not fall victim to the rhetoric of holism.

Our legitimate interest in the quality of our patients' lives is rooted in our wish to understand the real influence of our treatment upon them. Except in a gross and obvious sense (where medicine is spectacularly successful or disastrously unsuccessful) it is very difficult to determine this. Quality of life is but a distant reflection of quality of care and is consequently a very poor lens through which to view our care. Where we have very positive or dismally negative effects on our patients' lives, we do not need an instrument to measure it. The question is: should we be developing more refined instruments to pick up smaller changes in quality of life in elderly patients with seizures in the hope that with sufficient numbers of patients we can relate this to some element or variable in our treatment? The forgoing discussion has indicated that the answer to this question is by no means clear.

CONCLUSION

The importance of seizures in older people is now well-established and there is a need to research more intensively into the problems of this increasingly important group of patients. At present there is remarkably little research into quality of life issues in older people. If we are to identify and deal with the concerns and difficulties experienced by older people with seizures we certainly need to look beyond the seizure count. This is concordant with the holistic wisdom that is conventional in geriatric medicine. When it comes, however, to assessing the impact of our specific treatments, and comparing one treatment with another, we must recognise the limitations of 'higher level' outcome measures in individuals who may have considerable co-morbidity and other medical and non-medical problems. A deeper understanding of the impact of seizures on quality of life and of the differential impact of different treatment strategies is required but it is important to define the contribution they may make to improving our approach to care. The very things that make older people with seizures different from young people with seizures may themselves make the role of quality of life measures in evaluating management more difficult to determine.

References

Baker, G.A., Jacoby, A., Buck, D., Brooks, J., Jones, L.A., Potts, P., Chadwick, D.W. (2000) The quality of life of older people with epilepsy: findings from a UK community study. (in submission).

Craig, I., Tallis, R.C. (1991) General practitioner knowledge and management of elderly onset epilepsy. *Care of the Elderly* 3(2), 69–72.

Craig, I., Tallis, R.C. (1994) Impact of valproate and phenytoin on cognitive function in elderly patients: results of a single-blind randomised comparative study. Epilepsia 35(2), 381–390.

Fine, W. (1967) Posthemiplegic epilepsy in the elderly. *British Medical Journal* i, 199–201.

Godfrey, J.W., Roberts, M.A., Caird, F.I. (1982) Epileptic seizures in the elderly: diagnostic problems. *Age and Ageing* **11**, 29–34.

Harrington, M., Hodkinson, H. (1987) Anticonvulsants and bone disease in the elderly. *Journal of the Royal Society of Medicine* 80, 425–427.

Hauser, W.A., Kurland, L.T. (1975) The epidemiology of epilepsy in Rochester, Minnesota: 1935 to 1967. *Epilepsia* **16**, 1–66.

Hauser, W.A., Annegers, J.S., Kurland, L.T. (1991) Prevalence of epilepsy in Rochester, Minnesota: 1940–1980. *Epilepsia* **32**, 429–445.

Hauser, W.A., Annegers, J.S., Kurland, L.T. (1993) Incidence of epilepsy and unprovoked seizures in Rochester, Minnesota: 1935–1984. *Epilepsia* **34**, 453–468.

Langhorne, P., Williams, B.O., Gilchrist, W., Howie, K. (1993) Do stroke units save lives? *Lancet* **342**, 395–398

Linzer, M., Pontinen, M., Gold, D.T., Divine, G.W., Felder, A., Brooks, W.B. (1991) Impairment of physical and psychosocial function in recurrent syncope. *Journal of Clinical Epidemiology* **44**, (10) 1037–1043.

Meador, K.M., Loring, D,W., Huh, K., Gallagher, B.B., King, D.W. (1990) Comparative cognitive effects of anticonvulsants. *Neurology* **40**, 391–394.

Murphy, J., and Isaacs, B. (1982) The post-falls syndrome: a study of 38 elderly patients. *Gerontology* **28**, 265–270.

Norris, J, W., Hachinski, V,C. (1982) Mis-diagnosis of stroke. *Lancet* **i**, 328–331.

Ramsay, R.E., Rowan, A.J., Salter, J.D., Collins, J., Nemire, R., Ortiz, W.R., and the VA Coop Study Group. Effect of age in epilepsy and its treatment: results from the VA Cooperative Study Epilepsia 35(Suppl 8), 91.

Sander, J.W.A.S., Hart, Y.M., Johnson, A.L., Shorvon, S.D. (1990) National General Practice Study of Epilepsy: Newly diagnosed epileptic seizures in the general population. *Lancet* **336**, 1267–1270.

Tallis, R.C. (1991) Assessing the outcome of rehabilitation In: Royal College of Physicians *Horizons in Medicine 3*, Royal College of Physicians: Transmedica Publications, 128–138.

Tallis, R.C. (1992) Rehabilitation of the elderly in the 21st century. *Journal of the Royal College of Physicians, London* 26(4), 413–422.

Tallis, R.C. (1993) Through a glass darkly: Measuring quality of care through quality of life in elderly patients with epilepsy. *Round Table Proceedings*, Oslo: RSM Publications, 79–96.

Tallis, R.C., Hal, l.G., Craig, I., Dean, A. (1991) How common are epileptic seizures in old age? *Age and Ageing* **20**, 442–448.

Vellas, B., Cayla, F., Bocquet, H., De-Pemille, F., Albarede, J.L. (1987) Prospective study of restriction of activity in old people after falls. *Age and Ageing* **16** (3), 189–193.

Wallace, H., Shorvon, S., Tallis, R.C. (1998) Age-specific incidence and prevalence rate of treated epilepsy in an unselected population of 2,052,922 and the age-specific fertility rates of women with epilepsy. *Lancet* **352**, 1970–1973.

Chapter 9

EPILEPSY AND LEARNING DISABILITY: IMPLICATIONS FOR QUALITY OF LIFE

Colin A. Espie and Mike Kerr

Epilepsy has wide-ranging effects, both on the lives of people with learning disabilities and on their carers. The particularly high prevalence of epilepsy in this population stresses the importance of the condition. As in the general population, the impact of epilepsy, and thus the aims of treatment, goes beyond the immediate effect of seizures. In fact, epilepsy influences many of the areas of functioning regarded as central to the quality of life of people with learning disabilities (Blunden, 1988), namely, physical health through seizures, premature death, accidents and unwanted effects of treatment; material well being through reduced employment opportunities and choice; social well-being through reduced community integration and resettlement from hospital (Bond *et al.*, 1991); and emotional well being through social stigma, behavioural effects of medication and the complex association of epilepsy with behavioural disorder.

It is this complexity of outcome that can leave clinicians and others struggling to assess their own roles and effectiveness. Furthermore, this struggle is often heightened by the inherent communication difficulties of people with learning disabilities. We will discuss here a structure for how quality of life in people with learning disability who have epilepsy may be assessed in clinical practice, and the theoretical underpinning of this assessment. It will be clear, we hope, that through the effective management of epilepsy in this population, substantial health gain may be possible for the individual, his or her family and for others involved in caring.

EPILEPSY AS A CO-MORBIDITY IN PEOPLE WITH LEARNING DISABILITY

Epidemiological data on epilepsy in people with learning disabilities are greatly influenced by both the source and level of ability of the sample population. These two factors are often, and perhaps rightly, felt to be connected, as the least able may be more likely to find themselves in a more institutional care setting.

This is well illustrated by a survey in an institution for people with learning disabilities which yielded a prevalence of epilepsy of 32%

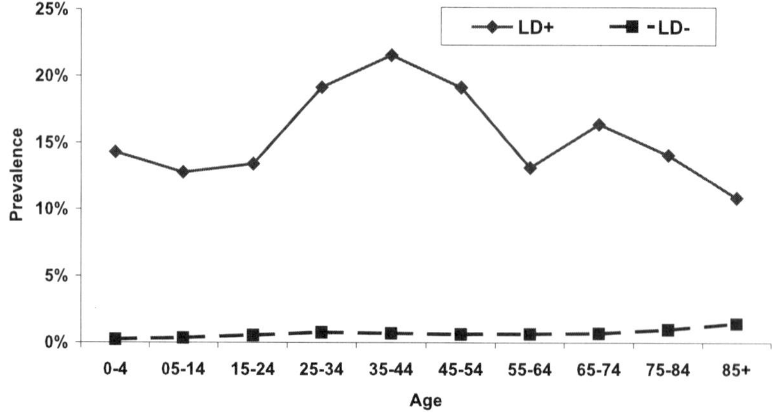

FIGURE 1 PREVALENCE OF EPILEPSY FOR POPULATIONS WITH AND WITHOUT LEARNING DISABILITY

(Mariani *et al.*, 1993), while a large community-based questionnaire survey of health needs yielded one of 22% (Welsh Office, 1996). These data can be compared with an estimate of the prevalence of epilepsy in the general population of between 0.4 and 1% (Chadwick, 1994). This large differential in risk is illustrated in Figure 1, which shows the relative prevalence of epilepsy in a population of people in the United Kingdom identified through health service contact data (Morgan CL, *personal communication*).

Figures enabling us to separate out the differential effects of declining IQ in the context of physical disability are available from surveys in populations of people with cerebral palsy: here there is an undoubted increase in likelihood of seizure disorder with decreasing IQ (Sussova *et al.*, 1990).

SPECIAL ISSUES — COMMUNICATION, BEHAVIOUR AND CARER SUPPORT

The assessment and management of epilepsy in people with learning disabilities is shaped to a large extent by other difficulties commonly presenting in this population. The three areas that most affect the clinician are: concomitant communication disorder, behavioural disturbance and carer support needs.

Communication

Clinicians typically rely on patient self-report at clinic appointments. Information on the nature of the seizures themselves, their frequency and patterning, and their impact and intrusiveness upon daily living is gathered verbally, often supported by written or charted records which the patient keeps up to date. The clinician is able to ask about aura experiences, level of consciousness, post-ictal recovery, inter-ictal states and perceived effectiveness, as well as side effects of medication. However, in working clinically with people with learning disabilities such interview information may be very limited. Both receptive understanding and expressive speech are likely to be impaired, increasingly so in relation to level of intellectual disability. Similarly, thought processes tend to be concrete rather than abstract, so even the person with mild learning disability may experience difficulty with concepts such as time, improvement or deterioration and compliance. We have been surprised to find how relatively little people with mild learning disability knew or understood about their epilepsy, although pleased that a structured programme of training could lead to increased knowledge (Clark *et al.*, 2000).

Much reliance has to be placed, therefore, upon reports from family and staff carers. Clearly, there are advantages to speaking with people who have been eyewitnesses of seizures, especially if they have known the individual for some time and can differentiate typical and atypical behaviours. Also, carers can usually report on overt seizure frequency. However, it is inevitable that important data are unavailable to the clinician, for example, about subjective well-being, cognitive effects and the emotional consequences of seizures. Inferences and attributions made by carers have to be carefully considered for two principal reasons. First, concerns expressed by family may be different from those of staff, either in nature or in magnitude. We have recent data indicating that family concerns about epilepsy are consistently one standard deviation above the mean for staff carers (Espie *et al.*, 1999a). Second, clinical experience suggests that people with learning disabilities are often accompanied to clinics by different people at each visit, making consistency and continuity in information and in healthcare problematic.

Behaviour

The diagnosis of epilepsy is in most cases made clinically, that is, underlying neurological and electrophysiological abnormality is inferred from behaviour. The accurate interpretation of behaviour, is therefore, fundamental. The International League Against Epilepsy (ILAE) classification (ILAE Commission, 1989) provides behavioural descriptors for each of the principal seizure types, but it should be borne in mind that the person with learning disability may present a less than textbook picture. Seizures may be affected by other background neurological abnormalities and their expression influenced by, for example, poor motor function and impoverished general arousal (Espie *et al.*, 1999b). Partial seizures may be difficult to differentiate from 'normal behaviour', and particularly from the wide range of stereotypies exhibited in this population (Paul, 1997). Absence seizures may be missed altogether or greatly underestimated, particularly in severely disabled, relatively passive populations.

Behaviours associated with possible triggering situations or emotions, and reported post-ictal phenomena are best evaluated as part of a functional analysis to determine their specific association with seizure activity (Iwata *et al.*, 1990; Espie and Paul, 1997). It is not uncommon for complex partial seizures and post-ictal confusion to be misinterpreted as 'purely behavioural' (e.g. 'acting out') and, conversely, for challenging behaviour to be attributed to epilepsy. Although it has been thought that epilepsy, particularly with temporal lobe focus, can result in displays of emotionality and aggression, this is by no means inevitable and such behaviour may have other root causes such as overstimulation or boredom.

Non-epileptic seizures (NES) represent a particular assessment challenge, particularly as it has been suggested that these present more frequently in people with learning disabilities than in other populations. Many people with NES also have epilepsy, thus raising the possibility of learned, maladaptive behaviour (Betts and Boden, 1992, Rowan and Gates, 1999). Contextual information is important in this differential diagnosis — when, how and where seizures present, and whether or not there is any other evidence of illness behaviour.

The complexity of appraisal here emphasises the range of skills required, such as may be found in a multidisciplinary team where there is neuropsychiatry, clinical psychology and epilepsy nurse specialist expertise.

Carer support

The anxiety and distress commonly associated with epilepsy may be experienced more acutely by carers than by people with learning disabilities. This can be a major factor and should be recognised as an integral part of assessment and management. Lifelong emotional bonds are not easily set aside and many family carers have had powerful conditioning experiences associated with life-threatening events, hospital admissions and refractory seizures. Similarly, staff in day centres and residential houses can be relatively inexperienced in dealing with epilepsy. Operational policies about the individual's care such as the administration of rectal diazepam, albeit necessary, can raise alarm. The inherent unpredictability of most seizures means that in many instances people are not specifically geared to cope with an event.

Epilepsy may be the principal health concern about an individual. However, the high prevalence of a wide range of other health problems (Espie and Brown, 1998) also contributes to carer strain. Furthermore, at various stages in the person's life, care arrangements will be altered for example by a move from family care to supported living, leaving school or as a result of new respite arrangements. These can be particularly stressful times for all those involved in the caring process and, of course, can lead to the person with epilepsy being more unsettled.

QUALITY OF LIFE

The concept of quality of life in people with a learning disability

It is perhaps no surprise that a concept which remains to some degree elusive in the field of epilepsy has proved to be equally so in the heterogeneous field of learning disability (Felce and Perry, 1995). It is worth considering the key components of a good quality of life before examining the impact research has had on investigating this. The work of O'Brien (1987) has been heavily influential, defining five 'accomplishments' which can be said to reflect the individual's quality of life (Table 1). Recognition of the importance of the 'accomplishments' model has influenced both researchers of quality of life and developers of services. However, the themes have been difficult to measure within research settings. Felce and Perry (1997) reviewed the literature on quality of life research and considered that five key domains could be subsumed under the quality of life mantle (Table 1). We reflected earlier in the chapter on how epilepsy and its management could so readily impact on any, or all, of these domains in any given individual.

Quality of life measures have been employed in evaluation, often when considering changes in service provision such as in the move away from institutional care. The evaluation measures have mirrored the domains above, though assessment of the concept of physical well-being has lagged behind. Much of the work has focused on social well-being through measurement of interaction with others, as in direct observation (Felce, 1988), or through assessing involvement in the community.

TABLE 1 QoL CONCEPTS FOR PEOPLE WITH LEARNING DISABILITIES

ACCOMPLISHMENTS	KEY QoL DOMAINS
• PRESENCE IN THE COMMUNITY	• PHYSICAL WELL-BEING
• COMPETENCE	• MATERIAL WELL-BEING
• CHOICE/DIGNITY	• SOCIAL WELL-BEING
• RESPECT	• EMOTIONAL WELL-BEING
• INVOLVEMENT	• PRODUCTIVE WELL-BEING

A constant challenge in the disability field is the balance between objective and subjective approaches to quality of life. This is particularly true when dealing with those with more profound disability and a consequent reduced ability to communicate. Goode (1997) has pointed out the difficulties of subjectivity in this group, and how subjective data have often been liable to inference and interpretation from observers. Again the importance of the balance between the subjective and objective is highlighted by the individual's own life experiences. Importantly, the subjective 'good' quality of life described by an individual with a learning disability may merely reflect a low level of expectation based on previous life experience.

In summary, the field of learning disability is faced by many of the difficulties experienced in any health field in defining quality of life. Furthermore, inherent difficulties in communication have led to increased focus on objective measurement, with the search for subjective measures remaining elusive.

The impact of epilepsy on quality of life

There is now a considerable literature on this topic. However, the literature is small in specific relation to people with learning disabilities. It cannot be assumed that epilepsy threatens the same aspirations for people with learning disabilities as it does for the general population. For example, holding a driving licence, having children, getting married and being able to pursue the career of your choice are all goals which are restricted by limited intellectual capacity and limited functional independence. Even with complete seizure control, the majority of people with learning disabilities would not achieve these. It is equally important, however, not to presume that epilepsy has little additional impact. Studies we conducted some time ago demonstrated that both continuing, refractory seizures and anti-epileptic drug polytherapy independently contributed to poorer psychosocial outcome in people with learning disability and epilepsy, when compared with matched controls of people with learning disability and no epilepsy (Espie *et al.*, 1989; Gillies *et al.*, 1989).

OUTCOME MEASUREMENT

The research base

Traditionally, the gold standard in the treatment of epilepsy has been the achievement of 'seizure free outcome' although, increasingly, there is emphasis on psychosocial outcome and quality of life. This wider emphasis is particularly important in learning disabilities both because of the complexity in the spectrum of individual need and the failure to achieve a seizure-free outcome in a high proportion of cases. Indeed, stabilisation on as few drugs as possible, preferably monotherapy, with a reduced but 'acceptable' frequency of seizures may be the optimal goal at present (Bourgeois, 1991; Richens, 1995; Brodie and Dichter, 1996).

We have completed recent review papers on the subject of outcome measurement (Kerr and Espie, 1997; Espie *et al.*, 1997). There are a number of domains of measurement which should be considered as part of the outcome picture. These will be summarised briefly and reference will be made to what we regard as useful measures.

Seizure Frequency

Seizure diaries should have behavioural descriptions of each of the main seizure types with which the individual presents. Such diaries should be the responsibility of the main carer but it is also a distinct advantage if diaries remain with the person with epilepsy across care settings (family home, day centre, respite service and so on). Each carer involved can then chart events as they occur simply by checking what they have seen against the behavioural descriptors. This system is preferred to the use of diagnostic categories which are likely to be unfamiliar to a sizeable proportion of carers (Espie and Paul, 1998).

Cognitive function

There is no validated, standardised measure for this population. Subtests from intellectual assessments may be used, but are likely to be insensitive for the majority of people with learning disabilities. Assessment of selective and sustained attention is more fundamental than learning and memory. People with severe learning disabilities can complete simple vigilance tasks such as visual reaction time. Observer ratings of 'concentration' and 'fatigue' have been found to correlate reasonably with formal vigilance measurement and behaviour state assessment (Espie *et al.*, 1999b).

Psychosocial functioning

The best available measures are the AAMR Adaptive Behaviour Scales (Nihira *et al.*, 1993) and the Vineland Adaptive Behaviour Scales (Sparrow *et al.*, 1984). Although the full versions of these scales are time consuming to complete, they provide a useful profile of functional status in terms of personal, domestic and community independence.

Behaviour

The analysis of behaviour patterns in terms of antecedent, setting conditions and possible reinforcers is best conducted by means of functional analysis (Espie and Paul, 1998). Behavioural diaries are also useful to quantify the frequency and intensity of behaviour. The best available formal measure is the Aberrant Behaviour Checklist (Aman *et al.*, 1985). This yields a number of subscale scores and has been validated as an outcome measure in drug trials.

Career functioning

Since the ability of the carer to cope may be critical to management and outcome, it can be useful to obtain a measure of carer stress. The Caregiver Strain Index is particularly recommended (Robinson, 1983) and it is relatively brief and easy to administer. Although originally developed for another population, it is now undergoing validation for use with carers of people with learning disability and epilepsy.

Global Indices

The Epilepsy and Learning Disabilities Quality of Life Questionnaire (ELDQoL; Jacoby *et al.*, 1995) was developed from interviews with parents of children with Lennox-Gastaut Syndrome and the physicians treating them. The ELDQoL is completed by carers and comprises three sub-scales (seizure severity, behaviour and mood) and single items relating to seizure-related injury, overall health and quality of life. Internal consistency by coefficient alpha ranges from 0.71 to 0.84 and the scale takes around 20 minutes to complete. Test re-test reliability is also reasonable at 0.67 to 0.84.

The Epilepsy Outcome Scale is another new scale, derived directly from reported concerns of carers of people with learning disabilities

(EOS; Espie *et al.*, 1998). It comprises four subscales reflecting concerns about seizures, drugs for epilepsy, risk of injury, and impact on daily life. A carer, taking around 8–10 minutes, completes the EOS. Mean alpha for the EOS total score is 0.92 and test re-test reliability is 0.86. Further development of the EOS is underway, including the development of a version for administration directly to people with mild learning disabilities.

Clinical application

A suggested clinical protocol is incorporated in Table 2. Seizure diary recording would run continuously with assessment on the Epilepsy Outcome Scale at six monthly intervals. The Vineland Adaptive Behaviour Scales, Aberrant Behaviour Checklist and Caregiver Strain Index need only be completed annually. Although even this limited set

TABLE 2 AN ASSESSMENT PROTOCOL FOR USE IN CLINICAL PRACTICE WITH PEOPLE WITH EPILEPSY AND LEARNING DISABILITIES

ASSESSMENT DOMAIN	RECOMMENDED TOOL	COMPLETED BY	RECOMMENDED INTERVAL
SEIZURES	SEIZURE DIARIES WITH WRITTEN DESCRIPTIONS OF EACH SEIZURE TYPE, AS BEHAVIOURALLY OBSERVED. SPACE FOR DAILY ENTRIES	ALL CARERS INVOLVED	CONTINUOUS
COGNITIVE FUNCTIONING	VISUAL ANALOGUE SCALES (0–10 CM) FOR RATING VARIABLES OF CONCERN (E.G. CONCENTRATION)	MAIN CARER	ANNUALLY (AND AT TIMES OF DRUG CHANGE)
PSYCHOSOCIAL FUNCTIONING	VINELAND ADAPTIVE BEHAVIOUR SCALES (EXPANDED FORM); SECTIONS ON 'DAILY LIVING SKILLS'	EPILEPSY NURSE SPECIALIST WITH MAIN CARER	ANNUALLY
BEHAVIOUR	ABERRANT BEHAVIOUR CHECKLIST (HOSPITAL OR COMMUNITY VERSION AS APPROPRIATE)	MAIN CARER	ANNUALLY
CARER COPING	CAREGIVER STRAIN INDEX (SAME CARER TO COMPLETE EACH TIME)	MAIN CARER	ANNUALLY
GLOBAL INDEX	EPILEPSY OUTCOME SCALE (SAME CARER TO COMPLETE EACH TIME)	MAIN CARER	EACH 6 MONTHS (AND AT TIMES OF DRUG CHANGE)

of measurement may seem quite ambitious, and potentially time consuming for the clinician, it should be borne in mind that many of the scales are completed by carers and do not, therefore, require direct clinical time. For example, the Vineland scales could be completed by an epilepsy nurse specialist in consultation with carers.

It is important to stress that this protocol should not replace taking a good history and sensitive clinical interviewing. Formal scales will not necessarily pick up on highly specific issues of concern and these must not be overlooked.

TREATMENT ISSUES — THE EVIDENCE BASE FOR MAXIMISING QUALITY OF LIFE

Epilepsy management and, in particular, the use of pharmacological interventions has largely been assessed within the criteria of clinical effectiveness, with the double-blind randomised controlled trial now the norm for new pharmacotherapies. This scientific rigour has not, unfortunately, been applied — except for some notable exceptions — to the learning disability population. The reasons for this are varied, including the problems of co-morbidity, fears over ethical implications and the relative difficulty in recruitment. This situation has led to a continued trend to open trials and retrospective case note evaluations, with a paucity of randomised controlled trials.

With regard to people with intellectual disability, we are therefore left with something of a clinical effectiveness dilemma. If we practice purely by gold standard approaches we are left with precious few interventions. We must therefore apply knowledge on interventions gained in the general population to this special population, but the validity of these findings in this population remains unproven — particularly when assessing quality of life outcomes. The latter course of action is, of course, a clinical necessity. In this section we will discuss the clinical effectiveness background to therapeutic interventions for people with intellectual disability — stressing where data on the broader quality of life outcomes exists. Studies looking at this population have been divided into assessing practice, usually antiepileptic drug reductions through cohort or intervention studies, and pharmacological interventions to control seizures.

Several intervention studies have been performed assessing drug reduction or 'rationalisation'. Fischbacher showed in a study, which was neither controlled nor randomised, that reduction of at least one anticonvulsant was feasible for many patients (Fischbacher, 1982).

Importantly he recognised the value of outcomes beyond seizure frequency, suggesting an associated behavioural improvement in this population. Other studies were not associated with quality of life outcomes and the clinician unfortunately cannot be guided to the true outcomes of drug reduction as yet.

The majority of data on pharmacological interventions are open to methodological criticism and hence interpretation is difficult. With few exceptions, good quality of life data is missing. A survey in Australia using an open non-randomised assessment of add-on lamotrigine in a childhood population (Buchanen, 1996) showed a 50% improvement in seizure control in 74% of children, with an associated improvement in quality of life, based on clinical judgement. Unfortunately clinical judgement remains a necessarily subjective concept.

Further studies investigating cohorts of individuals with intellectual disability are not available. However, pharmacological research has focused on two epilepsy syndromes strongly associated with intellectual disability, West syndrome (infantile spasms) and the Lennox Gastaut syndrome. West syndrome (Dulac *et al.*, 1994) is a developmental age defined (within the first year of life) syndrome, making interpretation of the impact of the intervention on further development problematical.

Studies in the Lennox Gastaut syndrome represent the most vigorous studies allowing us some insight into quality of life outcomes. The Lennox Gastaut syndrome is characterised by multiple seizure types including atypical absences, a characteristic EEG finding of slow spike and wave activity, and a frequent association with intellectual disability. Two of the novel anticonvulsants, topiramate and lamotrigine have been evaluated in this syndrome.

Lamotrigine has been subject to the most rigorous quality of life evaluation in the Lennox Gastaut population. The compound has been investigated through a randomised placebo controlled add-on design (Motte *et al.,* 1997). Importantly, the study used a specifically designed quality of life scale and parental global health evaluation, in addition to the usual seizure frequency measures. In terms of seizure efficacy the study was successful, with a significant reduction in atonic seizures and in total seizures. The impact on quality of life measures was interesting. Parent/carer assessment showed an improvement in global health. Outcome on the ELDQoL showed significant improvement in mood and reduced seizure severity (Jacoby *et al.*, 1996). No difference in side effect profile was seen as compared with placebo.

A study of topiramate recruited 98 patients with the Lennox Gastaut Syndrome with an age range of 2 to 42 years. Primary successful outcome points were deemed to be either a combination of a significant reduction in atonic (drop) attacks and parental global evaluation of seizure severity or, a percent reduction of all seizure types. Some attempt was therefore made to evaluate the impact on quality of life through these parental evaluations. The methodology applied was a randomised placebo controlled add-on design. The population had quite severe seizures, all having at least 60 seizures per month. Results showed a statistically significant median reduction in drop attacks (placebo increase by 5%, topiramate decrease by 15%; $p = 0.04$) and in parent evaluation of seizure severity (placebo 28% improvement, topiramate 52%). There was no statistically significant decrease in overall median seizure frequency (Glauser 1997). Parental global seizure severity was the only chosen measure of quality of life in this study.

It would appear therefore that as yet there is little to guide the clinician into appropriate medication choice related to quality of life outcome. It is therefore likely that choice will be made on perceived differences in side effects between compounds. The majority of compounds have not had adequate trial methodology applied — many because they were developed before such methodology existed. The more recent studies on lamotrigine and topiramate have shown that both randomised controlled trial methodology and quality of life recording can be applied to this population.

CONCLUSION

Epilepsy has a profound effect on the quality of life of individuals with learning disability and their carers. Clinically relevant tools to assess both the abilities of individuals and their quality of life do exist. The challenge for clinicians will be to apply these in every day clinical practice.

References

Aman, M.G., Singh, N.N., Stewart, A.W., Field, C.J. (1985) The Aberrant Behavior Checklist: a behavior rating scale for the assessment of treatment effects. *American Journal of Mental Deficiency* **89**, 485–491.

Betts, T., Boden, S. (1992) Diagnosis, management and prognosis of a group of 128 patients with non-epileptic attack disorder: Part I. *Seizure*, **1**, 19–26.

Blunden, R. (1988). Pragmatic features of quality services. In: Janicki, M.P. Krauss, M.W., Seltzer, M.M. (eds.) *Community residences for persons with developmental disabilities: Here to stay* Baltimore: Paul H Brookes, 117–121

Bond, S. Smith, M. Pitcairn, K., Fowler, P. (1991) *Community Resettlement from Hospital of People with a Mental Handicap: Volume 4, an Overview of the Study*. Newcastle upon Tyne: Centre for Health Services Research.

Bourgeois, B.F.D. (1991) Relationship between anticonvulsant drugs and learning disabilities. *Seminars on Neurology* **11**, 14–19.

Brodie, M.J., Dichter, M. (1996) Antiepileptic drugs. *New England Journal of Medicine* **334**, 168–175.

Buchanen, N. (1996) The efficacy of Lamotrigine on seizure control in 34 children, adolescents and young adults with intellectual and physical disability. In: Loiseav, P. (ed.) Lamotrigine: a brighter future. Royal Society of Medicine Symposium Series No. 24. London: RSM, 89–102.

Chadwick D. (1994) Epilepsy *Journal of Neurology, Neurosurgery, and Psychiatry*. **57**, 264–277.

Clark, A., Espie, C.A., Paul, A. (2000) Adults with learning disabilities: Knowledge about epilepsy before and after a psychoeducational package (*in submission*).

Dulac, O. Chugani, H., Bernardini, B (eds.). (1994). Infantile spasms and West Syndrome. London: W.B. Saunders.

Espie, C.A., Brown, M. (1998) Health needs and learning disabilities: an overview. *Health Bulletin* **56**, 468–476.

Espie, C.A., Paul, A. (1997) Epilepsy and learning disabilities In: Goldstein, L.H., Cull, C. (eds.) *The Clinical Psychologist's Handbook of Epilepsy*. London Routledge, 184–202.

Espie, C.A., Pashley, A.S., Bonham, K.G., Sourindhrin, I., O'Donovan, M. (1989). The mentally handicapped person with epilepsy: A comparative study investigating psychosocial functioning. *Journal of Mental Deficiency Research* **33**, 123–135.

Espie C.A., Kerr M, Paul, A., O'Brien G, Betts T, Clark J., Jacoby A., Baker G. (1997) Learning disability and epilepsy: A review of available outcome measures and position statement on development priorities. *Seizure*, **6**, 337–350.

Espie, C.A., Paul, A., Graham, M., Sterrick, M., Foley, J., McGarvey, C. (1998) The Epilepsy Outcome Scale: the development of a measure for use with carers of people with epilepsy plus intellectual disability. *Journal of Intellectual Disability Research* **42**, 90–96.

Espie, C.A., Watkins, J., Branford, D., Paul, A. (1999a) *Measurement and psychometric properties of the Epilepsy Outcome Scale*. Epilepsia, Supp. 2, S185.

Espie, C.A., Paul, A., McColl, J.H., McFie, J., Amos, P., Gray, J., Hamilton, D.S., Jamal, G.A. (1999b) Cognitive functioning in people with epilepsy plus severe learning disabilities: a systematic analysis of predictors of daytime arousal and attention. *Seizure* **8**, 1–8.

Felce, D. (1988). Evaluating the extent of community integration following the provision of staffed residential alternatives to institutional care. *Irish Journal of Psychology*. **9**. 346–360.

Felce, D., Perry, J. (1995). Quality of life: Its definition and measurement. *Research in Developmental Disabilities* **16**(1), 51–74.

Felce, D., Perry, J. (1997). Quality of life: a multidimensional, multielement framework. In: Brown, R. (ed.) *Quality of life for people with disabilities* Cheltenham: Stanley Thorn, 56–71

Fischbacher, E. (1982). Effect of reduction of anticonvulsants on wellbeing. *British Medical Journal*. **285**, 423–424.

Gillies, J.B., Espie, C.A., Montgomery, J.M. (1989) The social and behavioural functioning of people with mental handicaps attending Adult Training Centres: a comparison of those with and without epilepsy. *Mental Handicap Research* **2**, 129–136.

Glauser, T. (1997). A double blind trial of topiramate in Lennox Gastaut syndrome. *Epilepsia* **38** (Suppl. 1), 131.

Goode, D. (1997). Assessing the quality of life of adults with profound disabilities. In: Brown R (ed.) *Quality of life for people with disabilities*. Cheltenham: Stanley Thorn, 72–90

ILAE Commission on Classification and Terminology of the International League Against Epilepsy (1989) Proposal for revised classification of epilepsies and epileptic syndromes. *Epilepsia* **30**, 389–399.

Jacoby, A., Baker, G., Dewey, M. (1995) Development of an instrument to assess quality of life in children with epilepsy and learning disability. *Quality of Life Research* **4**, 442.

Jacoby, A., Baker, G.A., Bryant-Comstock, L., Phillips, S., Bamford, C. (1996) Lamotrigine add-on therapy is associated with improvement in mood in patients with severe epilepsy. *Epilepsia* 37(Suppl. 5), S202

Kerr, M., Espie, C. (1997) Learning Disability and Epilepsy (I) Towards Common Outcome Measures: Learning Disability and Epilepsy *Seizure* **6**, 331–336

Mariani, E., Ferini-Strambi, L., Sala, M., Erminio, C., Smirne, S. (1993) Epilepsy in institutionalised patients with encephalopathy: Clinical aspects and nosological considerations. *American Journal on Mental Retardation* **98**, 27–33.

Motte, J., Trevathan, E., Arvidsson, J., Barrerra, M.N., Mullens, E., Manasca, P. (1997) Lamotrigine for generalised seizures associated with the Lennox Gastaut syndrome *New England Journal of Medicine* **337**, 1807–1812.

Nihira, K., Leland, H., Lambert, N. (1993) *Adaptive Behavior Scales*. Austin, Texas, American Association on Mental Retardation.

O'Brien, J. (1987) A guide to personal futures planning In: Bellamy, G.T., Wilcox, B. (eds.) *A Comprehensive Guide to Activities Catalog: An Alternative Curriculum for Youth and Adults with Severe Disabilities*. Baltimore: Paul H. Brookes.

Paul, A. (1997) Epilepsy or stereotypy: diagnostic issues in learning disabilities. *Seizure*, **6**, 111–120.

Richens, A. (1995) Rational polypharmacy. *Seizure* **4**, 211–214.

Robinson, B.C. (1983) Validation of a caregiver strain index. *Journal of Gerontology* **38**, 344–348.

Rowan, A.J., Gates, J.R. (1999) *Non-epileptic seizures* (2nd edition). Oxford: Butterworth-Heinemann.

Sparrow, S.A., Balla, D.A., Cicchetti, D.V. (1984) *Vineland Adaptive Behavior Scale: Expanded Interview Edition*. Circle Pines, Minnesota: American Guidance.

Sussova, J., Seidl, Z., Faber, J. (1990) Hemiparetic forms of cerebral palsy in relation to epilepsy and mental retardation. *Developmental Medicine and Child Neurology*. **32**, 792–795.

Welsh Office (1996) *Welsh Health Survey, 1996*. Cardiff: Welsh Office.

CONTRIBUTIONS OF QUALITY OF LIFE ASSESSMENT TO PATIENT MANAGEMENT

Chapter 10

NON EST VIVERE, SED VALERE VITA EST*
A PHYSICIAN REFLECTS ON QUALITY OF LIFE

Tim Betts

Martial, Epigrammata 6, 70

Goring, one of the Nazi leaders, is alleged to have said, 'when I hear the word "culture" I reach for my pistol'. What should the clinician reach for when he or she hears the phrase 'Quality of Life?' Hopefully, neither a pistol nor the sickbag, but since it is a phrase often uttered with an air of liturgical reverence, as part of a mystic ritual used to impress the uninitiated, it can set the teeth on edge and cause irritation in other parts of the body.

I find the phrase particularly irritating when used:

a) to bolster the results of an otherwise unimpressive drug trial, as a cynical marketing exercise.
b) as empty 'management speak' to justify inaction or the latest cost cutting exercise.
c) as a mantra in discussions about the management of those about to die, when the correct phrase should, of course, be 'quality of death'.

So I enter into this discussion on Quality of Life (QoL) with some negative cognitions which hopefully will be changed by reading the other chapters in this book. In doing so I shall be asking several questions and the first and most obvious one is: How can I, as a physician, make sure that neither my patients' epilepsy, nor my treatment of it, impairs their quality of life more than is unavoidable?

The second question is whether or not QoL can be accurately and meaningfully defined. Third, if accurate definition is possible, can we accurately measure it in a *meaningful* way? The fourth question is whether being able to measure QoL can change medical practice; are such measures actually helpful to doctor and patient? Can scores obtained from QoL measures designed to look at changes in group means help me to recognise individual problems and identify solutions for a particular patient?

I shall need to be persuaded that any QoL measure is sufficiently precise and robust that I can rely on it and on the validity of any change in its score, particularly a short term change. Many published measures are those of fixed past events that are not amenable to change (except over a very long time period) and, relying on binary 'yes/no' answers, are not sensitive enough to detect subtle but important changes in treatment outcomes (Kellet *et al.*, 1997). Some measures, like emotional well-being and satisfaction, will change quickly with improved seizure control, but this raises the question of whether we could improve emotional well-being and satisfaction without necessarily improving seizure control. Measures of social and vocational functioning may be more resistant to change (Ferguson and Rayport, 1965); improving seizure control may not alter these aspects of life at all. In patients suffering severe seizures starting in childhood, their removal may make life more, rather than less, difficult (Ferguson and Rayport, 1965) because of the added adjustment difficulties of encountering new social situations well after their non epileptic peers have done so. Loss of the consideration given to the chronically ill may lessen quality of life. Needed relationships may end — a third of married subjects eventually divorced after successful surgery for epilepsy (Bladin, 1992). The successfully treated patient may have to face the 'burden of normality'.

Having been involved in many drug trials where QoL measures have been employed, I will need to be convinced that such scales measure more than just mood and morale; and that those that measure mood, used appropriately, are not repeated too often and too soon. There are hints in the literature that most drug trial scales do no more than this (Devinsky *et al.*, 1997). Since many QoL scales are rather tedious and complicated to fill in (judging by the experience of many of my patients during drug trials) could they not be simpler, easier to understand and yet be as reliable? Another important issue is whether it is possible to see any meaningful change over the relatively short life of a drug trial — the patient will still be unable to drive, may well not be seizure free, will still be overprotected, and will still suffer from impaired cognition since the original drug burden will not yet have been removed.

I am, therefore, going to concentrate on applying what I have read of QoL issues to the clinical environment and how we might improve our service to maximise both our own and our patients' quality of life.

INTO THE MEDICAL DOMAIN

Epilepsy is clearly a medical condition and often requires medical treatment. But I think my profession has over-medicalised it. Faced, for instance, with an increase in a patient's seizure frequency, we tend to reach for our prescription pad rather than looking to see whether stress, social upset or a change in lifestyle has been responsible. This is partly because unless the physician has had psychiatric training, the importance of a social and psychological history is often under-estimated; and partly because our patients assume that we only want to hear about medical facts and symptoms and so may somatise their emotional difficulties. They have, after all, entered the medical domain where they are required to assume a patient identity (Taylor, 1997) and obey unwritten but taken-for-granted rules which result in intrusions into intimacy, loss of dignity, self-concept and control. This is at a time when, if they are given the diagnosis of epilepsy, their self image and feelings of mastery will be further compromised by their own cultural and family beliefs about the nature and causation of their condition (about which the physician may be totally ignorant). Cultural beliefs may, of course, contaminate QoL measures, although this does not seem to be a problem in the different communities of Western Europe (Baker *et al.,* 1997). Translating a QoL measure into another language may cause difficulty and needs to be done meticulously (Chaplin and Malgrem, 1999).

Failure to assess a person's seizure symptoms thoroughly and medically may lead to mistakes in attribution and failure to recognise a remediable cause. However, merely concentrating on this medical function prevents the patient (and the family) from telling their story and the doctor from putting their symptoms into a social, cultural and psychological context — an experience which is stultifying and non educational for the doctor. For me, job satisfaction is about understanding and engaging with both the emotional and physical aspects of a patient's illness and giving priority to neither in the long term (though in the short term of course, such prioritising may be necessary).

There is developing interest in the narrative of a medical history, both for patients to put their experiences into context and for the physician to understand that context (Greenhalgh, 1999). I try to make sure in my clinic that the patient and, if necessary, the family have ample opportunity to 'tell their story' and know it will be listened to. Without being able to do this, many people feel disillusioned with medical care and may turn to alternative and complementary practitioners, at a time when conventional medicine still has much to offer.

Psychiatrists have long known of the importance of the life event chart in teasing out puzzling presentations so that somatic symptoms are tabulated against changes in life style and emotional events. Psychiatrists have, of course, long pondered on quality of life and are slightly amused by its sudden discovery by their medical colleagues — and the cloud of psychologists and social workers that now seem needed at every consultation. Leaving the assessment of patients' social and psychological needs to psychologists and social workers (worthy as they are) turns the physician into a mere medical technician; so does leaving it all to the nurse, particularly as this demeans his or her particular medical skills.

To produce a life events chart for somebody with an illness which they have had for a very long time (like epilepsy) can be time consuming and tedious and needs careful and meticulous reading of old notes and letters. This may require that a member of the epilepsy team spends half a day going through the patient's old medical records in great detail, but is often time well spent. It is interesting when going through patients' notes to discover how often their stories change, depending on whom they are talking to or being managed by (I am not talking about deliberate deceit here: that is another fascinating story) and also how important results of investigations are often overlooked.

It is often very difficult, just by talking to the patient or their general practitioner, to discover the results of previous investigations. Patients may see investigations as just part of a ritual that has to be gone through to get advice (Taylor, 1997) and may not understand their purpose and importance. Even if they do, they may not be told the result — or may be told it in terms that they cannot understand. For example, a patient of mine had had a CT (computerised tomography) scan and had asked her previous consultant for the result. The sum total of her knowledge was the consultant's statement that, 'it didn't show me what I was expecting to find.' Often, when patients are told that their MRI (magnetic resonance imaging) scan is normal, they express disappointment because they conceptualise the scan as a way of reaching inside their brain and determining the cause of their seizures. Sometimes, if not told the result of a test, they conclude that it must have been normal, 'because no one told me anything.' This can be both a snare and a delusion.

Likewise, it can be very difficult to tell what kind of imaging a patient has had. If the patient describes a very noisy claustrophobic experience, then the clinician can reasonably assume that it was an MRI scan. But it is unlikely that the patient will know the result; and even if known, the description of the abnormality given to the patient will often be unhelpful. Yet defects in communication may leave the patient extremely anxious and uncertain for a considerable period of time.

The issue of photosensitivity provides a useful illustration of the importance of telling patients the results of their investigations. Many patients, although they are neither photo nor pattern sensitive, have never been told that they are not, or what that implies. They therefore continue to avoid TV sets, electronic games and computers in particular; and so deny themselves job opportunities. Equally importantly, they are not armed with the necessary information to refute the misconceptions of many employers that having epilepsy means you cannot work with computers.

I think it is extremely important that patients are told the results of their investigations and, indeed, have copies of the reports if they wish. They could also have copies of the actual investigation itself. It is equally important that their general practitioner receives a copy of the result of the investigation together with an interpretation of the meaning of the result (for example, what is meant by the term 'neuronal migration disorder'). It is also important that both patient and practitioner know the limitations of the investigation; that, for example, a normal CT scan does not exclude a remediable cause for the epilepsy.

In paediatric practice, it is common for the parents to receive a copy of the letter sent to the general practitioner. There seems to be no reason why this practice cannot be extended to adult patients also. Some general practitioners do already, as a matter of routine, show all letters received from hospital practitioners to their patients (though they don't always indicate that this has been done). In my own clinic, we intend to start copying letters to patients routinely, but will also carefully audit the effect this has both on the patient and on the quality of letter writing.

OUT OF THE MEDICAL DOMAIN

For a variety of reasons already referred to above, the hospital setting may not always offer patients the opportunity to bring and discuss their own agenda about their epilepsy. It might be better for some, particularly those with a learning difficulty or physical handicap, if the initial consultation were carried out in their own home, where they will feel more comfortable. This will also allow the assessment team a chance to decide what elements of the clinic process are necessary for the patient and to plan investigations, in particular any special help or sedation the patient needs to get through them. It is possible, of course, to bring the investigation to the patient and an EEG carried out in the patient's own home may be more useful than one carried out in the clinic where he or she may be frightened and uncooperative. Alternatively, it may be possible after a home visit to plan a gradual introduction to the necessary investigations and to de-sensitise the patient to any fears that they may have.

Visiting the patient's home also has the advantage that those doing the assessment can talk to vital witnesses who never come to the hospital and begin to assess the psychological and social impact that seizures may be having on the patient at home. Home consultations also provide an opportunity to look at family reactions to the seizures and to assess the degree of over-protection; and to assess the degree of risk seizures pose within the home, so that the appropriate precautions can be decided upon. It is interesting that general practitioners are expected to gain experience in hospital practice; it should be equally important for hospital practitioners to have some experience of domiciliary practice.

WHERE QUALITY OF LIFE MEASUREMENT IS NEEDED

QoL measures have been used in the assessment of patients undergoing surgery. One lesson I have learnt from the QoL literature is that early surgery rapidly restores QoL to normal, whereas late surgery, after years of fruitless medical therapy, does not. As one might expect, the most significant changes in QoL occur in those patients who become completely seizure free, though in one study (Kellet *et al.,* 1997) there was an intermediate effect in those patients who achieved almost, but not complete seizure control. This may have been because that study used disease-specific, rather than generic, instruments to measure QoL. In post-surgical studies, emotion and well-being change almost immediately, but vocational and social functioning take longer. Indeed, Sperling *et al.* (1995) showed that it was over two years before the impact of surgery on such domains could reasonably be assessed.

It has been shown that candidates who exhibit good or poor psychological adjustment before surgery continue to do so after surgery, independent of seizure outcome (Hermann *et al.,* 1992). Pre-surgical status appears to be a stronger prognostic indicator of the success of surgery (regarding psychosocial outcomes) than seizure frequency. Rose *et al.,* (1996) reported that a high degree of 'neuroticism' before surgery resulted in poorer psychosocial adjustment after surgery, even if the patient became seizure free — suggesting that pre-existing personality variables also influence post-operative adjustment. Patient expectations prior to surgery may also predict patient satisfaction after surgery. Patients who are overly optimistic about the outcome of surgery may experience psychosocial difficulty post-operatively if they do not attain absolute seizure relief. If patients anticipate complete seizure freedom, they are less likely to be satisfied by mere seizure reduction (Wheelock *et al.*, 1998). These findings suggest the need for careful pre-surgical evaluation of people undergoing surgery to identify those who may need education about the likely outcome so that they do not become unduly optimistic; and to identify those with psychological needs, such as undue anxiety, for pre-treatment therapy and post-treatment rehabilitation.

Some surgeons try to identify patients who are already anxious or depressed or potentially psychotic before surgery, in order to avoid operating on them, but this, I think, is wrong. Surgery is designed to stop patients having seizures, because seizures are potentially dangerous and can lead to loss of life. Post-operative anxiety and depression (which is surprisingly common even in those who do not seem so predisposed) or psychoses are treatable conditions and should not prevent patients from having surgery to control their seizures. QoL measures should be used to help to identify those who have special needs and may need intensive rehabilitation after surgery, not used to exclude them from the procedure.

There are several other areas of epilepsy care which could be illuminated by QoL measures and would seem to me to be ones where clinicians often have little empathy or understanding of the needs of the patients whom they are treating. The first is young children and patients who have learning difficulties so severe that they cannot be their own advocates. People who are learning disabled may respond particularly adversely to conventional drug treatment and it has been suggested that for many of them the limited objective of reducing the frequency of the more damaging seizures is more important than achieving complete seizure control (Betts, 1998). We need to determine if this is actually true and to develop measures (which may well need to be behavioural rather than verbal) to determine the best treatment outcomes for patients in this category.

The second area where QoL measures might help to shape therapy is for adolescent patients with epilepsy. Many adult physicians have preconceived ideas (extrapolating backwards from dim memories of their own adolescence!) about the needs of adolescents with epilepsy. The adolescent with epilepsy often leaves paediatric care (where parental concerns may seem more important) and is plunged into adult care without any transition period. There has been very little assessment of the needs of adolescents with epilepsy. There is need for an instrument which embraces emotional well-being and satisfaction with care, and not just vocational and social functioning (Austin *et al.*, 1993), and which identifies the vulnerable adolescent most in need of targeted services. We need an instrument that measures over-protection!

There is also a growing interest in the needs of women with epilepsy, because epilepsy occurring in women particularly effects their sexual development and sexuality, the menstrual cycle, contraception, fertility, reproduction, the puerperium, the mother and child relationship and the climacteric (Betts and Crawford, 1998). We need QoL measures that reflect these particular events in a woman's life cycle so that we can shape our medical care to meet her needs and to measure her emotional well being and satisfaction with what we do. As with patients undergoing surgery and adolescents with epilepsy, we need to identify the most vulnerable women, who need particular care.

CONCLUSION

My own view is that QoL research has become diverted down a slightly sterile path of measuring short term and probably meaningless changes within the context of drug trials, when they could most usefully be directed at helping physicians and others target packages of care to the right person at the right time. They should emphasise the fact that for disorders like epilepsy purely medical care is not enough, and that if the clinician does not also provide emotional, psychological and social care, he has failed to provide effective therapy. Treating seizures is important (and may be life saving); treating the whole patient is even more important. If we are to save the patient's life with medication or surgery, it is important to consider the quality of that saved life.

However, QoL measures, though important in research, must not become a substitute for good interviewing skills, information giving or home assessments, and they should never become a recipe for inaction or complacency.

In conclusion, I have tried to show that 'Quality of Life' can be an empty sterile phrase and that physicians need to be reassured about its validity and utility. There are things that physicians can do in terms of providing good information, making sure patients understand their condition and are well informed, have a chance to tell their story and to be assessed not in the clinic, but at home. The true value of QoL measures is to help physicians shape and target therapy to those who need it. There are still areas where we have little understanding of the emotional and social needs of our patients and where specific QoL measures would help.

ACKNOWLEDGEMENTS

I am grateful to two of my Special Study Module Students, Sarah Cluskey and Ruth Haley, for tutorial discussions around this topic and for literature searches.

References

Austin, J., Dunn, D., Levstek, D. (1993) First seizures: concerns and needs of parents and children. *Epilepsia* **34** (Suppl. 6), S24.

Baker, G., Jacoby, A., Buck, D., Stalgis, C., Monnet, D. (1997) Quality of life in epilepsy: a European study. *Epilepsia* **38**, 353–362.

Betts, T. (1998) *Epilepsy, Psychiatry and Learning Difficulties*. London: Martin Dunitz, 96–98.

Betts, T., Crawford, P. (1998) *Women and Epilepsy*. London: Martin Dunitz.

Bladin P. (1992) Psychosocial difficulties and outcome after temporal lobectomy. *Epilepsia*, 33, 898–907.

Chaplin, J., Malgrem, K. (1999) Cross cultural adaptation and use of the Epilepsy Psychosocial Effects Scale: comparison between the psychosocial effects of chronic epilepsy in Sweden and the United Kingdom. *Epilepsia* **40**, 93–96.

Devinsky, O., Baker, G., Cramer, J. (1997) Quantitative measures of assessment. In: Engel, J., Pedley, T. (eds.) *Epilepsy: A Comprehensive Textbook*. Philadelphia: Lippincott-Raven, 1107–1113.

Ferguson, S., Rayport, M. (1965) The adjustment to living without epilepsy. *Journal of Nervous and Mental Disease* **140**, 26–37.

Greenhalgh, T. (1999) Narrative based medicine: narrative based medicine in an evidence based world. *British Medical Journal* **318**, 323–325.

Herman, B., Wyler, A., Soames, G. (1992) Pre-operative psychological adjustment and surgical outcome are determinants of psychosocial status after anterior temporal lobectomy. *Journal of Neurology, Neurosurgery and Psychiatry* **55**, 491–496.

Kellet, M., Smith, D., Baker, G., Chadwick, D. (1997) Quality of life after epilepsy surgery *Journal of Neurology, Neurosurgery and Psychiatry* **63**, 52–58.

Rose K., Derry, P., McLachlan, R. (1996) Neuroticism in temporal lobe epilepsy: assessment and implications for pre and post operative psychosocial adjustment and health related quality of life. *Epilepsia* **37**, 484–491.

Sperling, M., Saykin, A., Roberts, F., French, J., O'Connell, M. (1995) Occupational outcome after temporal lobectomy for refractory epilepsy. *Neurology* **45**, 970–977.

Taylor, D. (1997) Broader aspects of treatment. In: Engel, J., Pedley, T. (eds.) *Epilepsy: A Comprehensive Textbook*. Philadelphia: Lippincott-Raven, 1115–1119.

Wheelock, I., Peterson, C., Buchtel, H. (1998) Pre-surgery expectations, post-surgery satisfaction and psychosocial adjustment after epilepsy surgery *Epilepsia* **39**, 487–494.

Chapter 11

CAN QUALITY OF LIFE ASSESSMENTS CONTRIBUTE TO EVERYDAY CLINICAL PRACTICE?

Harry W. McConnell and Peter J. Snyder

While the majority of the chapters in this volume refer to Quality of Life (QoL) indices from the perspective of looking at 10, 100, or perhaps 1,000 patients in a research setting, this chapter will focus on the meaning of such a concept and of these measures for the individual patient in the clinic setting. What is useful in measuring a given patient population may not be useful for that individual patient. Indeed, what measures should be chosen for an individual patient are time- and situation- dependent, and the issues of concern may vary considerably even from one clinic visit to the next.

At the heart of this argument is consideration of the relative contributions of 'evidence-based medicine', 'narrative-based medicine' and 'hypothesis-based medicine' in everyday clinical practice, with respect to the care and decisions made about an individual patient. Interactions between a clinician and a patient must utilise both the 'art' and 'science' of medicine. The clinical method draws on narrative skills to integrate the overlapping stories of patients, their carers and laboratory results (Greenhalgh, 1999) as well as upon the clinician's knowledge of clinical trials and other sources of 'objective evidence'. Hypothesis-based medicine implies that data collected from both the narrative-interpretative paradigm and from objective evidence-based sources can be combined to form an hypothesis about the problem faced by the patient, and thus about the best approach to solving it. In the majority of clinical situations faced by an epileptologist, there is insufficient truly 'evidence-based' medicine to clearly suggest a treatment. Decisions about which treatment in epileptology are largely informed by clinical trials, which are sometimes influenced more by marketing concerns than by real clinical need. An eclectic approach to the treatment of epilepsy is therefore not only desirable, but essential.

THE PHYSICIAN-PATIENT ENCOUNTER

How does all this concern the clinician assessing the QoL of a patient with epilepsy in a clinical situation? The term 'quality of life' refers to a number of aspects of care that have not traditionally been addressed, on a routine basis, in a typical clinic appointment at an epilepsy centre. These include independence, locus of control, self-esteem, the ability to reach one's potential, job security, emotional well being, acceptance in society, and personal growth. In recent years more attention has been paid to issues concerning QoL in patients with epilepsy (Trimble and Dodson, 1994). It is the task of the physician to ensure not only that the seizures are treated as effectively as possible, but that associated QoL issues are addressed. It is important to remember that the principal reason for which seizures are a focus of direct attention in an epilepsy clinic is not their treatment *per se*, but rather the hypothesis that their successful treatment will positively affect the QoL of the patient. The relative importance of controlling seizure frequency is different for every patient because seizures affect the lives of each patient differently (Baker, 1995). For some patients, for example, seizure severity is a much more relevant measure than seizure frequency (Baker *et al.*, 1993; 1994). For others it is the type of seizure that is more important — a patient with drop attacks and with simple partial seizures, for example, may be relatively unconcerned about the frequency of the latter, but have a greatly impaired QoL as a result of the former. While seizures themselves carry clearly defined potential risks with respect to morbidity and mortality (Spitz, 1998), the main focus for the patient is more often the effect of the seizures on how they live, on their psychological well-being and on their family and work environment.

Research into QoL in epilepsy has focused on the need to address the subjective view of the patient. Calman (1984) defined quality of life as 'the gap between a person's expectations and their achievements', which is necessarily a subjective view of the patient and not necessarily indicative of the objective level of their social functioning, nor of the many relevant medical and environmental factors. It may be largely dependent on the patient's current affective state and any psychiatric co-morbidity (McConnell and Snyder, 1998). It is therefore important also to assess the patient's mood state as part of the routine clinical interview, independent of any QoL measures applied. If the clinical assessment of QoL in patients with epilepsy is to take all these various factors into account, it should include not only use of standard questionnaires (either paper-based or computer-assisted), but also narrative evidence obtained from the patient in the course of the clinical interview and from family members or carers.

The assessment of a patient's seizures, including their phenomenology and classification, should always take into account information from the patient, an eye-witness and neurophysiological data. In the same way, the assessment of QoL must take into account psychological, social and clinical data obtained from patients themselves, their social supports and from other 'evidence-based' sources. The role of questionnaires for the assessment of QoL in a clinic setting should not therefore be seen as decreasing the amount of clinician time necessary to treat that patient. QoL questionnaires can best be viewed as a catalyst for a fruitful interview to assist with the overall clinical management of the patient, and in so doing will most probably increase, rather than decrease, the amount of time spent talking with the patient. QoL questionnaires provide a numerical measure of the patient's subjective QoL that can be compared from visit to visit. What is important here is not the overall scores for any given patient, but rather the specific subscores of various QoL indices directly relevant to that patient. QoL questionnaires do not allow the clinician to make evidence-based decisions; nor do they substitute for a clinical history or narrative account. Rather, they represent a subjective means by which the clinician leads the interview in a direction that is relevant to that patient on that day.

It is important to recognise that factors for assessing QoL will be different for children, young and older adults (Jacoby, 1997); that medical and surgical factors themselves play a role in the patient's QoL (Duncan, 1990; Rougier *et al.*, 1997; Vickrey *et al.*, 1993); as do the important effects of family (Hartshorn and Byers, 1994; Hoare, 1988); and social factors (Gibson, 1991; Fisher *et al.*, 1998), amongst the most important of which are likely to be stigma, driving and employment issues (Scambler, 1989). For many patients, particularly those with intractable complex partial seizures (Johannessen *et al.*, 1995), the effects of antiepileptic medications (AEDs) (Wagner *et al.*, 1995) and impaired cognitive functioning (Perrine *et al.*, 1995; Prevey *et al.*, 1998) are the most important issues. The individual factors important for a given individual will vary greatly and need to be considered on an individual basis (Gilliam *et al.*, 1997). Furthermore, they may change for an individual patient over time. It is the interaction behind the patient-physician dialogue that brings all these issues to the forefront in the clinical encounter (Elwyn and Gwyn, 1999). With the advent of managed care and other reforms in the health care industry, it is important that 'quality of life' is not simply a buzzword but rather is viewed as an essential and measurable element in the care of patients with epilepsy.

Paradoxically, a recently developed computer programme was designed to reduce rather than increase the amount of time spent by a neurologist with a patient in an epilepsy clinic! The patient is asked to complete a computer-based questionnaire, the result being an automatically generated clinic visit progress note, for insertion into their medical chart. This programme has been proposed as a cost-effective alternative for routine epilepsy clinic appointments (Doller *et al.*, 1993) as the physician only has to check the progress note for obvious inaccuracies, a mere seven minutes of patient contact time being required to complete this chore. Clearly, however, seven minutes does not allow sufficient time to adequately assess the behavioural, psychosocial, and QoL issues that may impinge on an individual with epilepsy. These complex issues must not be ignored, and seizure frequency should not be adopted as the 'holy grail' in the treatment of epilepsy, in the name of efficiency or cost-effectiveness. The 'seizure-only' treatment of epilepsy represents false economy (McConnell and Snyder, 1998).

It is also salutary to note that in one recently reported study of epilepsy care (Wagner *et al.*, 1997) use of a standardised health status questionnaire, the SF-36, though it lengthened consultation time and provided the clinicians with new information about their patients, apparently had little influence on patient management. Indeed, SF-36 data were considered by the clinicians as useful to patient management in under 10% of their encounters with patients and prompted a change in therapy in only little over 10%. Patients' perceptions also appeared unaffected by the use of their SF-36 results. There were no differences in reported levels of satisfaction with either the doctor or the consultation between patients for whom SF-36 data were available and those for whom they were not.

CURRENTLY AVAILABLE FORMAL ASSESSMENTS OF QoL FOR USE IN THE CLINICAL SETTING

In both medical and surgical settings, there is a growing trend towards monitoring patients' QoL as a measure of treatment outcome, rather than merely limiting evaluation to seizure frequency and severity. The introduction of formal measures of QoL helps to give primacy to the patient's point of view. Epileptology as a whole has lagged far behind other disciplines in using formal QoL assessments as outcome measures and has only 'jumped on the bandwagon' in recent years. Measures of QoL are now becoming more common in trials of AEDs (Cochrane *et al.*, 1998; Kline Leidy *et al.*, 1998) though there are still a paucity of QoL data available on the newer AEDs.

The concept of QoL includes (but is not limited to) the core domains of psychological, social, occupational, and physical well being. Measures of QoL attempt to quantify — from the perspective of the individual with epilepsy — any perceived limitations across these core domains as a result of the epilepsy. The development of psychometric instruments for this particular purpose has a relatively recent history. In 1980, Dodrill and colleagues published the Washington Psychosocial Seizure Inventory (WPSI), which was designed to evaluate the extent of psychosocial dysfunction and specifically standardised on that population (Dodrill *et al.*, 1980 and see Chapter 5 in this volume). The last 12–15 years has seen the development of many other measures of QoL specifically designed for patients with epilepsy (see Chapter 5). The theoretical and practical issues pertaining to the use of such measures have been widely reviewed by Baker, *et al.*, (1994), Fallowfield (1994), Trimble and Dodson (1994), Spencer and Hunt (1996), and Cramer (1994) and are further discussed in other chapters in this volume.

With the development of these new measures, there has followed many cross-sectional and short-term longitudinal studies of QoL in patients with epilepsy (see Chapters 6 and 12). These studies have focused primarily on: the psychosocial outcomes of antiepileptic drug withdrawal (Jacoby *et al.*, 1992); the behavioural and QoL effects of newer AEDs (see review of McConnell and Duncan, 1998); assessment of QoL in community samples of people with epilepsy (Jacoby *et al.*, 1996;); comparison of QoL of specific patient populations (e.g., low versus high seizure frequency: Jacoby *et al.*, 1996; Baker *et al.*, 1997); the assessment of cognitive factors in relation to QoL (Perrine *et al.*, 1995); and the assessment of surgical outcome (Hermann, 1994).

If we accept that quality of life should be assessed not only in the research arena, but also in the day-to-day management of patients with epilepsy, then it is important that easily interpretable measures are available with which to follow the clinical progress of individual patients. Tables 1 and 2 detail a selection of measures developed for research purposes which could also be useful in everyday clinical practice, and their potential limitations.

THE FUTURE

With so many different measures of QoL now available to the clinician, it is important that these tools not be misused. Rather, the validity and

TABLE 1 EPILEPSY-SPECIFIC MEASURES OF QUALITY OF LIFE FOR CLINICAL USE

ASSESSMENT TOOL	COMMENTS ON CLINICAL USE WITH EPILEPSY PATIENTS
EPILEPSY FOUNDATION (USA) CONCERNS INDEX (KLINE LEIDY *ET AL.*, 1998)	NEW TOOL ASSESSING 20 ITEMS SPECIFICALLY CONCERNING PEOPLE WITH EPILEPSY. ITS CLINICAL AND RESEARCH ROLES ARE YET TO BE ELUCIDATED, BUT ITS SIMPLICITY AND SPECIFICITY FOR EPILEPSY SUGGEST THAT IT MAY FIND A ROLE CLINICALLY AS A USEFUL ADJUNCT TO OTHER GENERIC HEALTH RELATED QoL MEASURES.
EPILEPSY SURGERY INVENTORY (ESI-55) (VICKREY *ET AL.*, 1992)	MOST USEFUL QoL MEASURE FOR FOLLOWING PATIENTS CLINICALLY AFTER EPILEPSY SURGERY. IMPORTANT TO OBTAIN BASELINE PRIOR TO SURGERY.
LIVERPOOL QUALITY OF LIFE ASSESSMENT SCALES (BAKER *ET AL.*, 1994)	VERY USEFUL AS CLINICAL MONITOR, ESPECIALLY SEIZURE SEVERITY AND ADVERSE EVENTS PROFILE SCALES; MAJOR ADVANTAGE IN THAT INDIVIDUAL SUBSCALES CAN BE EASILY ADMINISTERED SEPARATELY. ALSO HAS THE ADVANTAGE OF BEING AVAILABLE IN PAPER AND ELECTRONIC FORMATS. MOST WIDELY USED AND VALIDATED QUESTIONNAIRE IN UK AND EUROPE
QUALITY OF LIFE BY CONSTRUCT ANALYSIS (REPERTORY GRID METHOD) (KENDRICK AND TRIMBLE, 1994)	THE ONLY STANDARD EPILEPSY-SPECIFIC QoL MEASURE THAT REQUIRES THE CLINICIAN TO TALK WITH THE PATIENT; EASY TO PERFORM IN A CLINICAL SETTING AS AN EXTENSION OF A CLINICAL INTERVIEW; MORE USEFUL FOR CLINICAL SITUATIONS IN SPECIALIST CENTRES THAN IN THE GENERAL PRACTICE SITUATION.
QUALITY OF LIFE IN EPILEPSY (QOLIE) QUESTIONNAIRES (89, 31 AND 10 ITEM VERSIONS) (DEVINSKY *ET AL.*, 1995)	WIDELY USED IN USA; 10 ITEM SCALE TOO SIMPLISTIC TO BE OF CLINICAL RELEVANCE; 89 ITEM SCALE TOO LONG TO BE OF USE IN A BUSY CLINICAL SETTING; MAJOR ADVANTAGE IS THE USE OF THE SF-36 AS A BASE FOR RESEARCH PURPOSES AND LARGE NUMBER OF SUBSCALES; MAJOR DISADVANTAGE IS THAT THE SPECIFIC SUBSCALE RELATED TO ADVERSE DRUG EFFECTS IS UNFORTUNATELY POOR (3 QUESTIONS ONLY OF LIMITED CLINICAL USE)
WASHINGTON PSYCHOSOCIAL INVENTORY (WPSI) AND THE ADOLESCENT PSYCHOSOCIAL INVENTORY (APSI) (DODRILL *ET AL.*, 1980)	OLDEST OF QoL-RELATED QUESTIONNAIRES WHICH HAS RECENTLY BEEN RESCORED AS A QoL INDEX. MAJOR ADVANTAGE IS THE ADOLESCENT VERSION OF THE FORM AND ITS PREVIOUS WIDESPREAD USE; MAJOR DRAWBACK IS THE LACK OF ATTENTION TO MEDICATION ISSUES AND ADVERSE EFFECTS.

reliability of each measure must be firmly established in the patient population for which their use is intended. There are many different types of epilepsy and many different perspectives on QoL — this must be reflected in future development of these scales.

Future quality of life measures must focus on individual priorities of lifestyle. Currently QoL measures are entirely research focused — looking at the effect of an intervention such as a novel pharmacological treatment on large numbers of patients. This bears no relation to an

TABLE 2 QUALITY OF LIFE MEASURES DEVELOPED FOR OTHER MEDICAL AND PSYCHIATRIC SETTINGS

ASSESSMENT SCALE	COMMENTS ON CLINICAL USE IN PATIENTS WITH EPILEPSY
SF-36 (WARE AND SHERBOURNE 1992)	THIS IS ONE OF THE MORE WIDELY USED QUALITY OF LIFE INDICES AND HAS BEEN VALIDATED ACROSS MANY ILLNESSES. IT HAS THE ADVANTAGE OF EXISTING IN BOTH PAPER AND IN ELECTRONIC FORMS AND FORMS THE BASIS OF THE QOLIE QUESTIONNAIRES.
NOTTINGHAM HEALTH PROFILE (HUNT *ET AL.*, 1981)	INCLUDED WITHIN THE LIVERPOOL ASSESSMENT SCALES AS A VALIDATED MEASURE WITHIN THE DOMAINS OF PHYSICAL FUNCTIONING; CONTAINS MANY QUESTIONS ABOUT PHYSICAL PROBLEMS NOT RELATED TO EPILEPSY
PSYCHOSOCIAL ADJUSTMENT TO ILLNESS SCALE (PAIS) (WILHELMSEN *ET AL.*, 1994)	HAS BEEN VALIDATED IN CANCER PATIENTS, RENAL FAILURE, BURNS AND IN HYPERTENSION BUT NOT IN AN EPILEPSY POPULATION. THE PAIS IS OF POTENTIAL USE IN AN EPILEPSY POPULATION, BUT NEEDS TO BE VALIDATED FOR CLINICAL USE IN PATIENTS WITH EPILEPSY
SICKNESS IMPACT PROFILE (SIP) (BERGNER *ET AL.*, 1976)	A GENERIC 136 ITEM QUESTIONNAIRE MEASURE OF ILLNESS EFFECTS ON RECREATION, WORK, EATING AND SLEEPING, SOCIAL INTERACTION, EMOTIONS AND OTHER FACTORS. IT HAS BEEN USED IN A VARIETY OF ILLNESS SITUATIONS, PARTICULARLY IN MEDICAL SITUATIONS AND IN CHRONIC PAIN. ITS MAIN DRAWBACK IN THIS POPULATION IS THAT IT CONTAINS MANY QUESTIONS ABOUT PHYSICAL PROBLEMS NOT RELATED TO EPILEPSY. IT IS USEFUL FOR COMPARING CHRONIC CONDITIONS. THE SIP HAS, HOWEVER, BEEN STANDARDISED IN ONE STUDY LOOKING AT EPILEPSY SPECIFICALLY (LANGFITT, 1995). THE SCALE IS THEREFORE OF USE AS A RESEARCH TOOL TO COMPARE EPILEPSY WITH OTHER ILLNESSES, BUT NOT AS A CLINICAL TOOL TO MANAGE PATIENTS WITH EPILEPSY.
WHOQOL (SKEVINGTON AND TUCKER 1999)	WORLD HEALTH ORGANISATION QUALITY OF LIFE MEASURE WHICH HAS THE ADVANTAGE OF BEING STANDARDISED IN DIFFERENT COUNTRIES AND IN DIFFERENT CULTURAL SITUATIONS, BUT HAS NOT BEEN LOOKED AT IN EPILEPSY PER SE AS A TARGET POPULATION. USEFUL AS A RESEARCH TOOL TO COMPARE THE EFFECTS OF ILLNESS ACROSS CULTURES, BUT NOT AS A CLINICAL TOOL FOR THE MANAGEMENT OF PATIENTS WITH EPILEPSY.

individual's quality of life and for this reason such measures have largely been ignored by clinicians. This is a real shame given that fiscal pressures in many hospital settings mean the clinician's time with patients is becoming more and more reduced. There is a real opportunity here for taking into account an individual's needs and priorities with respect to QoL and using measures geared to the clinical setting and, hence, to the individual patient. Static paper-and-pencil QoL measures for the masses could even be replaced with dynamic online rating scales, individualised for a given patient and even for a given specific clinical situation. Data warehousing techniques and new network protocols will facilitate a new concept of QoL rating scales and the static pencil and paper test could soon be replaced by tools used by all clinicians on a daily basis which are entirely patient-driven.

The patient's clinician must be willing to pay close attention, on an ongoing basis, to the impact of the patient's seizure disorder on the various aspects of QoL listed above regardless of whether this includes the application of QoL measures. This is best done within the context of a multidisciplinary team. QoL measures should never be an excuse to not speak with a patient. QoL must not become merely a 'buzz-word' for pharmaceutical companies. Speaking with patients enables early detection of social, psychological, and occupational difficulties, and so targeted patient and family education and the early initiation of appropriate behavioural and pharmacological interventions. This is likely to dramatically increase the QoL of the patients with whose care physicians are entrusted.

References

Baker, G.A. (1995) Health-related quality-of-life issues: Optimising patient outcomes. *Neurology* **45** (Suppl. 2), S29-S34.

Baker, G.A., Smith, D.F., Dewey, M., Jacoby, A., Chadwick, D.W. (1993) The initial development of a health-related quality of life model as an outcome measure in epilepsy. *Epilepsy Research* **16**, 65–81.

Baker, G.A., Jacoby, A., Smith, D., Dewey, M., Johnson, A.L., Chadwick, D.W. (1994) Quality of life in epilepsy: The Liverpool initiative. In: Trimble M.R., Dodson W.E. (eds.) *Epilepsy and Quality of Life*. New York: Raven, 135–150.

Baker, G.A., Jacoby, A., Buck, D., Stalgis, C., Monnet., D. (1997) Quality of life of people with epilepsy: A European study. *Epilepsia* **38**, 353–362.

Bergner, M., Bobbitt, R.A., Pollard, W.E. (1976) The sickness impact profile: validation of a health status measure. *Medical Care* **14**, 57–67.

Calman, K.E. (1984) Quality of Life in Cancer Patients — an hypothesis. Journal of Medical Ethics, **10**, 124–127.

Cochrane, H.C., Marson, A.G., Baker, G.A., Chadwick, D.W. (1998) Neuropsychological outcomes in randomised controlled trials of antiepileptic drugs: a systematic review of methodology and reporting standards. *Epilepsia* **39**, 1088–1097.

Cramer, J.A. (1994) Quality of life for people with epilepsy. *Neurological Clinics* 12(1), 1–13.

Devinsky, O., Vickrey, B.G., Cramer, J., Perrine, I.L., Hermann, B., Meador, K., Hays, R.D. (1995) Development of the quality of life in epilepsy inventory. *Epilepsia* **36**, 1080–1104.

Dodrill, C.B., Batzel, L.W., Queisser, H.R., Temkin, N. (1980) An objective method for the assessment of psychological and social problems among epileptics. *Epilepsia* **21**, 123–135.

Doller, H.J., Hostetter, W., Krishnamur, K., Homan, R.W. (1993) Epileptologist's assistant: A cost-effective expert system. *Proceedings of Annual Symposium for Computers in Applied Medical Care,* 384–388.

Duncan, J. (1990) Medical factors affecting quality of life in patients with epilepsy. In: Chadwick, D. (ed.) *Quality of Life and Quality of Care in Epilepsy*: Royal Society of Medicine, Round Table Series No.23. London: RSM, 80–91.

Elwyn, G., Gwyn, R. (1999) *Narrative based medicine:* Stories we hear and stories we tell: analysing talk in clinical practice. *British Medical Journal* **318**, 186–188.

Fallowfield, L (1994) An overview of quality of life measurements. In: Trimble, M.R., Dodson, W.E. (eds.) *Epilepsy and Quality of Life*. New York: Raven Press,49–64.

Fisher, R.S., Parks-Trusz, S.L., Lehman, C. (1998) Social issues in epilepsy. In: Shorvon, S., Dreifuss, F., Fish, D., Thomas, D. (eds.) *The Treatment of Epilepsy* Oxford: Blackwell, 357–369.

Gibson, P.A. (1991) Update on epilepsy: psychosocial issues. *Journal of Clinical Research and Pharmacoepidemiology* **5**, 323–329.

Gilliam, F., Kuzniecky, R., Faught, E., Black, L., Carpenter, G., Schrod, R. (1997) Patient-validated content of epilepsy-specific quality-of-life measurement. *Epilepsia* **38**, 233–236.

Greenhalgh, T. (1999) Narrative based medicine: Narrative based medicine in an evidence based world. *British Medical Journal* **318**, 323–325.

Hartshorn, J.C., Byers, V.L. (1994) Importance of health and family variables related to quality of life in individuals with uncontrolled seizures. *Journal of Neuroscience and Nursing* **26**, 288–297.

Hermann, B.P. (1994) Quality of life after epilepsy surgery. In: Trimble, M.R., Dodson, W.E. (eds.) *Epilepsy and Quality of Life*. New York: Raven Press, 227–248.

Hoare, P. (ed.) (1988) *Epilepsy and the Family: A Medical Symposium on New Approaches to Family Care*. Manchester, UK: Sanofi UK Ltd.

Hunt, S.M., McEwan, J., McKenna, S.P. (1981) *The Nottingham Health Profile: User's Manual.* Edinburgh: University of Edinburgh.

Jacoby, A. (1997) Age-related considerations in quality of life of people with epilepsy. In: Engels, J., Pedley, T.A. (eds.) *Epilepsy: a comprehensive textbook*. New York: Raven Press, 1121–1130.

Jacoby, A., Johnson, A.L., Chadwick, D.W. (1992) Psychosocial outcomes of antiepileptic drug discontinuation. *Epilepsia* 33, 1123–1131.

Jacoby, A., Baker, G.A., Steen, N., Potts, P., Chadwick, D.W. (1996) The clinical course of epilepsy and its psychosocial correlates: findings from a UK community study. *Epilepsia* 37(2), 148–161.

Johannessen, S.I., Gram, L., Sillanpää, M., Tomson, T. (eds.) (1995) *Intractable Epilepsy*. Petersfield, UK: Wrightson Biomedical Publishing Ltd.

Kendrick, A.M., Trimble, M.R. (1994) Repertory grid in the assessment of quality of life in patients with epilepsy: the quality of life assessment schedule. In: Trimble, M.R., Dodson, W.E. (eds.) Epilepsy and quality of life. New York: Raven Press Ltd., 151–164.

Kline Leidy, N., Rentz, A.M., Grace, E.M. (1998) Evaluating health-related quality of life outcomes in clinical trials of antiepileptic drug therapy. *Epilepsia* 39, 965–977.

McConnell, H.W., Duncan, D.A. (1998) Behavioural Effects of Antiepileptic Drugs. In: McConnell H.W., Snyder P.J. (eds.) *Psychiatric Comorbidity in Epilepsy. Basic Mechanisms, Diagnosis, and Treatment.* Washington, D.C.: American Psychiatric Press, Inc., 205–244.

McConnell, H.W., Snyder, P.J. (eds.) (1998) *Psychiatric Comorbidity in Epilepsy. Basic Mechanisms, Diagnosis, and Treatment*. Washington, D.C.: American Psychiatric Press, Inc.

Perrine, K., Hermann, B.P., Meador, K.L., Vickrey, B.G., Cramer, J.A., Hays, R.D., Devinsky, O. (1995) The relationship of neuropsychological functioning to the quality of life in epilepsy. *Archives of Neurology* 52, 997–1003.

Prevey, M.L., Delaney, R.C., Cramer, J.A., Mattson, R.H. (1998) Complex partial and secondarily generalized seizure patients: cognitive functioning prior to treatment with antiepileptic medication. *Epilepsy Research* 30, 1–9.

Rougier, A., Claverie, B., Pedespan, J.M., Marchal, C., Loiseau, P. (1997) Callosotomy for intractable epilepsy: overall outcome. *Journal of Neurosurgical Sciences* 41, 51–57.

Scambler, G. (1989) *Epilepsy* London: Tavistock.

Skevington, S.M., Tucker, C. (1999) Designing response scales for cross-cultural use in health care: data from the development of the UK WHOQOL. *British Journal of Medical Psychology* 72(1), 51–61.

Spencer, S.S., Hunt, P.W. (1996) Quality of life in epilepsy. *Journal of Epilepsy* 9, 3–13.

Spitz, M.C. (1998) Injuries and death as a consequence of seizures in people with epilepsy. *Epilepsia* 39, 904–907.

Trimble, M.R., Dodson, W.E. (eds.) (1994) *Epilepsy and Quality of Life*. New York: Raven Press.

Vickrey, B.G., Hays, R.D., Brook, R.H., Rausch, R. (1992) Reliability and validity of the Katz Adjustment Scales in an epilepsy sample. *Quality of Life Research* 1, 63–72.

Vickrey, B.G., Hays, R.D., Spritzer, K.L. (1993) Methodological issues in quality of life assessment for epilepsy surgery. In: Chadwick D.W., Baker G.A., Jacoby A. (eds.) *Quality of Life and Quality of Care in Epilepsy: Update 1993*. Royal Society of Medicine, Round Table Series No.31. London: RSM, 27–39.

Wagner, A.K., Keller, S.D., Kosinski, M., Baker, G.A., Jacoby, A., Hsu, M.A., Chadwick, D.W., Ware, J.E. (1995) Advances in methods for assessing the impact of epilepsy and antiepileptic drug therapy on patients' health-related quality of life. *Quality of Life Research* 4, 115–134.

Wagner, A.K., Ehrenberg, B.L., Tran, T.A., Bungay, K.M., Cynn, D.J., Rogers, W.H. (1997) Patient-based health status measurement in clinical practice: a study of its impact on epilepsy patients' care. *Quality of Life Research* 6, 329–341.

Ware, J.E., Sherbourne, C.D. (1992) A 36-item short-form health survey (SF-36) I: Conceptual framework and item selection. *Medical Care* 30, 473–483.

Wilhelmsen, I., Bakke, A., Tangen, Haug, T., Endresen, I.M., Berstad, A. (1994) PAIS-SR in a Norwegian material of patients with functional dyspepsia, duodenal ulcer and urinary bladder dysfunction. Clinical validation of the instrument. *Scandinavian Journal of Gastroenterology* 29(7), 611–617.

Chapter 12

USE OF QUALITY OF LIFE ASSESSMENT AS AN OUTCOME MEASURE IN CLINICAL RESEARCH

Gus A. Baker

Historically, in trying to assess whether or not a particular treatment is beneficial, health providers have depended on clinical end points based on anatomical, physiological and biochemical markers. Recently the limits of such measures have been acknowledged, because of their failure to address issues seen by patients themselves as important and relevant to their day to day functioning. As a result there is increasing emphasis on the need to describe the outcomes of treatment in ways that make sense to both health professionals and to patients (Schipper *et al.*, 1996)

In this chapter, I will consider the aims of treatment from the viewpoint of the patient, the health provider, and society as a whole. I will discuss the limitations of the traditional clinical end-point for epilepsy, seizure frequency, in assessing how successfully or otherwise these aims are met; and the application of currently available non-clinical outcome measures as an alternative means of doing so. I will comment on the interpretation of findings from studies which have employed such measures and their implications for the treatment and management of epilepsy; and I will end with a brief discussion of ongoing issues in utilising patient-based outcome measures.

AIMS OF TREATMENT

There is a significant body of evidence from our own and other studies that patients' expectations of their treatment are relatively simple — to be seizure free, or at least have seizures well-controlled, without any medication side-effects. Those patients who achieve such goals are inevitably more likely to report a better quality of life than those who continue to have seizures with or without side-effects (Jacoby *et al.*, 1992; Baker *et al.*, 1997). For patients who, realistically, are unlikely to be rendered seizure free, issues such as reducing the severity of seizures, minimising the side-effects of medication and maximising physical functioning, mental health, and social and role functioning become important targets (Smith *et al.*, 1995).

For healthcare providers, rendering patients seizure-free with minimal medication side-effects and subsequently improving their quality of life is also likely to be seen as the most important target of the management and treatment of epilepsy. However, while freedom from seizures is the ideal, it is not always achievable and patients' experiences of living with their continuing condition, and of its treatment, should be of equal concern. In a situation of limited health care resources, the question of the cost-effectiveness of different available treatments cannot be ignored. The recently licensed antiepileptics (AEDs) are considerably more expensive than the older ones; and healthcare providers are therefore likely to be interested in whether or not they represent good value for money.

For society the targets of treatment can be viewed as those which maximise the ability of the individual with epilepsy to lead an independent and fulfilling life, while minimising the costs in respect of any resource utilisation required in the care of their condition. These costs include: direct medical costs such as hospital care, drugs and investigations and non-medical costs such as residential care; and indirect costs due to loss of economic productivity, including both unemployment and underemployment (Cockerell *et al.*, 1994; Jacoby *et al.*, 1998). Such costs have been shown to be higher for newly diagnosed patients than those with established epilepsy (Cockerell *et al.*, 1994) and for patients with poorly controlled seizures than for those in whom seizures are well-controlled (Jacoby *et al.*, 1998).

In principle, there is no reason why these various treatment targets cannot be compatible, though it has become increasingly clear that patients' own concerns about the impact of their illness often bear little relation to those aspects that preoccupy their clinicians; and, likewise, that their views about what constitutes a good health outcome are not necessarily the same as those of health professionals and policy makers (Guyatt *et al.*, 1993).

LIMITATIONS OF CLINICAL END POINTS

Seizure frequency is the commonest and often used endpoint for the assessment of the efficacy of treatment for epilepsy (Porter, 1986). In antiepileptic drug trials, a good outcome is reported if an individual patient achieves a reduction in seizure frequency of at least 50% without any serious adverse drug effects, though this cut-off has recently been accepted as not particularly satisfactory from the point of view of patients. Consequently, investigators are currently much more likely to express success in terms of the number of patients who achieve a 75% or even a 100% reduction in seizure frequency.

Seizure frequency has also traditionally been regarded as the principal measure of efficacy in the assessment of the outcome of surgery for patients with intractable epilepsy; outcome is usually determined by the proportion of patients rendered seizure free (Rausch and Crandall, 1982). Recently a number of initiatives have led to investigators widening the assessment of the efficacy of surgical intervention to consider other variables including social adjustment, psychological and neuropsychological functioning, as well as the degree to which surgery met the expectations of the individual patient and their family (Vickrey *et al.*, 1992, 1993; Wilson *et al.*, 1998).

There are several reasons why seizure frequency alone is an inadequate measure for assessing the efficacy of treatment for epilepsy, and these include that:

- even a 75% reduction in seizure frequency may not be a therapeutic success, if the patient remains disabled by the seizures
- infrequent but unpredictable seizures or severe (tonic-clonic) seizures can be more disabling than frequent but unpredictable or mild (simple partial) seizures
- double-blind placebo controlled cross-over studies designed to assess the efficacy of novel antiepiletic drug trials have often insufficient power to detect even a 50% reduction in seizure frequency; and if no other measures are used, important information may be ignored
- comparative studies of active drugs often do not detect significant differences in efficacy using assessment of seizure frequency only, possibly because too few variables are considered
- clinical experience dictates the severity of seizures may be equally important to the patients and that anti-epileptic drugs which act by inhibiting seizure spread may influence seizure severity by modifying what the patient experiences during their seizures
- a study that relies on seizure frequency alone may fail to detect any positive or negative psychological or neuropsychological changes directly attributable to the therapy under investigation.

As a response to these limitations, a considerable amount of effort has been given in the last decade to widening the assessment of the efficacy of the management and treatment of epilepsy. This has included the development of measures designed to address the specific issue of seizure severity (Mattson *et al.*, 1985; Baker *et al.*,1991,1998; Duncan and Sander, 1991) and of quality of life measures aimed at assessing the wider effects of the management and treatment of epilepsy (Trimble and Dodson, 1994).

CURRENT INITIATIVES IN ASSESSMENT

Measures of Seizure Severity

With regard to the former, there are three documented initiatives, one of which, the Liverpool Seizure Severity Scale (LSSS) has already been described in detail earlier in this volume (see Chapter 5). The LSSS was designed to be completed by patients themselves, as a means of documenting their perceptions of the ictal and post-ictal effects of seizures, and of seizure control. It was developed initially to assess the effects of lamotrigine in a double blind placebo controlled cross-over study, but has been used in many other antiepileptic drug trials subsequently. Recent modifications to the LSSS were directed at criticisms that patients who experience more than one seizure type find themselves in difficulty when asked to complete it. In the modified version, they are asked to complete the scale both for their most severe and least severe seizures. There is also a carers' version of the LSSS, for patients unable to complete it for themselves because of physical or cognitive problems (Baker *et al.*, 1998).

The other two initiatives in this group involve assessments designed to be completed by clinicians rather than patients; though one, the National Hospital Severity Scale (NHSS), has subsequently been modified to make it suitable for patient completion (Duncan and Sander, 1991). The NHSS is an 11 item scale, incorporating a weighting system which produces scores for different seizure types, according to the frequency of the occurrence of a particular feature of the attack. Though evidence of its validity and reliability has been reported by the authors, evidence of its sensitivity has yet to documented.

The third initiative is the Veterans Administration Composite Rating Scale (Mattson and Cramer, 1985), generally regarded as the first real attempt to measure seizure severity. Its authors developed the scale with the intention of quantifying the frequency and severity of seizures and the systemic, neurotoxic and behavioural effects of antiepileptic drugs. Mattson and colleagues (1985) describe four major components of the scale, which includes a seizure rating based on the frequency and severity of the seizures, modified by the functional impairment caused by them and by the presence of sub-optimal blood serum levels. Scores

TABLE 1 ITEMS COMMON TO THE THREE SEIZURE SEVERITY SCALES

ITEM		ITEM	
1	SEIZURE TYPE	7	PREDICTION OF SEIZURES
2	SEIZURE DURATION	8	STOPPING SEIZURES
3	POST-ICTAL EVENTS AND DURATION	9	TONGUE BITING AND INCONTINENCE
4	AUTOMATISMS	10	OTHER INJURIES
5	SEIZURE CLUSTERS	11	PRECIPITATING FACTORS
6	CYCLIC AND DIURNAL PATTERNS	12	RECOVERY TIME

on all four components are compared to produce a composite score. Unfortunately evidence of reliability and validity is limited and the complexity of the scale is such that it is time consuming to administer and difficult to interpret (Smith *et al.,* 1995).

Table 1 lists items common to the various seizure severity scales but not exclusive to any one. While there is some agreement between the authors of these scales as to what constitutes seizure severity, there is also some disagreement as to the boundaries of measurement.

Quality of life measures

The main approaches to quality of life outcome assessment in epilepsy have been described in detail in Chapter 5 of this volume and so will not be repeated here. In summary, however, they may be categorised as: those that have involved the development of an entirely novel QoL measure, such as the WPSI (Dodrill *et al.,* 1980) or the Social Effects Scale (Chaplin *et al.,* 1990); those that have involved use of a previously developed generic profile with customised additions, such as the Epilepsy Surgery Inventory (Vickrey *et al.,* 1992, 1993) or the QOLIE-89 (Devinsky *et al.,* 1995); those that involve use of a battery of previously validated scales addressing specific QoL domains together with additional disease-specific questions, such as in the Liverpool QoL Battery (Jacoby, 1992; Baker *et al.,* 1999); and, finally, the patient-generated approach adopted by Kendrick and Trimble (1994).

A number of more recent initiatives are worth drawing to the reader's attention, the first of which involves the work of the group based in Liverpool, of which this writer is a part. The original Liverpool QoL Battery was developed for application in studies involving patients with established epilepsy. Acknowledging that the issues of importance might differ for different patient groups, the Group has gone on to develop NEWQoL, the Quality of Life in Newly Diagnosed Epilepsy Instrument.

Inevitably there is considerable overlap between NEWQoL and the original battery, but use of the word 'epilepsy' has been avoided following qualitative work that illustrated clearly that many people with new-onset seizures do not necessarily regard themselves as having epilepsy. No measure of seizure severity is included in NEWQoL, since patients experiencing few seizures were found to have difficulty with this concept. Changed self-concept, ambition limitations and self-perceived change in health were all identified as important domains for patients with recent onset seizures, so NEWQoL incorporates questions on all of these. An independent assessment of the psychometric properties of NEWQoL (Abetz *et al.,* in press) concludes that scaling assumptions were generally met satisfactorily and it represents a potentially useful tool to assess functioning and well-being in this particular group of people with epilepsy.

Another measure not covered earlier, also the work of the Liverpool Group, is ELDQoL, the Epilepsy and Learning Disability QoL Questionnaire (Baker *et al.,* 1996; Jacoby *et al.,* 1996). Since those with accompanying learning disability represent a sub-group of patients with epilepsy in whom measuring QoL is particularly complex, ELDQoL was developed from first principles (Baker *et al.,* 1994) and comprises a 66-item instrument, with subscales to assess seizure severity (14 items), drug-related side effects (18 items), mood (14 items) and behaviour (9 items), as well as single items relating to experience of seizure-related injuries, health, and QoL overall. The measure is intended for completion by a parent or other informal carer. ELDQoL has been shown to have good content and construct validity, is reliable and is acceptable to carers. There is also some evidence, from a recent randomised study, of its responsiveness to change (Jacoby *et al.,* 1996).

One other measure of interest here is the Side-Effect and Life Satisfaction Scale (SEALS, Gilham *et al.,* 1996). Though somewhat limited as a measure of QoL, its authors claim that the SEALS Inventory fills a gap, particularly in the context of clinical trials, for 'a more compact, more behaviourally orientated scale' than those discussed above. SEALS is a 50-item self-report questionnaire originally developed by Brown and Tomlinson (1982) and further standardised by Gilham and her colleagues (1996). Principal components analysis at the stage of its initial development suggested an underlying scale structure of five factors which the authors called 'mood and irritability', 'general cognitive difficulties', 'satisfaction', 'fatigue' and 'interpersonal'. Five factors were also produced in the later validation study by Gilham, though they do not match the original five, being identified in the second analysis as 'cognition', 'dysphoria', 'temper', 'tiredness' and 'worry'. The authors admit that further work is required to confirm that it is reasonable to adopt the more recent structure. However, SEALS does appear clinically sensitive, with patients experiencing chronic intractable seizures having significantly poorer scores on two of the five factors — cognition and dysphoria — than patients who were newly diagnosed, and better scores on worry.

REPORTED USE OF QoL ASSESSMENTS AS OUTCOMES IN CLINICAL TRIALS

Recently, there has been considerable emphasis on the use of patient-based measures, including QoL, as indicators of outcome in clinical trials of new pharmacological therapies for epilepsy. A selection of some of the epilepsy specific QoL measures developed for use in clinical trials are presented in Table 2.

The first trial of a novel antiepileptic to employ such an approach was that by Smith *et al.*, (1993), which examined the efficacy of lamotrigine as add-on treatment in adults with intractable epilepsy. The battery of QoL measures applied in the study has been described earlier in this volume. Sixty-one subjects completed the battery on entry to the trial and at the end of the treatment. Small but significant differences in patients' perceptions of the severity of their seizures were demonstrated between those on lamotrigine and those not; in addition, patients treated with lamotrigine reported significant improvements in affect balance and sense of mastery compared to those on placebo. An interesting finding from the study was that of the 61 patients completing the study, 41 elected to continue taking lamotrigine after the end of the trial, despite the fact that only 10 had achieved a greater than 50% reduction in seizure frequency — the then standard marker of efficacy in such trials. A comparison of those opting to continue with those not opting to do so revealed that the former had a significantly better physical and psychological profile during the active phase of the trial. These results also confirmed anecdotal evidence of the mood-enhancing effect of the active compound and its ability to reduce seizure severity.

A limited QoL evaluation was carried out by Dodrill *et al.*, (1996) as part of a trial of another novel antiepileptic, gabapentin. Adult patients with medically refractory partial seizures were randomised to one of three different dosing regimens (600, 1,200 or 2,400mg/day) added initially to other AED medication. Concurrent AEDs were then tapered over a 10-week period, until gabapentin monotherapy was achieved in

TABLE 2 A SELECTION OF EPILEPSY SPECIFIC QoL MEASURES DESIGNED FOR CLINICAL TRIALS

TITLE	AUTHORS	NUMBER OF ITEMS	SCORING	RELIABILITY	VALIDITY	SENSITIVITY	USES
ELDQoL	BAKER AND JACOBY	66	LIKERT	INTERNAL CONSISTENCY TEST/RETEST	CONTENT, FACE AND CONSTRUCT	ESTABLISHED IN ONE STUDY	CLINICAL TRIALS
LIVERPOOL QoL BATTERY	BAKER *ET AL.*	VARIABLE	GENERALLY LIKERT	INTERNAL CONSISTENCY TEST/RETEST	CONTENT, FACE AND CONSTRUCT	ESTABLISHED IN ONE STUDY	CLINICAL PRACTICE/ CLINICAL TRIALS
NEWQoL	JACOBY AND BAKER	33	LIKERT	INTERNAL CONSISTENCY, TEST/RETEST	CONTENT, FACE AND CONSTRUCT	CURRENTLY BEING ASSESSED	CLINICAL TRIALS
QUALITY OF LIFE IN EPILEPSY INVENTORY	THE QOLIE GROUP	89, 31 & 10	LIKERT	INTERNAL CONSISTENCY, TEST/RETEST	CONTENT, FACE AND CONSTRUCT	CURRENTLY BEING ASSESSED	CLINICAL PRACTICE/ CLINICAL TRIALS
SEALS	GILLHAM *ET AL.*	100	LIKERT	INTERNAL CONSISTENCY, TEST/RETEST	CONTENT, FACE AND CONSTRUCT	ESTABLISHED IN A SINGLE CLINICAL TRIAL	CLINICAL TRIALS
WASHINGTON PSYCHOSOCIAL SEIZURE INVENTORY	DODRILL *ET AL.*	132	DICHOTO- MOUS	INTERNAL CONSISTENCY, TEST/RETEST	CONTENT, FACE AND CONSTRUCT	ESTABLISHED IN SEVERAL STUDIES	CLINICAL PRACTICE/ CLINICAL TRIALS

as many cases as possible. QoL was assessed prior to randomisation and at study exit, the measures employed being the Profile of Mood States, the WPSI and a visual analogue mood rating scale. In addition, patients underwent a range of neuropsychological tests. Two hundred and one patients completed the QoL testing. Patients treated with gabapentin showed statistically significant improvements, independent of any reduction in seizure frequency, and more favourable changes were noted when two rather than one concurrent AED was discontinued.

The SEALS Inventory has been used to evaluate lamotrigine and carbamazepine monotherapy in the treatment of 256 patients with newly diagnosed epilepsy (Gilham *et al.*, 1996). SEALS was completed at baseline and subsequent assessment points during the double-blind study. For each of the five SEALS sub-scales, patients on lamotrigine showed a significantly greater change in a positive direction than those on carbamazepine, after controlling for baseline seizure frequency, change in seizure frequency, age and gender.

Within the framework of clinical trials, a group of patients for whom QoL assessments may be particularly relevant is those with complex epilepsies, in whom complete seizure freedom or even a substantial reduction in seizure frequency is unlikely. A recent double-blind study of lamotrigine as add-on therapy for patients with a clinical diagnosis of the Lennox-Gastaut Syndrome included the ELDQoL (see above) to assess their quality of life. Based on the responses of their main carers, who completed the questionnaire at baseline and end of treatment, there were improvements in seizure severity and in the rate of seizure-related injuries for the treated patients compared to those on placebo, though the differences were not statistically significant; and there was a marked improvement in mood for treated patients. Carers were also asked to make a retrospective rating, at the end of the trial, of 12 different aspects of the patient's functioning and to indicate whether, since entry to the study, there had been an improvement, no change or a deterioration. The numbers improving were high for all 12 aspects in the group on lamotrigine, compared to controls, the differences being statistically significant for severity of attacks and sociability.

Because of interest in the potential added value of QoL assessments, several clinical trials of novel antiepileptics are currently under way which incorporate them as secondary measures of outcome. At present, only two countries, Australia and Canada, require pharmacoeconomic data before a new drug can be registered and QoL data are seen as supportive only. Nonetheless, since the pharmaceutical companies start from the premise that their drug is better than the others available and it is incumbent on them to produce evidence to that effect, interest in QoL outcomes seems unlikely to fade rapidly.

The UK Medical Research Council study of antiepileptic drug withdrawal (AEDWS Group, 1991; Jacoby *et al.,* 1992) was a clinical trial that concerned itself with evaluating two alternative management strategies, rather than with the assessment of a specific pharmacological agent. It was the first published trial in epilepsy to incorporate a comprehensive QoL assessment, an early version of the Liverpool battery. The aim of the study was to compare slow withdrawal versus continuation of AEDs in patients whose epilepsy was in remission. The primary clinical outcome measure for the study was the percentage of patients surviving seizure-free under the two policies; QoL was assessed as a secondary outcome, using a battery which included the Nottingham Health Profile (Hunt *et al.,* 1981), the Affect-Balance Scale (Bradburn, 1969), measures of self-esteem (Rosenberg, 1965), Mastery (Pearlin and Schooler, 1978) and perceived stigma (Jacoby, 1994), a social activities index (Anderson, 1992) and a global QoL item (Andrews and Withey, 1976). Single items were also included about employment status and social relationships.

Results of this pragmatic trial showed that the risk of a seizure recurrence associated with the policy of slow withdrawal was substantial compared to that of continuing on AED medication — so the conclusion from the clinical data alone was that continuation was to be preferred. To explore the psychosocial outcomes of the two policies, a series of regression models were fitted to the data which showed that, in contrast, the effect of randomisation to AED withdrawal was small and non-significant across all the QoL domains considered. The models highlighted that this lack of QoL risk was attributable to the fact that the QoL costs of having a seizure were balanced by similar QoL costs of taking AEDs, the latter being ones often under-estimated by clinicians but of considerable importance from the point of view of patients.

THE ISSUE OF STANDARDISATION

One issue with which QoL researchers in epilepsy, as in other disease areas, must grapple is that of the standardisation of assessments. The current lack of standardisation is made amply apparent by results of a recent systematic review, undertaken by this author and his colleagues, of methodology and use of quality of life and behavioural outcome measures in randomised controlled trials (RCTs) of antiepileptic drugs

TABLE 3 QoL AND BEHAVIOURAL TESTS USED IN MORE THAN THREE RCTs

NAME OF MEASURE	NUMBER OF CLINICAL TRIALS
MINNESTOTA MULTIPHASIC PERSONALITY INVENTORY	9
WASHINGTON PSYCHOSOCIAL SEIZURE INVENTORY	8
PROFILE OF MOOD STATES	6
HOSPITAL ANXIETY AND DEPRESSION SCALE	4
BECK DEPRESSION INVENTORY	3
CONNOR'S TEACHER SCALE	3
CONNOR'S PARENT SCALE	3
NEUROTOXICITY RATING SCALE	3

in patients with epilepsy. Trial reports were found by searching Medline and PsychLit 1966–1998 and hand-searching key journals. Inclusion and exclusion criteria were applied, and methodological, subject and treatment data and the quality of life and behavioural measures applied were extracted, using a standard proforma. In the initial analysis 51 reports met the inclusion criteria. Reporting of basic methodological issues such as randomisation method was poor. There has been no uniform approach to the use of behavioural or quality of life outcome measures or justification for their selection. A substantial number of different tests have been used (see Table 3).

In all, 58 measures were identified from 51 trials, ranging in focus across personality testing and assessment of emotional well-being, behaviour, health and overall QoL. The Minnesota Multiphasic Personality Inventory was the most commonly used, followed by WPSI and POMS. Only 10 measures in 17 trials were shown to be sensitive to change (see Table 4).

Poor reporting of methods and use of a plethora of measures create great difficulties for anyone wishing to make sense of currently available clinical trial data relating to outcome. If we are better to understand the QoL and behavioural outcomes of RCTs of antiepileptics, we need a much more rational and consistent approach to their application.

CONTINUING ISSUES IN THE USE OF OUTCOME MEASURES IN EPILEPSY

As I hope I have shown, there is an increasing number of non-clinical measures for use in trials of treatment for epilepsy, though at this stage in the development game some are better validated than others. It may be that ultimately certain measures come to be seen as 'gold standard' ones. Recently, an attempt to identify potentially useful measures was made by a group of experts (Trimble and Dodson, 1994) who rated on

TABLE 4 MEASURES SHOWN TO BE SENSITIVE TO CHANGE

NAME OF MEASURE	NUMBER OF CLINICAL TRIALS	SENSITIVITY
MINNESTOTA MULTIPHASIC PERSONALITY INVENTORY	9	5
WASHINGTON PSYCHOSOCIAL SEIZURE INVENTORY	8	1
PROFILE OF MOOD STATES	6	2
HOSPITAL ANXIETY AND DEPRESSION SCALE	4	1
BECK DEPRESSION INVENTORY	3	1
CONNOR'S TEACHER SCALE	3	2
CONNOR'S PARENT SCALE	3	1
NEUROTOXICITY RATING SCALE	3	1
MIDDLESEX HOSPITAL QUESTIONNAIRE	2	2
LIVERPOOL QoL BATTERY	1	1

five different dimensions eleven generic and epilepsy-specific QoL instruments. In line with current thinking on QoL assessment, the raters concluded that scales that were 'essentially 'subjective', driven by patients' needs and assessing items selected by patients, would seem to be preferred.' As further information becomes available, it will be important to review and revise this initial list, but the rationale for it will, I think, have considerable appeal for non-experts in the outcomes field. Some degree of consensus about which are the most useful QoL measures for epilepsy will also allow for standardisation across studies, which in turn may facilitate between-trial comparisons of QoL data and meta-analyses of different study results.

There are two other key issues for the future which should be highlighted here, the first being that of the cross-cultural applicability of QoL measures. Almost all the currently available QoL measures were developed either in the UK or the US, requiring cross-cultural validation if they are to be employed elsewhere. To date, cross-cultural adaptation of QoL measures has largely been limited to forward-backward translation, a process with which a number of problems have been identified (Leplege and Verdier, 1995). True validation involves technical and conceptual, as well as linguistic issues (Meadows *et al.*, 1995). To judge the suitability of a measure for use across cultures, four broad criteria have been proposed (Flaherty *et al.*, 1988): *content equivalence*, which refers to the relevance of each item in a QoL measure to all cultures concerned; *semantic equivalence*, which concerns the retention of the meaning rather than literal translation of item wording; *conceptual equivalence*, which concerns the question of whether or not there are universal meanings attached to terms fundamental to subjective QoL assessment; and *technical equivalence*, which relates to whether methods of data collection differentially affect results in different cultures. Given that many clinical trials in epilepsy are now international in focus, such scientific rigour is increasingly accepted as a basic requirement for their use.

The other issue which needs to be further addressed is the real relevance of changes in QoL scores. The importance of the concept of the 'minimally important difference'(Jaeschke *et al.*, 1989) is emphasised by results from recent clinical trials of novel treatments. As yet, there is little evidence available about the meaningfulness to patients or health providers of the statistically significant changes on QoL dimensions detected in reported clinical trials. Relevant information will accrue over time as results from further trials enter the public domain and so allow QoL profiles associated with particular clinical features of epilepsy and particular treatments or management strategies to be more precisely defined.

CONCLUSIONS

Quality of life assessment is a relevant measure of efficacy in clinical trials. In epilepsy its use is spreading and its importance as an indicator of the benefits of treatment is being increasingly recognised. While there remains a paucity of studies that have utilised QoL measures, in those where they have been applied valuable additional information has been obtained. Unfortunately, however, the application of QoL measures has not been uniform and a standardised approach has yet to be achieved. Further, researchers continue to develop new tools rather than relying on ones that already exist. This has contributed to a situation where few measures have been well validated and used extensively, making it difficult to make sense of information about the outcomes of treatment for epilepsy. This is in the interests of neither clinicians nor their patients. Realistically, it is unlikely that consensus will be reached on a 'gold standard' QoL measure or set of measures. This should not prevent those measures that have been well validated being applied routinely in a uniform way.

References

Abetz, L., Jacoby, A., Baker, G.A., McNulty, P. (2000) Patient-based assessments of QoL in newly diagnosed epilepsy patients: validation of the NEWQOL. *Epilepsia*, in press.

Anderson, R. (1992) The aftermath of stroke. Cambridge: Cambridge University Press.

Andrews, F.M., Withey, S.B. (1976) *Social indicators of well-being: Americans' perceptions of life quality*. New York: Plenum Press.

Antiepileptic Drug Withdrawal Study Group (1991) A randomised study of antiepileptic drug withdrawal in patients in remission of epilepsy. *The Lancet* 337, 1175–80.

Baker, G.A., Jacoby, A., Berney, T., Dewey, M., Hosking, G., Forret, E., Chadwick, D.W. (1994) Development of an instrument to assess quality of life in children with epilepsy and learning disability. (Abstract) *Epilepsia* 35(Supp 7), 47.

Baker, G.A., Jacoby, A., Buck, D., Stalgis, C., Monnet, D. (1997) Quality of life of people with epilepsy: a European study. *Epilepsia* **38**, 353–362.

Baker, G.A., Jacoby, A., Smith, D., Dewey, M., Johnson, A.L., Chadwick, D.W. (1994) Quality of life in epilepsy: the Liverpool initiative. In: Trimble, M.R., Dodson, W.E. *Epilepsy and Quality of Life*. New York: Raven Press, 15–150.

Baker, G.A., Smith, D.F., Dewey, M., Morrow, J., Crawford, P.M., Chadwick, D.W. (1991)The development of a seizure severity scale as an outcome measure in epilepsy. *Epilepsy Research* **8**, 245–251.

Baker, G.A., Smith, D.F., Jacoby, A., Chadwick, D.W. (1998) Seizure severity scale revised. *Seizure* 7(3), 201–206.

Bradburn, N.M. (1969) *The structure of psychological well-being*. Chicago: Aldine.

Brown, S.W., Thomlinson, L.L. (1982) Anticonvulsant side effects: a self-report questionnaire for use in community surveys. *British Journal of General Practice* **18**, 147.

Chaplin, J.E., Yepez, R., Shorvon, S., Floyd, M. (1990) A quantitative approach to measuring the social effects of epilepsy. *Neuroepidemiology* **9**, 151–158.

Cockerell, O.C., Hart, Y.M., Sander, J.W.A.S., Shorvon, S.D. (1994) The cost of epilepsy in the United Kingdom: an estimation based on the results of two population-based studies. *Epilepsy Research* **18**, 249–260.

Devinsky, O., Vickrey, B.G., Cramer, J., Perrine, K., Hermann, B., Meador, K., Hays, R.D. (1995) Development of the quality of life in epilepsy inventory. *Epilepsia* **36**, 1089–1104.

Dodrill, C.B., Arnett, J.L., Hayes, A.G., Garofalo, E.A., Griner, M.J. (1996) Gabapentin monotherapy: quality of life evaluation during a double-blind, multicenter study in patients with medically refractory partial seizures. *Epilepsia* **37**, S10.

Dodrill, C.B., Batzel, L.W., Queisser, H.R., Temkin, N. (1980) An objective method for the assessment of psychological and social problems among epileptics. *Epilepsia* **21**, 123–135.

Duncan, J., Sander, J.W.A.S. (1991) The Chalfont seizure severity scale *Journal of Neurology, Neurosurgery and Psychiatry* **54**, 873–876.

Flaherty, J.A., Moises Gaviria, F., Pathak, D. *et al.* (1988) Developing instruments for cross-cultural psychiatric research. *Journal of Nervous and Mental Diseases* **176**, 257–262.

Gilham, R., Baker, G., Thompson, P., Birbeck, K., McGuire, A., Tomlinson, L., Eckersley, L. (1996) Standardisation of a self-report questionnaire for use in evaluating cognitive, affective and behavioural side effects of anti-epileptic drug treatments. *Epilepsy Research* **24**, 47–55.

Guyatt, G., Feeny, D.H., Patrick, D.L. (1993) Measuring health-related quality of life. *Annals of Internal Medicine* **118**, 622–629.

Hunt, S., McEwan, J., McKenna, S.P. (1981) *The Nottingham Health Profile: Users' Manual*. Edinburgh: University of Edinburgh.

Jacoby, A. (1994) Felt versus enacted stigma: a concept revisited. Social Science and Medicine 38, 261–274.

Jacoby, A., Baker, G., Bryant-Comstock, L., Phillips, S., Bamford, C. (1996) Lamotrigine add-on therapy is associated with improvement in mood in patients with severe epilepsy. *Epilepsia* **37**, S202.

Jacoby, A., Johnson, A.L., Chadwick, D.W.(1992) Psychosocial outcomes of antiepileptic drug discontinuation. *Epilepsia* **33**, 6, 1123–1131.

Jacoby, A. (1992) Epilepsy and the quality of everyday life. Findings from a study of people with well-controlled epilepsy. *Social Science and Medicine* **43** (6), 657–666.

Jacoby, A., Buck, D., Baker, G.A., McNamee, P., Graham Jones, S., Chadwick, D.W. (1998) Uptake and costs of care for epilepsy: Findings from a U.K. regional study. *Epilepsia*, **39** (7), 776–786.

Jaeschke, R., Singer, J., Guyatt, G. (1989) Measurements of health status: ascertaining the minimally important difference. *Controlled Clinical Trials* **10**, 407–415.

Kendrick, A.M., Trimble, M.R. (1994) Repertory grid in the assessment of quality of life in patients with epilepsy: The quality of life assessment schedule. In: Trimble M.R., Dodson, W.E. *Epilepsy and quality of life*. New York: Raven Press Ltd, 151–164.

Leplege, A., Verdier, A. (1995) *The adaptation of health status measures: methodological aspects of the translation process*. Oxford: Rapid Communications.

Mattson, R.H., Cramer, J.A., Collins, J.F., Smith, D.B., Delgado-Esqueta, A.V., Browne, T.R., Williamson, P.D. (1985) Comparison of carbamazepine, phenobarbitol, phenytoin and primidone in partial and secondarily generalised tonic-clonic seizures. *New England Journal of Medicine* **313**, 145–151.

Meadows, K., Bentzen, N., Touw-Otten, F. (1995) Cross-cultural issues: an outline of the important principles in establishing cross-cultural validity in health outcome measurement. In: Hutchinson A., Bentzen, N., Konig-Zahn, C. *Cross cultural health outcome assessment: a user's guide*. European Research Group on Health Outcomes (ERGHO), Groningen, The Netherlands, 34–40.

Pearlin, L., Schooler, C. (1978) The structure of coping. *Journal of Health and Social Behaviour* **19**, 2–21.

Porter, R.J. (1986) Antiepileptic drugs: efficacy and inadequacy. In: Meldrum, B.S., Porter, R.J. (eds.) *New anti-convulsant drugs. Current problems in epilepsy* Vol 4. London: John Libbey, 3–16.

Rausch, R., Crandall, P.H. (1982) Psychological status related to surgical control of temporal lobe seizures. *Epilepsia* **23**, 191–202.

Rosenberg, M. (1965) *Society and the Adolescent Self-image*. Princeton: Princeton University Press.

Schipper, H., Clinch, J., Olweny, C.L.M. (1996) Quality of life studies: definitional and conceptual issues. In Spilker, B. *Quality of life and pharmacoeconomics in clinical trials*. 2nd ed. New York: Lippincott Raven, 11–24.

Smith, D.F., Baker, G.A., Davies, G., Dewey, M., Chadwick, D.W. (1993) Outcomes of add-on treatment with Lamotrigine in partial epilepsy. *Epilepsia* **34**, 312–322.

Smith, D.F., Baker, G.A., Jacoby, A., Chadwick, D.W. (1995) The contributions of the measurement of seizure severity to quality of life research. *Quality of Life Research* **4**, 143–158.

Trimble, M.R., Dodson, W.E. (1994) *Epilepsy and quality of life*. New York: Raven Press Ltd.

Vickrey, B.G., Hays, R.D., Graber, J., Rausch, R., Engel, J., Brook, R.H. (1992) A health-related quality of life instrument for patients evaluated for epilepsy surgery. *Medical Care* **30** (4), 299–319.

Vickrey, B.G., Hays, R.D., Spritzer, K.L. (1993) Methodological issues in QOL assessment for epilepsy surgery. In: Chadwick, D.W., Baker, G.A., Jacoby, A. *Quality of life and quality of care in epilepsy*: Update 1993. London: Royal Society for Medicine, 27–39.

Wilson, S.J., Saling, M.M., Kincade, P., Bladin, P.F. (1998) Patients' expectations of temporal lobe surgery. *Epilepsia* **39**(2), 167–174.

Chapter 13

QUALITY OF LIFE AS AN OUTCOME MEASURE: A PHARMACEUTICAL INDUSTRY PERSPECTIVE

Pauline McNulty, Stefan K.F. Schawabe and Dennis D. Gagnon

Before the 1990s there was a limited choice of drug treatments available for patients with epilepsy. Carbamazepine and phenytoin were used mainly for treating patients with partial seizures, while sodium valproate was the drug of choice for primary generalized epilepsies. Other treatment options included phenobarbital, primidone, ethosuximide and the benzodiazepines.

All of these established (or traditional) antiepileptic drugs (AEDs) — though effective — have significant disadvantages associated with their use. Two of the main first-line agents, carbamazepine and valproate, are still the most widely prescribed drugs today. Carbamazepine can, however, cause double vision, dizziness, and nausea (Brodie and Dichter, 1996) as well as a range of idiosyncratic reactions, the most common being skin rash (Anon, 1989). This drug can also induce its own metabolism (Macphee *et al.*, 1987) and interacts with many other drugs, including the oral contraceptive pill (Brodie, 1992). Common adverse reactions associated with valproate include dose-related tremor, weight gain, and alopecia (Brodie and Dichter, 1996). More rarely, valproate has been associated with fatal cases of liver failure (Powell-Jackson, 1984). Both drugs are teratogenic and have been associated with foetal defects, such as spina bifida. Of the other AEDs, phenytoin has a narrow therapeutic window and careful monitoring of plasma drug concentrations is required, while phenobarbital can cause sedation and depression in adults and hyperactivity and aggression in children, and tolerance can develop with continued use of the benzodiazepines. Most of the traditional AEDs can also impair cognition, affecting memory, performance, and mood (Kälviäinen *et al.*, 1996).

In addition to the systemic and cognitive adverse effects experienced by at least half of patients receiving traditional AEDs (Schmidt, 1982; Pellock, 1994), administration of these drugs can be further complicated by their often complex pharmacokinetic and pharmacodynamic properties.

DEVELOPMENT OF THE NEW ANTIEPILEPTIC

Clinical Development of New AEDs

Most of the traditional AEDs were discovered by chance rather than design, and most reached the market without undergoing well-controlled, double-blind, randomised clinical trials. After a long period of inactivity in drug development in this field, the 1990s saw a flurry of new treatment options. The discovery of new AEDs, developed primarily to be better tolerated and less toxic than the traditional therapies, has been approached in three ways (Sabers and Gram, 1996):

- from screening programmes of potential antiepileptic compounds
- modification of the chemical structure of known AEDs
- rational drug development based on better understanding of the basic pathophysiology of epilepsy and the basic mechanisms of drug activity.

Between 1993 and 1996, three new AEDs, felbamate, lamotrigine, and gabapentin, were approved for use in the USA, the first such drugs to be approved since valproate in 1978 (Dichter and Brodie, 1996). These three new AEDs, and others, such as topiramate, tiagabine, and vigabatrin, are now in use throughout the world. The United States Food and Drug Administration (FDA) has deemed zonisamide to be approvable and others, including oxcarbazepine and levetiracetam, are currently under consideration.

The development of new AEDs has been accompanied by the more stringent evaluations of efficacy and safety that are now required by the various international regulatory agencies before marketing approval is granted. However, the study of new AEDs is a complex undertaking. In many other therapeutic areas, a patient entering a clinical trial is randomised to treatment with the new or standard therapy or a placebo. The dangers associated with potential undertreatment or inappropriate treatment of epilepsy often make this approach ethically unacceptable.

Consequently, new AEDs are studied first in placebo-controlled, add-on trials in patients whose seizures do not respond to currently available treatments (Pledger and Schmidt, 1994). These patients can experience many seizures per day (usually partial seizures with or without secondarily generalized seizures) and are among the most difficult patients to treat. The new AED or placebo is added to the patient's existing medication regimen and the change in seizure frequency resulting from the new AED is measured and compared with placebo.

The chances of a patient becoming seizure-free in this setting are remote. Thus, other primary measures of efficacy are chosen, such as the percentage reduction in seizure rate or, sometimes, the reduction from baseline in seizure count of at least 50% (seizures are usually monitored over baseline and treatment periods, each lasting from 8 to 12 weeks). Additional objective measures of efficacy can include, for example, a reduction of 75% or more in seizures from baseline and the number of seizure-free days. Non-efficacy measures may include physician-rating scores and other clinical benefits, such as greater tolerability, improved safety and better functional capacity and quality of life measures.

This approach to evaluating new AEDs in adjunctive polytherapy trials has been seen as insensitive because interactions with concomitant treatments may mask the true efficacy of a new compound. Furthermore, the toxicity of a new AED may be overestimated, especially if the toxicity of the new drug is similar or additive to that of the concomitant therapy (Sabers and Gram, 1996). However, add-on trials have been able to demonstrate the efficacy of most of the newer AEDs (Pledger and Schmidt, 1994).

AEDs that are effective in the adjunctive setting often go on to be developed as monotherapy for newly-diagnosed patients. Subsequent clinical development can be extended to special patient populations, such as children, or to distinct epilepsy syndromes (Kramer *et al.*, 1993).

Clinical investigations of new AEDs as monotherapy can be undertaken by direct comparison with an established AED, either in a parallel-group or cross-over study design. Such trials are likely to show equivalent efficacy between the new and the traditional AED. A primary endpoint in this setting may be the time to first seizure after a specified period of treatment (Brodie *et al.*, 1995). Other major endpoints might be the time to withdrawal for any reason or, sometimes, the time to withdrawal due to unwanted or intolerable adverse effects.

While equivalence trial designs are accepted by health authorities in many countries, the FDA is unwilling to consider results from such studies as proof of efficacy (Leber, 1989; Pledger and Schmidt, 1994). Their rationale is that a result showing no differences between a new and an established AED could be interpreted as neither of the drugs having any clinical benefit (Leber, 1983), both being effective, or the trial simply being unable to demonstrate a difference that really exists. The FDA therefore insists on double-blind studies that demonstrate superiority of the new AED (i.e. a statistically significant difference) compared with a control treatment.

The attenuated active-control design, which compares a high dose of a new AED with a low dose of a standard AED, is a recognised alternative to direct comparisons with standard AED regimens (Pledger and Kramer, 1991). The low-dose control should protect patients from status epilepticus. Another approach is to study patients in whom AED treatment has been temporarily discontinued before surgery so that neurodiagnostic monitoring can be performed. Treatment duration in such trials must be short, but the design permits an ethical, in-patient comparison of the new AED with placebo (Pledger and Kramer, 1991).

The pre-surgical and the attenuated active-control designs are not suitable for examining long-term effects of new AEDs, but they do allow early evaluations of new treatments as monotherapy.

Efficacy and Safety of the New AEDs

Reviews of the efficacy and tolerability of some of the newer AEDs have been published (Dichter and Brodie, 1996; Marson *et al.*, 1996; Wilson and Brodie, 1996; Marson *et al.*, 1997; Shorvon and Stefan, 1997), but so far, few randomised studies have compared these AEDs directly. All of the recently approved drugs are more efficacious than placebo. Adverse reactions are often central nervous system effects, and the potential for interaction with other AEDs is generally lower than for most of the older AEDs. Broad comparisons between the new drugs using cross-study data usually do not provide conclusive evidence for major differences in efficacy or tolerability between these new drugs, although the precise spectrum of activity of the new AEDs is poorly defined (Marson *et al.*, 1997). An overview of the efficacy and tolerability for six of the most widely available new AEDs is given in Table 1.

Accumulating data suggest that these new drugs can provide benefits over the established agents, particularly in terms of compliance, pharmacokinetics, and tolerability. However, more patient data are needed for many of these new drugs before general conclusions can be drawn. Trials must be of sufficient duration to enable assessment of side effects after chronic treatment, maintenance of therapeutic benefits, and long-term risk-benefit. Brodie (1996) has suggested that over 100,000 patients need to be treated with a new AED before its true safety profile can be determined realistically. For example, felbamate, a promising new AED launched in the early 1990s, was found to cause the

TABLE 1 OVERVIEW OF NEW ANTIEPILEPTIC DRUGS

DRUG	INDICATION	THERAPY TYPE	ODDS RATIO (95% CONFIDENCE INTERVAL) FOR 50% RESPONSE	SIDE EFFECTS		AED INTERACTION POTENTIAL	
				PRINCIPAL	SERIOUS	NEW AED ON STANDARD AED	STANDARD AED ON NEW AED
FELBAMATE	PARTIAL AND SECONDARY GENERALIZED SEIZURES, LENNOX-GASTAUT SYNDROME	MONO AND ADJUVANT	NC	IRRITABILITY, INSOMNIA, ANOREXIA, NAUSEA, VOMITING, WEIGHT LOSS, SOMNOLENCE, HEADACHE	APLASTIC ANAEMIA, HEPATIC FAILURE	++++	+++
GABAPENTIN	PARTIAL AND SECONDARY GENERALIZED SEIZURES	ADJUVANT	2.29 (1.53, 3.43)	SOMNOLENCE, FATIGUE, ATAXIA, DIZZINESS, GASTROINTESTINAL UPSET		—	—
LAMOTRIGINE	PARTIAL, SECONDARY GENERALIZED, TONIC-CLONIC SEIZURES, ABSENCE	MONO AND ADJUVANT	2.32 (1.47, 3.68)	RASH, DIZZINESS, TREMOR, ATAXIA, DIPLOPIA, HEADACHE, GASTROINTESTINAL UPSET	STEVENS-JOHNSON SYNDROME, ERYTHEMA MULTIFORME, LYELL'S SYNDROME	—	++++
TIAGABINE	PARTIAL AND SECONDARY GENERALIZED SEIZURES	ADJUVANT	3.03 (2.01, 4.58)	CONFUSION, DIZZINESS, SOMNOLENCE, FATIGUE GASTROINTESTINAL UPSET, ANOREXIA,		—	++
TOPIRAMATE	PARTIAL AND SECONDARY GENERALIZED SEIZURES	ADJUVANT	4.07 (2.87, 5.78)	NON-SPECIFIC CNS CHANGES SUCH AS TREMOR, DIZZINESS, ATAXIA, HEADACHE, FATIGUE, COGNITIVE DISTURBANCES, RENAL CALCULI, GASTROINTESTINAL UPSET	NEPHROLITHIASIS	(+)	++
VIGABATRIN	PARTIAL AND SECONDARY GENERALIZED SEIZURES, INFANTILE SPASMS	ADJUVANT	3.67 (2.44, 5.51)	BEHAVIOURAL CHANGES, DEPRESSION, SEDATION, FATIGUE, WEIGHT GAIN, GASTROINTESTINAL UPSET	PSYCHOSIS, DEPRESSION	+	—

AED, ANTIEPILEPTIC DRUG; NC, NOT CALCULATED; 50% RESPONSE, PATIENT WITH A 50% REDUCTION IN SEIZURE FREQUENCY COMPARED WITH BASELINE; ODDS RATIO: THE HIGHER THE ODDS RATIO THE GREATER THE PROBABILITY OF A PATIENT RESPONDING TO TREATMENT WITH THE NEW AED COMPARED WITH PLACEBO; ++++, HIGHEST POTENTIAL FOR AED INTERACTION; +, LOW POTENTIAL FOR AED INTERACTION; –, MINIMUM OR NO POTENTIAL FOR AED INTERACTION; (+), MIXED EFFFECTS.

REFERENCES: DICHTER AND BRODIE, 1996; SABERS AND GRAM, 1996; MARSON *ET AL.*, 1997; SHORVON AND STEFAN, 1997 dangerous side effect of aplastic anaemia upon broad clinical use. This AED is now held in reserve for cases of epilepsy that do not respond to any other treatments.

Overall, advances in the treatment of epilepsy during the 1990s mean that physicians and patients now have a much wider choice of agents, and there is a greater potential for enhancing the quality of life of patients with this disorder.

MEASUREMENT OF QoL IN CLINICAL TRIALS

Quality of life (QoL) measures are increasingly being included in clinical trials as endpoints in addition to traditional efficacy and safety outcomes (Wiklund, 1996). QoL measures are useful in that they provide a metric of the benefit of new AEDs from the point of view of the patient and, sometimes, the caregiver. Capturing these important perspectives is precisely the reason that regulatory agencies are paying increased attention to QoL endpoints (Morris *et al.*, 1996). Additionally, because there is now a larger number of drugs from which to choose, many patients, physicians, and other medical decision-makers want to know how a particular drug will impact on QoL. These endpoints are, therefore, being included in clinical trials to enhance what is known about the clinical profile of a drug, both to satisfy regulatory requirements and to develop information to aid promotion.

To achieve these goals, pharmaceutical companies must establish that a new AED has a positive affect upon QoL (i.e. that a treatment effect exists). To this end, sponsors of a new AED must select QoL instruments with good psychometric properties, develop an adequate analysis plan prior to unblinding the study, and follow a well-designed research protocol (Fayers *et al.*, 1997; Bernhard *et al.*, 1998; Fairclough *et al.*, 1998). While guidelines for QoL research have been, and are being, published elsewhere (Smith, 1993; Beitz *et al.*, 1996; McCabe *et al.*, 1996; Staquet *et al.*, 1996; Leidy *et al.*, 1999), it is instructive to review some of these issues from the perspective of the pharmaceutical industry itself.

Establishing a Treatment Effect on QoL

Prospective, double-blind, randomised controlled trials (RCTs) in the clinical setting are the study design of choice to show treatment effects on QoL (Smith, 1993). The FDA has warned against using uncontrolled studies (such as open-label, community-based studies) in attempts to isolate treatment effects on QoL (Wiklund, 1996). Of course, patient selection for an RCT should not be so restrictive that generalisation of findings to the target population at large is precluded (Rittenhouse and O'Brien, 1996). An RCT design is especially important for adjunctive therapy trials, where randomisation of treatment regimens across subjects adjusts for confounding influences due to concomitant AED therapy. Whether the comparator treatment arm is a placebo or a low dose of another AED, the RCT design allows differences in QoL to be attributed to treatment with the new AED.

Modelling the underlying causal relationships between treatment with new AEDs and consequent effects upon QoL is fundamental to the design of clinical trials that include QoL endpoints. By a causal model, we mean the explicit conceptualisation of the relationships between clinical variables and QoL measures, such as that presented by Wilson and Cleary (1995; and see Chapter 4). New AEDs can affect QoL positively (via a reduction in the frequency or severity of seizures), as well as negatively (via side effects of therapy). Capturing the positive and negative effects of AED therapy in clinical trials requires careful selection of QoL instruments for inclusion in industry-sponsored clinical trials.

Disease-specific or generic instruments can be used to measure treatment effects of an AED on QoL. Disease- or condition-specific QoL instruments assess problems associated with a given disease or condition and tend to be more sensitive to changes related to efficacy in this setting. Generic instruments record levels of QoL as impacted by both efficacy and safety, and are widely applicable, to those patients with the specific disease, those with other diseases, and the general public, therefore allowing comparisons across disease areas. Additionally, instruments have been developed that record the impact of side effects of AED therapy from the perspective of the patient. Each of these instrument types have their own characteristics, requiring careful consideration before including any one of them in a clinical trial.

Measuring the Impact of Side-Effects of AED Therapy

In a study that included the administration of a patient-completed symptom checklist, the impact of some side effects from AED therapy on QoL were measured directly (Wagner *et al.*, 1995). Low scores were correlated with occurrences of unsteadiness, hand tremor, slow reaction, headache, and upset stomach.

An instrument that was specifically developed to capture the impact of AED side effects on QoL is the Neurotoxicity Scale (Aldenkamp *et al.*, 1995). This scale has shown significant differences in the cognitive domains of fatigue and slowing between subjects randomised to a benzodiazepine compared with others randomised to placebo. Another instrument designed to measure the impact of AED-induced side effects on epilepsy patients is the Side Effect And Life Satisfaction Inventory (SEALS; Gillham *et al.*, 1996). With the administration of SEALS to 923 patients with epilepsy, it was shown that patients taking vigabatrin and one other AED had poorer SEALS scores than those taking lamotrigine and one other AED. Patients taking two or more AEDs had poorer scores than those taking a single AED.

As well as reliability and validity, QoL instruments should show sensitivity to clinically relevant endpoints. In the Wagner *et al.* (1995) study cited above, side effects of AED therapy were significantly correlated to a number of generic and epilepsy-specific QoL scales. The generic scales, however, were best able to differentiate between groups of patients differing in the impact of 13 symptoms. Therefore, the inclusion of a stand-alone patient-based checklist of AED side effects in a clinical trial of a new AED may be superfluous if generic or disease-specific QoL measures are also included.

Whilst such symptom checklists are undoubtedly useful tools when viewed from the perspective of a sponsor of a new AED, certain concerns remain. Firstly, such instruments are not strictly measures of QoL — they measure symptoms, which in turn may or may not affect QoL (Wilson and Cleary, 1995). Secondly, the administration of a symptoms checklist could potentially exaggerate the reporting of adverse events. Pharmaceutical companies, in conjunction with regulatory agencies, have already developed sophisticated techniques for the recording and reporting of adverse events. Finally, if side effects of therapy do affect QoL, then it is probably best to measure that influence using QoL instruments based upon psychometric theory.

Disease-Specific Measures of QoL

Recent work has been performed showing that certain epilepsy-specific QoL instruments are sensitive to seizure frequency. The epilepsy-targeted scales of the Quality of Life In Epilepsy Inventory-89 (QOLIE-89), a QoL instrument containing disease-specific and generic scales, discriminated between seizure-free and low-seizure-frequency subjects and those subjects with moderate or high seizure frequency (Perrine *et al.*, 1995). In the Wagner *et al.* (1995) study discussed above, the epilepsy-specific QoL scales included in the battery were among the scales best able to discriminate among patients differing in time since last seizure, indicating that the epilepsy-specific scales may be responsive to changes in efficacy measures.

Using QOLIE-89 over a period of 24 weeks, QoL was measured in a double-blind, randomised, controlled study of adjunctive tiagabine therapy in patients who had inadequate seizure control with either phenytoin or carbamazepine monotherapy (Cramer *et al.*, 1998). Seizure worry was reduced across all treatment groups. Attention/ concentration, memory, and language skills also showed some sensitivity to clinical change. These data demonstrate the sensitivity of the instrument, as well as differences between the two treatments, during a brief time frame.

The Liverpool Battery comprises eight instruments or scales, and may be responsive to changes in the context of a clinical trial (Smith *et al.* 1993). This placebo-controlled, double-blind, cross-over study of lamotrigine in 81 patients with refractory partial seizures indicated significant differences between the lamotrigine group and placebo in the seizure severity, positive affect balance, and mastery scales. However, because most patients were able to identify their assigned drug, the validity of the reported treatment effects is indeterminate.

Generic Measurements of QoL

The Wagner *et al.* (1995) study found that many of the generic QoL scales included in the test battery were at least as sensitive to seizure frequency as the epilepsy-specific scales. The Short Form-36 (SF-36) (Ware *et al.*, 1993) performed especially well in discriminating between patients based upon seizure frequency. Other studies have shown that a generic QoL instrument can be sensitive to clinical measures. In a retrospective study of 300 patients recruited from the UK, Germany, and France, seizure frequency *and* severity were found to be significant predictors of seven out of ten scales in the Functional Status Questionnaire (Baker *et al.*, 1998).

These findings mean that generic QoL instruments may be adequate to demonstrate a positive impact upon QoL based upon improved efficacy. In that case, epilepsy-specific instruments may not be required. A reduction in the number of QoL endpoints helps avoid the problem of multiple comparisons, where the probability of finding a significant treatment effect is artificially increased. If one or more of the generic scales can show treatment effect, then the inclusion of epilepsy-specific scales only penalises the analyses by increasing the statistical requirements for demonstrating a treatment effect.

An added benefit of including a generic QoL measurement in industry-sponsored clinical trials is the capturing of the impact of side effects. Patients do not necessarily identify individual factors such as efficacy and individual side effects as leading to QoL changes, but may nonetheless perceive an impact upon QoL as a whole. Therefore, the generic instrument may be a very efficient way of measuring QoL when the balance between efficacy and side effects is important, as is the case in the treatment of epilepsy.

Health-State Utilities

Recent evidence suggests that measuring QoL with descriptive generic instruments may not entirely capture the patient's valuation of his or her health state. While generic instruments measure health status along various QoL constructs (the SF-36 measures eight separate constructs), individual patients may value these constructs differentially. As part of the Knee Replacement Patient Outcomes Research Team, researchers measured overall QoL of knee replacement patients using the SF-36 and also measured directly the utility of the patients' current states of health using the standard gamble technique for eliciting patient preferences (Bennett *et al.*, 1997). Interestingly, the derived utilities for the self-health states correlated more strongly with the physical SF-36 constructs, and generally failed to correlate with the mental constructs of the SF-36. This indicates that the interpretation of QoL results can benefit from a direct measurement of patient preferences.

More directly relevant to epilepsy, Stavem (1998) measured directly the current health-state patient preferences in 57 well-controlled epilepsy patients taking AEDs, using the time trade-off and standard gamble techniques. The means (and standard deviations) of the health-state utilities measured by the different techniques were 0.92 (0.11) and 0.93 (0.11) (where 1.0 represents perfect health) for the time trade-off and the standard gamble techniques, respectively. The standard deviations are much better than achieved by many generic QoL measures. With low standard deviations associated with the measurement of current health-state utilities, such measurement may be more sensitive to patient groupings and change in clinical status than are the generic QoL measures.

The direct measurement of current health-state utilities can discriminate between patients based upon seizure frequency. Eighty-one epilepsy patients were interviewed to derive health-state utilities using the time trade-off technique (Messori *et al.,* 1998). Patients were classified according to the following five categories: (1) presence of drug-related side effects; (2) at least 10 seizures per month; (3) two to nine seizures per month; (4) zero to one seizure per month; and, (5) no seizures during the past year. The following mean utilities (standard deviation, number of patients) were found for the five categories, from one to five: 0.40 (0.07, 9), 0.66 (0.08, 12), 0.79 (0.13, 30), 0.91 (0.09, 15), and 0.96 (0.04, 15).

From the recent work in measuring patient preferences in epilepsy patients, we see that low utilities are associated with the presence of drug-related side effects. Additionally, the time trade-off technique appears to be sensitive to seizure frequency. These are desirable properties for a measure that could be used to adjudicate between side effects and efficacy. It is encouraging that the variances are relatively low. These measures will be that much more useful in the context of RCTs if they can detect *changes* in utilities as associated with changes in side effects and efficacy. Only further experience with these measures will tell.

PERSPECTIVE OF REGULATORY BODIES ON QoL EVIDENCE

Although regulatory agencies do not require QoL evidence for new drugs, pharmaceutical companies are increasingly including this evidence as part of their submissions for drug approval and pricing/reimbursement decisions (Smith, 1993; Morris *et al.,* 1996; Wiklund, 1996; Patrick, 1998; Leidy *et al.,* 1999). A recent survey conducted by the Tufts Centre for the Study of Drug Development polled pharmacoeconomics/outcomes research departments; 45 department heads responded, representing nearly all of the major pharmaceutical companies (Caglarcan and Di Masi, 1998). The survey found that 33% of those responding submitted pharmacoeconomic analyses (including QoL) to the FDA as part of their new drug application submissions. Similarly, 55% of those responding submitted pharmacoeconomic analyses to government authorities outside the USA as part of registration. This proportion is expected to grow.

QoL information is especially relevant for palliative therapies (e.g. in many cancers), or for therapies used in treating chronic conditions such as epilepsy. QoL assessment in epilepsy being a relatively recent development, however, its use is becoming common in clinical trials of new AEDs, complementing standard measures of safety and efficacy (Jacoby, 1999). To date, only one AED includes QoL in the label, but there are a small number of drugs in other disease areas which have gained this type of approval in the USA (Burke, 1998). Parent-reported impressions of QoL in children with Lennox-Gastaut syndrome favoured felbamate compared with placebo according to the 'Clinical Studies' section of the Physicians' Desk Reference (1998) entry for the drug.

Guidelines exist for the use of pharmacoeconomic information in the pricing and reimbursement processes in Canada and Australia. Guidelines are also under consideration, or in development, in the USA, the UK, and the Netherlands (Commonwealth Department of Human Services and Health, 1995; CCOHTA, 1997; FDA, 1997; Anon, 1998; NHS Executive, 1999). Discussion and efforts in these countries point towards increased consideration of QoL in the regulatory approval and pricing/reimbursement processes, but there remain significant technical challenges to be overcome. Guidelines for protocol development and consistent reporting of QoL results from clinical trials are already available, though a consensus checklist for the collection and interpretation of QoL data does not currently exist (Staquet *et al.*, 1996; Fayers *et al.*, 1997).

Collaborative efforts by the pharmaceutical industry, QoL researchers, and regulatory agencies are attempting to define guidelines and standards for QoL assessment in clinical trials and the inclusion of this information in regulatory processes, but the efforts appear to be moving forward slowly. A recent meeting brought together QoL researchers and representatives of European regulatory agencies and the FDA with the aim of identifying and refining key regulatory issues regarding QoL studies (MAPI Research Institute, 1998). Resolution of these issues is clearly important.

Current perspectives of regulatory agencies in the USA and Europe on QoL evidence is discussed in more detail in the following sections.

USA

Although the use of pharmacoeconomic and QoL data was allowed in product labelling and advertising prior to 1997, the 1997 FDA Modernization Act was seen as an easing of the stance on health outcomes data (FDA, 1997). Although the various categories of health care economic information were not specifically mentioned in the

Modernization Act, it is clear that the FDA recognises QoL as an important outcome for many interventions. Indeed, since 1985 the Agency has recommended that all oncology trials include QoL as an endpoint (Johnson and Temple, 1985). It is expected that during 1999 the FDA will issue guidance on the use of QoL data to support drug submissions and product claims. Currently, it appears that data from a single well-designed RCT incorporating rigorous and valid QoL assessment may be sufficient to support such claims (MEDTAP Research News, 1999).

Public statements by FDA representatives have provided general guidance to the pharmaceutical industry by indicating that QoL data must be collected using reliable and validated instruments appropriate for the study designs and indications. The instruments must be administered consistently using established procedures. Furthermore, appropriate methods must be used to analyse data (Beitz *et al.*, 1996; Burke, 1998; MEDTAP Research News, 1999). Gemcitabine, a drug used in the treatment of advanced or metastatic pancreatic cancer, was the first drug approved by the FDA for marketing based primarily on its effect on 'QoL-like' outcomes rather than solely on efficacy or safety data (Anon, 1995). By March 1999, at least 17 drugs had QoL mentioned as part of their Physicians' Desk Reference (1998) entry (which is an exact copy of the product's US Government-approved labelling), mostly in the 'Clinical Studies' section of the entry. Two products, Serevent® and Camptosar®, have been cleared to allow the use of QoL for promotional purposes.

Ongoing discussions between the International Society for Pharmacoeconomic and Outcomes Research (ISPOR) and the FDA are intended to lead to the development of a consensus document on QoL issues. It will cover fundamental issues, such as terminology, types of QoL instruments, study design, and analysis. A working paper is currently available on the ISPOR Internet website (ISPOR, 1999).

The Pharmaceutical Research and Manufacturers of America (PhRMA) Health Outcomes Working Group (HOWG) is sponsoring similar activities also aimed at clarifying these issues. In addition, the FDA is collaborating with the International Society for Quality of Life Research (ISOQOL). ISOQOL recently set up a regulatory/policy committee with the primary aim of providing guidance to the USA and European regulatory agencies regarding QoL. A number of White Papers will be produced that will cover issues such as methods and statistical techniques in QoL research and their relevance to regulatory agencies.

Europe

Regulatory procedures in Europe are currently evolving with the introduction of centralised and decentralised registration procedures with mutual recognition. Most nations currently have their own approach to regulatory issues such as pricing, reimbursement, and advertising, and are likely to do so for some time. As the regulatory environment in Europe moves toward a pan-European regulatory process under the European Medicines Evaluation Agency (EMEA), the role of QoL in the approval process has not appeared thus far to be a critical agenda item. However, interested individuals and organisations in Europe have begun to make efforts to address regulatory issues regarding QoL.

The European Regulatory Issues on QoL Assessment (ERIQA) project is a working group of QoL researchers and pharmaceutical industry representatives that aims to establish principles and practices for the integration of QoL outcomes in the regulatory process (ERIQA Group, 1998). The efforts of this group have been outlined in two phases: first, existing guidelines will be reviewed to help establish a general set; and second, the group will attempt to define guidelines for a number of specific disease areas. The outcomes of this working group will be disseminated to representatives of European regulatory agencies. Collaborations with the PhRMA HOWG in the USA and ISPOR are ongoing.

THE FUTURE ROLE OF QoL ASSESSMENT IN AED CLINICAL TRIALS

At the turn of the 21st century, the epilepsy drug market is still dominated by traditional AEDs, some of which were developed 30 or 40 years ago. Newer AEDs that are efficacious but with improved safety profiles have been introduced into many countries over the past 10 years. To extol the benefits of these newer agents compared with the older agents, pharmaceutical companies have begun to embrace QoL as an outcome measure to provide additional information about the profile of a drug. QoL assessment has itself developed over the past 15 years, and several measures have been applied to the epilepsy disease area.

For industry-sponsored clinical trials of new AEDs, the primary goal with regard to QoL is to establish a positive treatment effect on QoL outcomes. In addition to supporting the regulatory submission, the QoL findings offer the company the potential to enhance the product labelling and subsequent promotion. To this end, the RCT is considered the study design of choice. The measurement of QoL needs to incorporate the impact of increased efficacy as well as the impact of therapy-related side effects, as each of the newer AEDs will have its own toxicology profile.

Symptom checklists can be valuable tools for measuring the impact of side effects, but some concerns remain about their use. While epilepsy-specific QoL measures can capture QoL effects due to the increased efficacy of a new AED, administration of generic QoL instruments can measure directly a patient's own balance between the impact of efficacy and side effects upon QoL. The inclusion of the direct measurement of current health-state utilities may be another way to balance the QoL impact of efficacy and side effects.

Currently, QoL data are not required for regulatory decisions; however, it appears that the pharmaceutical industry will continue to incorporate QoL assessment in clinical trials and these findings will be submitted to support drug submissions. Specifically, for new AEDs, the use of QoL assessment has become integral to many clinical trial programmes.

Current discussions and efforts in the USA and Europe have highlighted the need for collaborative efforts among pharmaceutical companies, QoL researchers, and regulatory agencies in order to develop guidelines and standards on the use and interpretation of QoL data. It appears universally agreed by all interested stakeholders that QoL endpoints are potentially important and relevant measures in many trials of new therapies. Furthermore, in specific disease areas such as epilepsy, QoL information could be an important factor for doctors and patients in treatment decision making. For such information to be considered as part of the regulatory submission for a new drug, however, QoL data must be held to the same standards as other clinical endpoints.

Guidance on the use of QoL in the regulatory process is likely to be forthcoming from the FDA and it is expected that the EMEA will issue similar guidance in the future. This guidance is likely to provide clarity on some of the key instrumentation, methodological, and analytical issues that have been identified and discussed thus far by interested stakeholders. However, given the complexity of this area, it is unlikely that the guidance will address adequately all of the issues at the first attempt. Ongoing discussions in groups such as ISPOR, ISOQOL, PhRMA HOWG, and ERIQA, in collaboration with regulatory agencies, will hopefully help resolve many key issues over time.

Working within its regulatory environment, the pharmaceutical industry has consistently produced high-quality clinical research and innovative products. Although challenges remain for successful incorporation of QoL data into the regulatory decision-making processes, the industry is committed to maintaining similarly high standards in providing credible and useful QoL information to support its products.

ACKNOWLEDGEMENTS

The authors would like to thank the following for their contribution to this chapter: Catherine Acquadro, Laurie Burke, Erol Caglarcan, Olivier Chassany, Katrin Conway, Diane Fairclough, Laura Glauda, Hind Hatoum, Bernard Jambon, Donald Patrick, Gordon Pledger, Dennis Revicki, Brian Rittenhouse, Margaret Rothman, Nancy Santanello, Jeffrie Strang, and Ben van Hout.

References

Aldenkamp, A.P., Baker, G., Pieters, M.S.M., Schoemaker, H.C., Cohen, A.F., Schwabe, S. (1995) The Neurotoxicity Scale: The validity of a patient-based scale, assessing neurotoxicity *Epilepsy Research* **20**, 229–239.

Anon. (1989) Carbamazepine update. *Lancet* **2**, 595–597.

Anon. (1995) FDA: Quality of life matters! *Annals of Oncology* **6**, 858.

Anon. (1998) Dutch Pharmacoeconomic Guideline Report. Prepared by the Dutch Sickness Funds Council for the Minister of Public Health, Welfare and Sport.

Baker, G.A., Gagnon, D., McNulty, P. (1998) The relationship between seizure frequency, seizure type and quality of life: findings from three European countries. *Epilepsy Research* **30**, 231–240.

Beitz, J., Gnecco, C., Justice, R. (1996) Quality-of-life end points in cancer clinical trials: The U.S. Food and Drug Administration Perspective. *Monograph of the National Cancer Institute* **20**, 7–9.

Bennett, K.J., Torrance, G.W., Moran, L.A., Smith, F., Goldsmith, C.H. (1997) Health State utilities in knee replacement surgery: the development and evaluation of McKnee. *Journal of Rheumatology* **24**, 1796–1805.

Bernhard, J,, Cella, D.F., Coates, A.S., Fallowfield, L., Ganz, P.A., Moinpour, C.M., Mosconi, P. (1998) Missing quality of life data in cancer clinical trials: serious problems and challenges. *Statistics in Medicine* **17**, 517–532.

Brodie, M.J. (1992) Drug interactions in epilepsy. *Epilepsia* **33** (Suppl. 1), S13-S22.

Brodie, M.J. (1996) Antiepileptic drugs, clinical trials, and the market place. *Lancet* **347**, 777–779.

Brodie, M.J., Dichter, M.A. (1996) Antiepileptic drugs. *New England Journal of Medicine* **334**, 168–175.

Brodie, M.J., Richens, A., Yuen, A.W.C. for the Lamotrigine/Carbamazepine Monotherapy Trial Group. (1995) Double-blind comparison of lamotrigine and carbamazepine in newly diagnosed epilepsy. *Lancet* **345**, 476–479.

Burke, L.B. (1998) Quality of life evaluation: the FDA experience. Quality of Life Newsletter. MAPI Research Institute, March 1998.

Caglarcan, E., Di Masi, J. (1998) The Role of Pharmacoeconomics in Pharmaceutical R&D Decision Making. DIA Conference, London, UK, October 13–15.

CCOHTA. (1997) Guidelines for economic evaluation of pharmaceuticals: Canada. 2nd Edition, March 1997. Ontario, Canada: Canadian Co-ordinating Office for Health Technology Assessment.

Commonwealth Department of Human Services and Health. (1995) Guidelines for the pharmaceutical industry on preparation of submissions to the Pharmaceutical Benefits Advisory Committee. Canberra: Australian Government Publishing Service.

Cramer, J., Bagnall-Ryan, J., Chang, J., Sommerville, K.W. (1998) Short-term change in quality of life when tiagabine (Gabitril®) or a standard medication is added to carbamazepine or phenytoin. Poster presented at the American College of Neuropsychopharmacology, Puerto Rico, December.

Dichter, M.A., Brodie, M.J. (1996) New antiepileptic drugs. New England Journal of Medicine 334, 1583–1590.

ERIQA Group. (1998) The European Regulatory Issues on QoL Assessment (ERIQA) project: establishing principles and practices for the integration of QoL outcomes in the regulatory process. MAPI Research Institute, Lyon, France.

Fairclough, D.L., Patterson, H.F., Cella, D., Bonomi, P. (1998) Comparison of several model-based methods for analysing incomplete quality of life data in cancer clinical trials. *Statistics in Medicine* **17**, 781–796.

Fayers, P.M., Hopwood, P., Harvey, A., Girling, D.J., Machin, D., Stephens, R. on behalf of the MRC Cancer Trials Office (1997) Quality of life assessment in clinical trials — guidelines and a checklist for protocol writers: the U.K. Medical Research Council experience. *European Journal of Cancer* **33**, 20–28.

FDA. (1997) Food and Drug Administration Modernization Act.

Gillham, R., Baker, G., Thompson, P., Birbeck, K., McGuire, A., Tomlinson, L., Eckersley, L., Silveria, C., Brown, S. (1996) Standardization of a self-report questionnaire for use in evaluating cognitive, affective and behavioral side-effects of anti-epileptic drug treatments. *Epilepsy Research* **24**, 47–55.

ISPOR Quality of Life Regulatory Guidance Issues (1999) *Development of a consensus document as a supporting document for FDA and other health regulatory authorities on health-related quality of life guidances.* [on line] www.ispor.org.

Jacoby, A. (1999) Assessing quality of life in patients with epilepsy. In: Mallarkey, G., Palmer, K.J. (eds.) *Issues in epilepsy* Auckland: Adis International, 171–189

Johnson, J.R., Temple, R. (1985) Food and Drug Administration requirements for approval and new anticancer drugs. *Cancer Treatment Reports* **69**, 1155–1159.

Kälviäinen, R., Äikiä, M., Riekkenen, P.J. (1996) Cognitive effects of antiepileptic drugs: incidence, mechanisms and therapeutic implications. *CNS Drugs* **5**, 358–368.

Kramer, L.D., Pledger, G.W., Kamin, M. (1993) Prototype antiepileptic drug clinical development plan. *Epilepsia* **34**, 1075–1084.

Leber, P. (1983) The implicit assumption of active control trials (a critical examination). *Controlled Clinical Trials* **14**, 133.

Leber, P. (1989) Hazards of inference: the active control investigation. *Epilepsia* **30**, S57–S63.

Leidy, N.K., Revicki, D.A., Geneste, B. (1999) Recommendations for evaluating the validity of quality of life claims for labeling and promotion. *Value Health* **2**, 113–127.

Macphee, G.J.A., Butler, E., Brodie, M.J. (1987) Intradose and circadian variation in circulating carbamazepine and its epoxide in epileptic patients: a consequence of autoinduction of metabolism. *Epilepsia* **28**, 286–294.

MAPI Research Institute (1998) *Quality of Life Newsletter*, March 1998.

Marson, A.G., Kadir, Z.A., Chadwick, DW. (1996) New antiepileptic drugs: a systematic review of their efficacy and tolerability. *British Medical Journal* **313**, 1169–1174.

Marson, A.G., Kadir, Z.A., Hutton, J.L., Chadwick, D.W. (1997) The new antiepileptic drugs: a systematic review of their efficacy and tolerability. *Epilepsia* **38**, 859–880.

McCabe, M.S., Shoemaker, D., Temple, R.J., Burke, G., Friedman, M.A. (1996) Regulatory perspectives on quality of life issues. In: Spilker, B. (ed.) *Quality of Life and Pharmacoeconomics in Clinical Trials.* 2nd edition. Philadelphia, PA, USA: Lippincott-Raven Publishers, 569–574.

MEDTAP Research News (1999) *Building a foundation for quality of life claims: interview with lead author Nancy Kline Leidy*, Ph.D. Bethesda, MD, USA, MEDTAP Research News, 1–2.

Messori, A., Trippoli, S., Becagli, P., Cincotta, M., Labbate, M.G., Zaccara, G. (1998) Adjunctive lamotrigine therapy in patients with refractory seizures: a lifetime cost-utility analysis. *European Journal of Clinical Pharmacology* **53**, 421–427.

Morris, L.A., Beckett, T.K., Lechter, K.J. (1996) A marketing perspective: theoretical underpinnings. In: Spilker, B. (ed.) *Quality Of Life and Pharmacoeconomics in Clinical Trials.* 2nd edition. Philadelphia, PA, USA: Lippincott-Raven Publishers, 541–548.

NHS Executive. (1999) *Faster access to modern treatment: how NICE appraisal will work.* A discussion paper. NHS Executive, Leeds, UK, January.

Patrick, D.L. (1998) Quality of life and pharmacoeconomic evaluation. *Quality of Life Newsletter*, MAPI Research Institute, March 1998.

Pellock, J.M. (1994) Standard approach to antiepileptic drug treatment in the United States. *Epilepsia* **35** (Suppl. 4), S11-S18.

Perrine, K., Devinsky, O., Meador, K.J., Hermann, B.P., Cramer, J.A., Hays, R.D., Vickery, B.G. (1995) The relationship of neuropsychological functioning to quality of life in epilepsy. *Archives of Neurology* **52**, 997–1003.

Physicians' Desk Reference (1998) Montvale, NJ: Medical Economics Company Inc.

Pledger, G.W., Kramer, L.D. (1991) Clinical trials of investigational antiepileptic drugs: monotherapy designs. *Epilepsia* **32**, 716–721.

Pledger, G.W., Schmidt, D. (1994) Evaluation of antiepileptic drug efficacy. A review of clinical trial design. *Drugs* **48**, 498–509.

Powell-Jackson, P.R., Tredger, J.M., Williams, R. (1984) Hepatotoxicity to sodium valproate: a review. *Gut* **25**, 673–681.

Rittenhouse, B.E., O'Brien, J.O. (1996) Threats to the validity of pharmacoeconomic analyses based on clinical trial data. In: Spilker, B. (ed.) *Quality of Life and Pharmacoeconomics in Clinical Trials*. 2nd edition. Philadelphia, PA: Lippincott-Raven Publishers, 1215–1223.

Sabers, A., Gram, L. (1996) Drug treatment of epilepsy in the 1990s: achievements and new developments. *Drugs* **52**, 483–493.

Schmidt, D. (1982) *Adverse effects of antiepileptic drugs*. New York, USA: Raven Press.

Shorvon, S., Stefan, H. (1997) Overview of the safety of newer antiepileptic drugs. *Epilepsia* **38** (Suppl. 1), S45-S51.

Smith, D., Baker, G., Davies, G., Dewey, M., Chadwick, D.W. (1993) Outcomes of add-on treatment with lamotrigine in partial epilepsy. *Epilepsy Research* **16**, 65–81.

Smith, N.D. (1993) Quality of life studies from the perspective of an FDA reviewing statistician. *Drug Information Journal* **27**, 617–623.

Staquet, M., Berzon, R., Osoba, D., Machin, D. (1996) Guidelines for reporting results of quality of life assessments in clinical trials. *Quality of Life Research* **5**, 496–502.

Stavem, K. (1998) Quality of Life in Epilepsy: Comparison of four preference measures. *Epilepsy Research* **29**, 201–209.

Wagner, A.K., Keller, S.D., Kosinski, M., Baker, G.A., Jacoby, A., Hsu, M.A., Chadwick, D.W., Ware, J.E. (1995) Advances in methods for assessing the impact of epilepsy and antiepileptic drug therapy on patients' health-related quality of life. *Quality of Life Research* **4**, 115–134.

Ware, J.E., Snow, K.K., Kosinski, M., Gandek, B. (1993) *SF-36 Health Survey: Manual and Interpretation Guide*. Boston, MA. The Health Institute, New England Medical Center.

Wiklund, I. (1996) Quality of life and regulatory issues. *Scandinavian Journal of Gastroenterology* **31** (Suppl. 221), 37–38.

Wilson, E.A., Brodie, M.J. (1996) New antiepileptic drugs. *Baillière's Clinical Neurology* **5**, 723–747.

Wilson, I.B., Cleary, P.D. (1995) Linking clinical variables with health-related quality of life: a conceptual model of patient outcomes. *Journal of the American Medical Association* **273**, 59–65.

IMPROVING QUALITY OF LIFE IN EPILEPSY

Chapter 14

LIVING WITH EPILEPSY: A PERSONAL ACCOUNT

Jan Follett

First of all I should explain that I have no medical training but have picked up some of the terms and words used in the treatment of my epilepsy. I live a normal life and always have done which is perhaps why I tend to forget I've got epilepsy. I know that I have left temporal lobe/ complex partial epilepsy. Only some of my fits are tonic clonic and since my neurologist changed my medication regime, my seizures have all been during sleep — which is good, though I now have the indignity of occasional incontinence to deal with! I have between 9–12 seizures a month brought on by stress, tiredness and monthly hormonal changes.

My epilepsy began with puberty and I remember it being just at night. I must admit I don't remember that much about it, as it never really affected my school life. I have short-term memory loss which is a nuisance but is prevalent with most neurological disorders. At that stage of my life, I don't think anybody knew I had epilepsy because I didn't have a day-time seizure until I was at Teachers' Training College years later. Epilepsy was never mentioned at home — remember, this is going back 33 years! Every morning my father put my tablets next to my breakfast spoon. I went to the local hospital, though I can't remember who I saw. My parents always came with me.

I decided that I wanted to be a teacher and persuaded my parents to let me go to college. I began to have seizures during the day, which I suppose had advantages — other students had to live in off-campus accommodation for two years out of three; but I was able to stay on campus throughout. I was a normal and typical student of the 1970s — long hair, smock, loon pants. I wasn't so naive as to take the recreational drugs that were being passed around surreptitiously. I was already taking enough drugs, and still having quite a lot of daytime seizures. My epilepsy has never been well controlled.

I trained to teach the deaf because I was fascinated by the idea of someone else with an invisible handicap. When I qualified, I taught at St Thomas' School for the Deaf in Basingstoke. Being in a special school, there was an assistant in each classroom and S was mine. This worked out nicely should I ever have a fit while teaching — fortunately however, I did not. To this day whenever I teach, I tell the children, 'I have epilepsy — it makes me fall on the floor sometimes. It's horrid! If that happens I want you to go straight to the library corner and sit down with a book.'

I married in 1981 to a lovely man who is really 'laid back' and singularly unimpressed with epilepsy! He was a merchant seaman, with his captain's ticket. He was also ship's doctor and so recognised the names of the anti-convulsants which were in my kitchen cupboard. When I told him that I had epilepsy, I fully expected him to end the relationship (as most boyfriends had) but he said 'I know, I recognised the tablets'. We are still married years later, with a daughter born in 1983.

About eight years ago I decided to undergo brain surgery. I was fed up having seizures everywhere. I had one in the hairdressers, one in the book-shop, one everywhere, or so it seemed! When I was walking along the pavement I always seemed to land in a puddle, which was bad enough, but people always summoned an ambulance and that meant coming home later on the bus in wet, soggy jeans! Ugh! Some ambulance drivers came to recognise me and would wait until I was completely recovered and could tell them my address properly (though I think this was a test, because they already knew it). I was really grateful when they took me home and didn't take me to the hospital. Of course, no-one wants epilepsy — which is why I considered the option of brain surgery. I was sent to a surgeon at the Maudsley Hospital in London to determine whether I was a suitable candidate for surgical treatment. Sadly, apparently I was not.

Epilepsy has never held me back in any intellectual capacity. It was after my disappointment over surgery that my husband suggested I embark on a course of study with the Open University. I remember saying that I wouldn't be able to do it, but he persuaded me to try. I began with a foundation course on Victorian culture and then developed an interest in philosophy. I found it a fascinating and relatively easy subject. One of the things that attracted me is that there are no right or wrong answers — as long as you can qualify your argument, you're okay! Now I can add 'BA Hons' to my name. I graduated last year

I would be lying if I said it was easy, but I was determined to study and the Open University was very helpful and understanding. Every student there has a counsellor as well as a tutor and there are a lot of students with handicaps and disabilities. The Open University demonstrates that it is still possible to obtain a degree if you have a fertile and enquiring mind.

A major problem with having epilepsy is that of short term memory loss. This was particularly difficult for me when studying for my degree. I should say that the Open University was very supportive. After I provided a doctor's letter, I was allowed extra time both for my assignments and my exams. I find it easier to remember something that I've listened to, so I was provided with a set of audio tapes from the Open University Office for Students with Disabilities, one for each set book in the course. Doing the degree has given me a lot of confidence and I would recommend it to anyone, with or without a disability.

Epilepsy is a great strain on the family. Not being able to drive is a serious limitation for me. It means that I can never be the one who transports our daughter and her friends to their various social activities. My husband acts as taxi driver to the family and I know he sometimes gets tired of this. I dislike being reliant on him. I want to drive myself. Not driving means I can never be totally independent and I resent that.

Other people's attitudes to epilepsy varies with their age. It's generally the fear of the unknown that seems to frighten people. The younger the person, the more understanding that person usually is. Children seem to have very little fear of epilepsy, whereas some older people cannot even say the word. I have older relatives who say I have 'funny turns' but cannot bring themselves to say 'fit' or 'seizure'. The stigma of epilepsy is awful. Epilepsy is often seen as a mental problem and not a physical one, which I find distressing. When you tell them you have epilepsy, some people just say 'Oh' but most, especially the older ones, look at you as if you've told them you've got a very serious infectious disease. One man, on hearing that I had epilepsy, came up to me and furtively whispered, 'I hear you've got the Big E then, I have too'. He couldn't bring himself even to say the word. It's very sad that there are still people who can't come to terms with their own condition.

Not surprisingly, epilepsy does nothing for one's opinion of oneself. Low self esteem and epilepsy seem to go hand in hand. It is vital to keep your mind alert and busy and it is also important to think positively and not give in to the school of thought which says: 'I can't do that, I've got epilepsy'. Most of the time I honestly forget I've got epilepsy, it's just a nuisance. Recently, one of the doctors that I see suggested I apply to British Epilepsy Association for election to its Council of Management. My first reaction, despite all I've been saying, was 'I couldn't do that! They wouldn't want me!' But I stood and wrote in my election statement how important I believe it is that epilepsy should not hold a person back. It must have worked because I was elected and have just completed my first year of office. Recently I received a phone call through BEA from someone who had trained as a teacher but lost confidence. She just needed encouragement from a fellow teacher who also had epilepsy.

I think I'm going to find my role on BEA Council very exciting, as I've got so many ideas. The difficult part will be to remember to take my own advice, think positively and not to let my epilepsy get me down. That's difficult but not impossible, especially after a seizure, when my brain feels as if it's been battered and the world looks out of focus. Days like that stop me from doing what I want to do because I can't study or write very well and so have to do something like housework, which I hate!

So for me, the key message is that it is very important not to let epilepsy rule your life. It is vital that you do what you want to do first and think about epilepsy second. It is the person who is important, not the hidden condition they suffer from. A person with epilepsy must learn to be strong, take the blows and go for it! It can be done!

Chapter 15

LIVING WITH EPILEPSY: A FAMILY PERSPECTIVE

Kathy Bairstow

I suppose we should not have been surprised when two of our three children started having convulsions within a few months of each other; after all, both their father, David, and I had had a few seizures during childhood and we knew that sometimes children could inherit certain conditions from their parents. Nonetheless, the diagnosis did come as something as a shock, as neither of us had had seizures for many years and so, I suppose, our own experiences had been filed away in our memory banks. In fact, I don't think either of us had thought our own medical histories were relevant until being questioned by the doctors after Jonathan's first convulsion. We were told that he had probably inherited a tendency to febrile convulsions (convulsions triggered by a rapid rise in temperature) and that he would grow out of them by the age of five. The same information was given to us after his younger brother, Philip, had a similar event. While Jonathan seemed to outgrow the tendency by the time he started school, as Philip got older he seemed more vulnerable to viruses and infections and eventually started to have seizures even when he didn't have a temperature. At this point he was given a diagnosis of epilepsy.

COMING TO TERMS WITH EPILEPSY

This diagnosis was even more of a shock! Epilepsy — what did that mean? It seemed to have an air of mystery about it and even in the hospital it was talked about in more hushed terms than mere 'febrile convulsions'. Not knowing anything about epilepsy, we began to worry about Philip's future. Did this diagnosis mean that he was brain damaged? Did it mean that he wouldn't be allowed to start at the local nursery school? Anyway, why did he have epilepsy? Was it David's fault or was it mine, or were we just not compatible as parents? These questions all seem a bit extreme now, but at the time, when we were responsible twenty-four hours a day for a young child with a potentially serious medical condition, they were important to us. Maybe, in a way, they were part of the process of coming to terms with epilepsy.

We were not given any explanation about epilepsy at the initial diagnosis, nor at the follow up appointment with the general practitioner. Our health visitor was our salvation at that point. She didn't know much about the different types of epilepsy and she couldn't offer any explanation as to why Philip's diagnosis had changed. However, she was a listening ear and did reassure us that there was absolutely no reason why Philip's development should be compromised or why he should not attend the local nursery and school. She also explained that it was essential that his medication be taken every day, and that eventually he might grow out of the epilepsy. The health visitor was also as puzzled as we were at the attitudes of the different general practitioners in the practice where we were registered: the older one told us to 'Go home, and get on with it', while the youngest one suggested an ambulance should be called every time a seizure occurred. So, at this time both Philip and I were given labels by the medical professionals, he as a 'known epileptic' and I as a 'neurotic mother' — labels that may be useful to medical professionals, but are not very helpful for the people so described!

MEDICAL MANAGEMENT

Following the diagnosis, our lives became a round of doctor and hospital appointments during which time Philip's anti-epileptic medication was increased and blood levels taken. It seemed then that whenever he had a seizure, the response was to increase his dosage. To parents with little understanding of such medical matters, this was rather alarming — we didn't understand that as he gained weight the medication also needed to be increased. We just thought his epilepsy must be getting worse, which was why he regularly needed more drugs.

Philip also seemed to become more aggressive around this time and often quite emotional. We wondered if he was becoming 'spoilt' by all the attention he had been given. He was also intolerant to various foods but, over a decade ago, that was not something to which most doctors gave credibility. However, following a private visit to an allergy specialist, it was confirmed that he was indeed intolerant to dairy produce, citrus fruits and many of the colourings and preservatives used so liberally in foods at that time. It came as a surprise to us that when these foods were eliminated from his diet, his general health improved. He still had slight co-ordination problems and less stamina than most of his peers, but seemed a much more content child than previously.

School was not the easiest place for Philip in the years following his diagnosis. This was because, while his first teacher had been very accepting of the fact that he might have seizures and had even agreed to administer his rectal diazepam, the other staff members were giving out different messages. The headmistress treated us in a very superior manner and was not at all supportive when we felt that Philip was falling behind. She thought we were keeping him away from school unnecessarily, yet also that he should be taken home from school even if he was only a little 'under the weather'. However, the dinner ladies were very good and one in particular nurtured Philip over the next year or two.

Interestingly, the fact that Philip had obvious health problems did not seem to bother his classmates, and though he never had a big circle of friends, he did have one or two special ones who remained friends until he entered secondary education. Philip's restricted diet posed some problems at school; so we would always try to provide him with foods that he was allowed so that he was no different from the others. Philip was generally sensible so far as his diet was concerned and, whenever anything was given to him by friends or neighbours, would always question whether he could have it. This provided a touch of humour during his preparation for his first Holy Communion when he asked the priest whether the 'bread' was wholemeal!

During the middle years of his childhood, Philip no longer had seizures when he was awake, which was wonderful for his school and social life. He knew that he could go along to Beavers and Cubs with his friends without any worries. David and I were working opposite shifts at that time. The decision to work these patterns had been taken when the boys were very young and was nothing to do with Philip's epilepsy. David worked during the week and I worked at the week-ends. It was a very good arrangement generally for the boys because they treated both parents as equal and if neither of us could be with them, they also had two grandmothers who were happy to look after them. However, for David and me it was quite a tiring time. Philip was still taking quite a high dose of medication, but only at bedtime. After his dosage he would fall asleep almost immediately but would often have seizures during sleep. As a result, he was also bedwetting and it was not unusual to have to change his bed three times a night. We discussed this with his doctors. They said that many boys were still bedwetting at a much older age and we shouldn't worry about it. We did worry a little because he had been dry before the medication was given and was embarrassed at this regression. The bedwetting also meant that he was reluctant to sleep over at his grandparents' house with his two brothers. The knock-on effect was that David and I rarely had time to ourselves or to socialise and gradually lost contact with our friends. The fact that we were looking after Philip during the night also meant that we were constantly 'on duty' and we both suffered periods of depression.

I don't think that David or I realised how near we came to breaking point. It was only when I visited a new general practitioner and voiced my concern over my own mental health that life began to change. While this general practitioner knew little about Philip's health problems, she realised that we were both worn out and needed more support. She had worked with Philip's paediatrician while a trainee and felt that, though he was experienced in many childhood conditions, he was not particularly interested in epilepsy. For this reason she suggested that Philip be referred to a professor of paediatrics in a local city.

This was a turning point in all our lives. Philip was around 7 or 8 by this time but still needed to be carried down the stairs at morning because he was so unsteady. He was embarrassed about this, but we thought it was simply because he was having so many seizures in his sleep. Following the consultation with the professor, we were told that many of his problems were due to intoxication caused by the high level and combination of his anti-epileptic medications. The medication was gradually reduced and the seizures became less. This meant that the rectal diazepam we had been giving him at night also became less and that he became less drowsy in the mornings. While he was still having occasional seizures, he was a changed boy. Suddenly he started to blossom — he was still immature in some ways compared to his peers, but he started to 'wake up' and make progress at school. He was a practical child and never happier than when he had a screwdriver in his hand. Previously he had been too shaky to put screws into wood. Now we were forever finding screws undone, but we didn't mind at all!

In the main, our other two boys had taken Philip's problems in their stride. Jonathan was always studious and enjoyed his own company and Michael very gregarious and had lots of friends. They had sometimes become impatient with Philip when they felt he was emotional or acting like a baby, but now they seemed to relate to him better and were pleased that he was becoming 'one of the boys', rather than someone with different needs to their own. Though we had tried to nurture the other two, David and I had always been conscious of the fact that Philip's needs had to be met and that sometimes the other boys were short-changed. The improvement in Philip's health following the change in medication was dramatic and it felt as though we could finally 'see the light at the end of the tunnel'. While the seizures did not stop completely at that time, our appointments with doctors and hospitals became less, as did our visits to school to keep them up to date with his health progress. This in itself was wonderful because, though we all had Philip's best interests at heart, we often felt that our attempts to get the best treatment for him meant that we had conflicting ideas as far as the medical and teaching professionals were concerned. For a long time it had seemed like them and us; now, with a change of doctor, that was no longer the case.

As a family we had tried not to let the epilepsy dominate our lives, although this was difficult at times. However, we learned a lot through our experiences, even though that learning process was not one embarked upon by choice. The boys, though still quite young, were quite knowledgeable about epilepsy and talked in a matter of fact way to their friends about why Philip needed his tablets and why he had to visit the hospital from time to time. Following a BBC Television children's programme appeal, they decided to sell their old toys and games to raise money for people with epilepsy. This was a lovely idea and became an annual event as every summer for about three years they held toy sales in our local area. The money raised was then donated to British Epilepsy Association. This was a wonderful experience for the boys and Philip, in particular, felt very important. It did wonders for his self-esteem when he was given a certificate by the Association and a picture of all three boys and their cousin appeared in the Association's magazine.

It is not possible to explain fully the impact epilepsy has had on our lives, only to say that at some points, particularly when Philip was having seizures every night, David and I felt desperate. In retrospect, that period was also very trying so far as our own relationship was concerned. However, now that some years have passed and Philip is seizure-free even without medication, we can be more philosophical. Yes, it is difficult having a child with such an unpredictable medical condition, but then parenting is always a difficult job. Most parents with three children born within three years would find life trying and we were no different from many. The important thing for us is that, as a family, we have more understanding of the needs of people with chronic medical conditions. For myself the experience led to employment as an advisor to people with epilepsy. It seems that every cloud does indeed have a silver lining!

PRESENT DAY

Philip is now 19 and working as a technician in micro-electronics. At the same time he is gaining qualifications that will eventually lead to a Higher National Diploma in Electronics. He is also learning to drive — no mean feat for a young man with such a challenging background!

Chapter 16

THE ROLE OF THE PRIMARY CARE PRACTITIONER

Simon J. de Groot

Almost all individuals in the United Kingdom are registered with a National Health Service General Medical Practitioner (GP), who has a responsibility to provide their general medical care. The doctor and patient generally have a long term relationship, the practitioner providing continuing personal care to the patient and his or her family over many years, and frequently over generations. If a patient moves area and changes GP, his medical records will be transferred as well. This structure of defined lists of patients along with life long records lends itself well to research into chronic diseases, particularly their epidemiology and natural history. In this chapter I will look at the ideal structure of general practice based care for epilepsy, then examine some of the community research looking at the actual provision of care. I will also look at the research into patients' perceptions of the quality of their care and, finally, at how a strategy for improvement can be developed.

In the UK, the average GP has just under 2000 patients registered on his or her personal list. From community studies (Goodridge and Shorvon, 1983) the prevalence of epilepsy measured in terms of those currently receiving treatment is five per 1000. The incidence of new cases is approximately five per 10,0000. This means that the average GP will have approximately ten patients on his list with active epilepsy and can expect to see only one or two new cases each year. It is not surprising, given these figures, that GPs express lack of familiarity and lack of confidence when it comes to dealing with epilepsy. In a survey of GPs in one UK city (Taylor, 1980), two thirds, while acknowledging their responsibility for the overall care for patients with epilepsy, reported difficulties in diagnosis, counselling and use of antiepileptic drugs. Despite this, given that most practitioners work within group practices with an average of 10,000 patients, epilepsy should be a commonly enough presenting condition for an interested GP to develop and maintain the appropriate knowledge and skills.

THE ROLE OF THE GP IN EFFECTIVE MANAGEMENT

In an ideal world, the GP will provide a structured approach to optimising management, including obtaining a detailed and accurate history, a physical examination, referring the patient to an epilepsy specialist for confirmation of the diagnosis and initiation of treatment, and management of the non-clinical aspects of the condition.

Initial Management

As the diagnosis in epilepsy generally relies on interpretation of the history, an accurate and full account (including, if possible, an eye witness account) is crucial. The GP is frequently best placed to obtain this. The history should include: as detailed description of the attack as possible, including state of consciousness; any prodromal features; any precipitating factors; the duration of the attack; the post ictal state and its length; age at the first attack; the frequency of attacks and whether these are stereotypical; the past medical history with particular reference to prenatal birth and perinatal history; history of head injury or CNS infection; and family history of epilepsy or other inherited CNS disease. The GP should conduct a physical examination to look for neurological signs and exclude other abnormalities.

New cases will generally need referral to secondary care to allay anxiety, confirm the diagnosis and arrange specialist investigation. Ideally, for routine referrals, the patient should be seen by a specialist with an interest in epilepsy within four weeks. Severe, prolonged or frequent seizures or focal neurological signs will require more urgent referral.

Generally, treatment is best initiated by the specialist rather than the GP. However, where there are delays in obtaining an expert opinion, or where there is no doubt about the diagnosis, or seizures continue and the patient wishes it, then consideration can be given to starting treatment. In the UK, it is unusual to initiate treatment after a single seizure; even when seizures are frequent, the patient may prefer not to take any medication if they are causing no distress (for example if they are occurring only at night).

Patients and their families will often be devastated by receiving a diagnosis of epilepsy. Patients may feel stigmatised as a result of the ignorance and fear of others. They will have many initial questions, for example related to safety at home, driving regulations, leisure activities and potential problems at school or work. Consequently, they have an immediate need for accurate information. The GP will be able to advise on many issues, but is unlikely to have the time to discuss all aspects fully. Ideally, there will be an 'in-house' epilepsy clinic with a trained nurse to whom the patient can be referred. Ideally, access will also be available to a specialist nurse working from the local specialist clinic. Many patients will also benefit from the support and information available through patient support organisations such as the British Epilepsy Association (see Chapter 20), which provide advice and information through leaflets, videos, patient information packs and helplines, as well as running local patient groups.

Continuing Care

The GP will be a key figure in the provision of long term continuing care for people with epilepsy. A patient's needs may change over time and with the course of their condition. The GP will be involved in instituting any changes in management which the hospital recommends, often reinforcing and further explaining the reasons. The GP also has a key role in sickness certification and the provision of reports for the UK Benefits Agency (through which patients apply for incapacity and disability benefits). The GP will act as the patient's advocate, it being generally accepted that he or she is best placed to give an opinion, by virtue of having long term knowledge of the patient.

Finally, general practice provides an excellent opportunity for research into epilepsy because of its maintenance of lifelong records for all patients. GPs should therefore maintain a register of their patients with epilepsy and, ideally, keep their records in an auditable form.

How then does the reality of primary care for epilepsy meet this ideal structure? To answer this question, I will report findings from a project in my local area into the actual provision of care, as well as into patients' perceptions of their condition and the care they received for it.

AN AUDIT OF EPILEPSY IN THE COMMUNITY

In 1996, Doncaster Medical Audit Advisory Group (Rogers and Taylor, 1996) conducted an audit and surveys of patients, practices and consultants in Doncaster. Doncaster is a small town in South Yorkshire, England, formerly a great mining and railway town, with a population of 290,000 people. With the contraction of heavy industry it is now developing more service industries. The audit provided a comprehensive review of the consequences of having epilepsy, and the services provided for it in Doncaster. The sample population of 875 patients approximates to half of the population believed to have epilepsy in Doncaster.

Doncaster is unusual in that unlike most areas of the UK it has for some time had specific services for those with epilepsy. It was, for example, the first area in the UK to develop the concept of the epilepsy liaison nurses. The liaison service was established in 1988 after an audit of his practice by a local GP demonstrated not only the extent of local need, but also that by intervention it was possible to improve care in terms of seizure control and reduced drug side effects (Taylor, 1980). In 1995, half of the Doncaster general practices agreed to participate in an epilepsy audit; and at the same time patients were surveyed about their epilepsy, their problems and needs and their perceptions of the local epilepsy service.

The objective of the general practice audit was to establish the level of recorded care together with a review of medication practices; and identify areas in which improvements needed to be made. The computerised and manual records of the 23 participating practices were retrospectively analysed against eleven clinical criteria (Table 1). Overall the practices achieved high levels of success for the audited criteria, with relatively high rates of recording, but it was notable that GP contact specifically for epilepsy was low in the preceding year. As a result, there was a low level of recording of recently given advice, recent seizure frequency and current problems. These findings echo those of similar community studies in other UK cities (Clifford, 1994; Brahama, 1995; Jacoby *et al.*, 1996), where between a third and a half of epilepsy patients had not been reviewed in the preceding year.

The objective of the survey of patients was to assess their quality of life and views about the quality of their care. Questionnaires were sent by post to all adults and the parents of all children identified from the

TABLE 1 AUDIT OF PRACTICE HELD RECORDS AGAINST SPECIFIED CLINICAL CRITERIA

AUDIT CRITERIA	NUMBER OF RECORDS WHERE RECORDED	PERCENTAGE OF RECORDS WHERE RECORDED
ONSET DATE RECORDED	827	95
SPECIALIST CONFIRMATION MADE AND RECORDED	739	84
EEG TAKEN, IF EVER	580	66
EYE WITNESS ACCOUNT RECORDED	807	92
GP CONTACT IN LAST YEAR MADE AND RECORDED	447	51
LAST SEIZURE DATE RECORDED	452	49
SEIZURE FREQUENCY RECORDED	405	46
GENERAL ADVICE GIVEN AND RECORDED	694	79
REFERRAL TO ENLS MADE AND RECORDED	212	24
SEIZURE DIARY PROVIDED	38	4
MONO- OR POLYTHERAPY	578	66

audited practices, who were currently on anti-epileptic medication and had not been seizure free over the last two years. The overall response rate was 84% (n = 444) for adults and 90% (n = 48) for parents. Many respondents commented that this was the first time someone had taken a genuine interest in their experiences.

Adults were asked how they felt epilepsy affected their everyday lives. The greatest perceived effect was on their overall health (46%), followed by their ability to work (41%). One important finding from our survey was that only one fifth of the adults were employed full-time, reflecting the findings of other surveys that unemployment is one of the major problems facing people with epilepsy. This is despite evidence from British Epilepsy Association that employees with epilepsy are less likely than other employees to have time off work and that most jobs are suitable for people with epilepsy. A quarter of our adults were on permanent sickness benefit, with about a half describing themselves as having long term health problems additional to epilepsy. One possible explanation for this low level of employment is that 62% of adults surveyed lacked any formal educational qualifications.

Fifty seven percent of adults and 42% of the parents of children described their epilepsy as very well controlled. Forty-one percent of adults had been seizure free in the preceding year, 25% had had one or less seizures a month. With regard to their treatment, a large number of patients (66%) were on monotherapy. Half considered that they had problems or side effects caused by medication, including difficulty concentrating, tiredness and memory problems. The adults were asked about any seizure-related injuries incurred in the preceding twelve months. The most frequently reported was head injury (by 13%). Over 10% of adults reported falling to the ground during a seizure.

Over half of the children surveyed were attending special school or receiving remedial help at school. Parents worried most about the uncertainty of their child's epilepsy — not knowing when an attack would happen (39%), and whether or not their child's epilepsy would effect his or her future (35%). Other worries included fear of injury during an attack (31%), possible drug side effects (27%), how much to restrict their child's activities (21%) and whether their child would grow out of epilepsy (21%).

The views of patients and the parents of children were largely positive about GP care. Seventy-two percent of adults and 78% of parents described care by their GP as excellent or good, few (only three percent each of patients and parents) considered it poor. Forty percent of adults

TABLE 2 DEPRESSION AND ANXIETY IN USERS AND NON-USERS OF THE LIAISON SERVICE

	CLINICAL ANXIETY			CLINICAL DEPRESSION		
	NORMAL	BORDERLINE	PROBABLE	NORMAL	BORDERLINE	PROBABLE
NOT REFERRED TO SERVICE IN LAST YEAR	177 (47%)	47 (13%)	83 (22%)	222 (60%)	48 (13%)	37 (10%)
REFERRED TO SERVICE IN LAST YEAR	28 (8%)	16 (4%)	22 (6%)	41 (11%)	41 (11%)	13 (3%)

and 20% of parents had consulted their GP specifically about epilepsy in the preceding year, though the majority only saw him or her to discuss a particular problem and not as part of a regular review. When they did consult their GP, it was most often with regard to medication issues rather than issues or advice relating to the impact of epilepsy. A large proportion (around a third) felt that their GP did not provide them with enough information about their epilepsy. The majority of adults considered their GP to be the main provider of their epilepsy care but a fifth expressed a preference for care to be shared between the GP and a hospital specialist. An important point emerging from the survey was that they saw the GP as better able to deliver personalised and continuous care. Fewer parents than adult patients expressed a preference for shared care, reflecting the perceived need for greater specialist involvement in the care of children.

The epilepsy liaison nursing service was widely used, a quarter of all adults and a third of all children having been seen by the service at some time. Older people were least likely to use the service. The patient survey highlighted that the majority derived great benefit from this contact; they reported improved understanding of epilepsy and medication issues, and interestingly, they also had lower rates of depression and anxiety compared with non-users of the service (Table 2).

IMPROVING PRIMARY CARE FOR EPILEPSY

Three barriers to effective primary care have been identified: organisational; general practitioner related; and patient related (Thapar, 1996). I will conclude by considering each of these in turn.

Organisational Barriers

The UK National Health Service has traditionally been demand-led. Only in recent years have programmes in disease prevention and health promotion, for example the cervical smear and breast screening programmes, been developed. Recently, effort has also been made to develop a structured programme for primary care through the development of care protocols and specialist clinics for the management of chronic diseases. It is clear that epilepsy has not been managed well by the traditional demand-led service. Patients have tended to accept sub-optimal care, rather than seeking improvement. Care for epilepsy could be improved by the implementation of a structured programme, that identifies relevant patients, most often via a search of repeat prescriptions for anti-convulsants. If there are sufficiently large numbers of patients, a specialist epilepsy clinic can be started. Whether or not this is feasible, there is a need for regular review. One partner and the practice nurse could perhaps develop a special interest. The practice could also enlist the help of a community liaison nurse. A specially developed protocol for new and existing cases would help optimise care and ensure all aspects of the clinical and psychosocial management were dealt with appropriately. Locally developed guidelines would be helpful (and a number have already been developed; Cumbria MAAG, 1992, Taylor *et al.*, 1995). Setting up a regular process of audit of care would identify important deficiencies. The resource implications of such a service are considerable, but so are the potentials for health gain.

It should perhaps be said that although general practitioners can do a great deal to improve their own services, satisfactory care for epilepsy can only be provided within a structure that includes adequate specialist services. In the UK, general practice is well placed to influence current service development through the commissioning and purchasing processes.

GP-related Barriers

General practitioners often feel uncomfortable with their own level of knowledge and skills when dealing with epilepsy. However, within the average group practice of 10,000 patients there are sufficient patient numbers for at least one of the partners to develop an interest and improve his knowledge. The Doncaster survey showed that patients were generally highly satisfied with their GP, but did express a wish for more and better information from him or her. Indeed greater provision of information, via the nursing liaison service, was shown to allay anxiety and improve health and understanding.

Patient-related Barriers

Finally, it is important for GPs to understand that many patients feel embarrassed or stigmatised by their condition and this may contribute to their failure to seek help for it. Increased awareness and public education about epilepsy may help to reduce its psychosocial sequelae.

CONCLUSION

General practice can provide the ideal setting for the care of people with epilepsy. The quality of this care can be improved by implementation of a planned structure, which includes both on-going support, education and information, and high quality clinical care. General practice also provides a valuable database for research into the epidemiology of epilepsy and the reality of living with this chronic condition.

References

Brahama, J. (1995) *An Audit of epilepsy in general practice*. Project report. Leeds: Leeds Medical Audit Advisory Group.

Clifford, R. (1994) *An audit on Epilepsy for General Practice*. Project Report. Gloucester: Gloucester Medical Audit Advisory Group.

Cumbria MAAG (Medical Audit Advisory Group). (1992) *Cumbrian standard for the management of patients with epilepsy*. Carlisle: Cumbria MAAG.

Goodridge, D.M.G. and Shorvon, S.D. (1983) Epileptic seizures in a population of 60,000. *British Medical Journal* **287**, 641–647.

Jacoby, A., Graham-Jones, S., Baker, G., Ratoff, L., Heyes, J., Dewey, M., Chadwick, D. (1996) A general practice records audit of the process of care for people with epilepsy. *British Journal of General Practice* **46**, 595–99.

Rogers, D., Taylor, M.P. (1996) *'Don't fit in front of your workmates' Living with Epilepsy in Doncaster*. Doncaster: Doncaster Medical Audit Advisory Group.

Taylor, M.P., Howell, S., De Groot, S.J., Hughes, Inglis, Hague, Boulter and Rittey C. (1995) *Doncaster epilepsy guidelines*. Doncaster: Doncaster Health.

Taylor, M.P. (1980) A job half done. *Journal of the Royal College of General Practitioners* **30**, 456–465.

Thapar, A.K. (1996) Care of patients with epilepsy in the community: Will new initiatives address old problems? *British Journal of General Practice* **46**, 37–42.

Chapter 17

THE CONTRIBUTION OF THE CLINICAL PSYCHOLOGIST

Laura H. Goldstein

This chapter will consider the specific contributions clinical psychologists can make to the improvement of the quality of life of persons with epilepsy. It is increasingly recognised that clinical psychologists have a major role to play in the assessment and treatment of people with epilepsy (Cull and Goldstein, 1997) and while clinical psychology interventions may be targeted at reducing the severity and frequency of epileptic seizures (see below), clinical psychologists can also contribute to improved quality of life in patients with epilepsy by assessing and remediating the cognitive and varied psychosocial difficulties that may accompany the disorder.

Clinical psychology practice is based on the careful assessment of the presenting problems of the individual patient, the results of which determine the treatment approach to be employed (see Lindsay and Powell, 1994 for an overview). Treatments now applied by clinical psychologists to their patients, both adult and child, have seen enormous developments over the past 20–30 years and, to some extent, this parallels the considerable developments in other treatments (neurosurgical, pharmacological) that are available for persons with epilepsy. The particular challenge for clinical psychologists working with patients with epilepsy is how best to contribute to the care of individuals who may be receiving different approaches to the treatment of their seizures, not all of which may be having a positive outcome.

Clinical psychology typically adopts the 'scientist-practitioner' model (Milne *et al.*, 1990) i.e. assessments and treatments are based on empirical evidence of their effectiveness, reliability and validity, having been derived from theoretical models of psychological functioning. In the field of epilepsy there is less information pertaining to the effectiveness of psychological interventions than exists in other fields (e.g. adult or child mental health) but careful assessment of the presenting and more general psychosocial problems in children and adults with epilepsy indicates where intervention approaches can be borrowed helpfully from other areas of work.

A widely used approach to the assessment of behavioural and psychosocial problems in adults and children is that of functional analysis. Different models of functional analysis exist (Goldstein, 1993) but common to all of these is an attempt to identify the settings in which problems occur and what events maintain the behaviour. Models of functional analysis therefore allow the clinician to generate a series of hypotheses about how the problem has developed and why it persists; such hypotheses then have treatment implications for the person concerned.

It is also widely accepted that people with epilepsy are at risk of having cognitive impairments, especially in the domains of memory and concentration. Whether these are a result of a combination of the underlying neuropathology, seizure activity, side effects of medication or associated mood disorder, they may well impact on people's everyday lives and restrict their educational and work opportunities. Clinical psychologists specialising in neuropsychology can assist in the delineation of such cognitive difficulties and can, through detailed assessment, identify the person's specific cognitive strengths and weaknesses. While identification of the latter may confirm what has been suspected beforehand, the identification of the former may then be used to devise cognitive rehabilitation programmes. This will be returned to later in the chapter, as will the important role of the clinical psychologist in predicting who will be at risk of developing severe cognitive impairment as a consequence of epilepsy surgery, with a view to the prevention of such an outcome.

TREATING PSYCHOLOGICAL DISTURBANCE ASSOCIATED WITH HAVING EPILEPSY

Given that people with epilepsy are at increased risk of a range of psychological difficulties such as anxiety, depression and low self-esteem (Fiordelli *et al.,* 1993; Cockerell *et al.,* 1996; Perini *et al.,* 1996; Baker, 1997) and may suffer from phobias related to seizure occurrence (Betts, 1992; Newsom-Davis *et al.,* 1998), it would seem appropriate for any attempt to improve the quality of life of the person with epilepsy to address these problems. This is further emphasised by the extensive community surveys that have documented the relationships between seizure severity/frequency and psychological difficulties (Baker *et al.,* 1996). Although it is well accepted that people with epilepsy may have difficulties with family and other interpersonal relationships (Ferrari *et al.,* 1983; Laaksonen, 1983) as well as with employment (Carroll, 1992;

Jacoby, 1995; Cooper, 1995; Troxell, 1997), it is now apparent that the psychosocial difficulties faced by people with newly diagnosed epilepsy may well differ from those whose epilepsy has become a chronic disorder (Chaplin *et al.,* 1992, 1993; Pershad and Siddiqui, 1992). Thus any psychological intervention undertaken to alleviate such problems may need to consider where, in the process of adjustment to having seizures, the person has reached (Chaplin *et al.,* 1993), in order to best facilitate further adjustment.

Disappointingly, relatively little systematic psychological intervention research has been published in this area, despite the scope for clinical interventions to alleviate psychological distress. Most of the work pointing to the role for psychological interventions in alleviating emotional problems in adults and children with epilepsy has been undertaken from a psychodynamic therapeutic perspective (see reviews by Taube and Calman, 1992; Miller 1994a, 1994b; Goldstein, 1997a; and *in press*). A range of complex psychological and psychosocial difficulties has been addressed, largely through single case studies, and for example such work has addressed issues such as the meaning of the seizures for the individual, denial of or the impact of having epilepsy and conflicts over dependence and independence. Case reports have documented the treatment of a range of specific difficulties such as anxiety and aggression (Tancredi and Guerini, 1992) poor self esteem (Grasso *et al.,* 1992) poor school and family relationships (Paladin *et al.,* 1989), feelings of depression, hopelessness and worthlessness and difficulties forming enduring relationships with the opposite sex (Dorwart, 1984), as well as the reduction of anxiety accompanying reflex epilepsy (Espadaler-Medina *et al.,* 1992).

Very limited information is available on the benefits of group therapy for individuals with epilepsy (Lessman and Mollick, 1978; Appolone and Gibson, 1980; Mathers, 1992). This generally suggests some benefits to group members, although not all patients necessarily benefit equally from the experience (Lessman and Mollick, 1978) and for some, the group intervention may be accompanied by an unwanted increase in seizure frequency (Mathers, 1992).

Cognitive behaviour therapy, which targets the person's thought patterns and behaviour, and which is based on the premise that thoughts affect emotional state (Beck *et al.,* 1979), has been used successfully in a wide range of studies of the treatment of anxiety and depression in adults without epilepsy (Andrews, 1990; Manning *et al.,* 1994; Mogg *et al.,* 1995; Kingdon *et al.,* 1996). It has also been effective in improving emotional and psychological well-being in adults with poorly controlled seizures (Upton and Thompson, 1992). Cognitive-behaviour therapy, applied on a group basis to adult patients with epilepsy, was found to produce an improvement in the therapists' global rating of the patients' well-being, as a result of treatment (Tan and Bruni, 1986). Gillham (1990), who applied brief cognitive-behavioural interventions to out-patients to improve seizure control, also reported a significant improvement in their psychological state.

Cognitive-behaviour therapy has also been effective in treating seizure phobia (Newsom-Davis *et al.*, 1998) and panic symptoms (Reisner, 1990) in individual patients. Progressive muscular relaxation (a more typical behaviour therapy approach) has been used to treat hyperventilation (Kiesel *et al.*, 1989) and has improved the sense of well being in patients who were taught this technique as a means of seizure control (Rousseau *et al.*, 1985). Anxiety related to the uncertainty in patients of the behaviour they exhibit during a seizure may be addressed by allowing them to view videotapes of their seizures (Sanders *et al.*, 1995).

Given the acceptance of difficulties faced by families with a child, young or grown-up, with epilepsy (Thompson and Upton, 1992) it is perhaps surprising that family therapeutic techniques have not been described for this patient group. The literature on the treatment of behavioural disorders of children with epilepsy is similarly limited (Cull, 1997). Most of the existing research focuses on psychological difficulties in families where a young child has epilepsy. However, the demonstration that families of adult children with seizures may also face considerable emotional strain suggests the potential benefit of interventions to address the particular sources of strain and mood disturbance. An understanding by clinicians of the long term impact of the content and method of delivery of a diagnosis of epilepsy, as well as an understanding of the popular myths and misconceptions about epilepsy that are likely to be held by family members, will also be important in dealing with psychosocial and psychological problems in patients with epilepsy and their families (Psenska and Holden, 1996). Similarly, an understanding of the types of uncertainty faced by parents of children with uncontrolled seizures will provide an indication of the ways in which clinicians can work towards assisting families to accept the diagnosis of epilepsy and provide the necessary information to enhance their ability to cope with it (Murray, 1993). This will prevent the families from coming to be viewed as a source of psychopathology for their children.

It is also worth noting that clinical psychologists possess the skills to assess the nature of parent-child interactions (Forehand and McMahon, 1981) and then apply interventions to alter any maladaptive patterns of interaction; the quality of such child-parent interactions and the relationship between them have been shown to predict the psychosocial adjustment of children with epilepsy in their school environment and in an independent problem-solving activity (Lothman and Pianta, 1993). There is also the potential for parents to be trained by clinicians to modify any maladaptive behaviour in their children (Callias, 1980). Clinicians can also offer parents advice on how to reduce the potentially detrimental effects of epilepsy on their children (Hoare and Kerley, 1992). This is likely to be particularly helpful in the early months following diagnosis and introduction of treatment, and if offered on an individual basis rather than via a group format.

Clinical psychologists, along with other professionals involved in the care of people with epilepsy, will be mindful of the increased suicide risk in people with this disorder (Mendez and Doss, 1992). No literature is available to indicate the potential contribution by clinical psychologists in attenuating such risk, but they will be able to appreciate the role of potent psychosocial stressors in their patients' lives that may put them at increased risk of committing suicide.

COGNITIVE BEHAVIOURAL TREATMENTS TO REDUCE SEIZURE OCCURRENCE

While treatment of seizure occurrence has been seen traditionally as the province of the medical profession, there is growing evidence that psychological approaches to seizure control can be effective, with the benefit of enabling the person to develop a sense of self-control over their seizure disorder, and possibly avoid the need for more invasive treatments.

Much of the emphasis of a psychological approach to seizure control stresses a learning theory model of seizure occurrence (Dahl, 1992). In this model, seizure occurrence is seen as an interaction between the person with epilepsy and their environment. Dahl (1992) suggested that while an initial seizure may not have been influenced by conditioning factors, subsequent early seizures might be susceptible to the processes of classical conditioning, whereby seizures come to be associated with particular setting events; via operant learning processes the consequences of having seizures then become associated with their occurrence so that over time positive consequences of having seizures will lead to increased seizure frequency. Any assessment of the pattern of a person's seizure occurrence needs to take such factors into account, especially if an intervention is to be designed and implemented.

There is now a growing literature demonstrating the effectiveness of cognitive-behavioural techniques in reducing seizure frequency for at least some people (children and adults) although as yet there is no clear view as to who is most likely benefit from such an approach (see Goldstein, in press, for an elaboration of these points).

Seizure frequency reduction has been achieved using progressive muscular relaxation (Rousseau *et al.*, 1985; Whitman *et al.*, 1990; Puskarich *et al.*, 1992) and using relaxation applied in high-risk-for-seizure-occurrence situations (Dahl *et al.*, 1987). Broadly cognitive-behavioural approaches have also been successful when applied on an individual basis (Gillham, 1990), although less so when applied to a small group of adults with epilepsy (Tan and Bruni, 1986). Multi-component approaches, including teaching people to be aware of, and where possible to avoid, seizure triggers or high-risk-for seizure-occurrence situations, (Dahl *et al.*, 1985, 1988; Reiter *et al.*, 1987; Gillham, 1990; Spector *et al.*, 1994; 1995) have also offered the possibility of seizure reduction, although only one long-term follow-up study has been reported (Dahl *et al.*, 1992).

A persisting weakness of these studies (Goldstein, 1990) is the failure to investigate the long term psychosocial benefit of reducing seizure frequency via psychological techniques. In addition, little has been written about the psychological factors that might mitigate against people either accepting or benefiting from a psychological treatment approach, and how people subsequently adjust to their reduced seizure frequency and greater self-control ability with respect to seizure occurrence.

Although beyond the scope of this chapter, clinical psychologists must be mindful of the possibility of their patients suffering from non-epileptic seizures, and the general psychological assessment framework of functional analysis is appropriate for the elucidation of the psychological factors that may underlie the origins and maintenance of seizures that have an entirely psychological cause (Goldstein, 1997b). A cognitive-behavioural approach to the treatment of non-epileptic seizures has been successful (Chalder, 1996).

NEUROPSYCHOLOGICAL ASSESSMENT AND REHABILITATION

It is well accepted that people with epilepsy may suffer from a range of cognitive problems (e.g. impairments in attention and memory) that can derive in greatest part from the neuropathology underlying their seizures, but also from the unwanted effects of anti-epileptic medication (Gillham and Cull, 1997) and ongoing subclinical epileptic activity (Binnie and Marston, 1992; Binnie, 1993). Such cognitive difficulties may restrict educational and vocational opportunities open to people with epilepsy, as well as having implications for other everyday activities (Goldstein and Polkey, 1992; Corcoran and Thompson, 1993). Careful delineation of such deficits can result, for example, in students with epilepsy being given more time during their examinations to allow for slowness in information processing, in much the same way that allowances can be made elsewhere, for example in cases of dyslexia. In addition the careful identification of cognitive strengths and weaknesses can assist individuals in the process of deciding upon appropriate courses of study and career paths to be followed.

Neuropsychological Contribution to Surgical Treatment of Seizures

The ability of clinical psychologists to assess the cognitive strengths and weaknesses of adults and children with epilepsy is well developed (Goldstein, 1991, 1997c; Fowler, 1997; Oxbury, 1997; Thompson, 1997) and there is increasing understanding of how differing neuropathology relates to cognitive abilities in epilepsy (McMillan *et al.*, 1987; Oxbury, 1997; Baxendale, 1998; Baxendale *et al.*, 1998). Perhaps one of the strongest contributions of clinical psychologists working with patients with epilepsy is the neuropsychological assessment of patients who are being considered for neurosurgical treatment of their seizure disorder. Here clinicians must not only provide a good description of the person's cognitive abilities, but must also be able to recognise when patients are at risk for developing severe cognitive impairment as a consequence of neurosurgery. To remove someone's seizures via a temporal lobectomy but permit them to develop a global amnesia for example would undoubtedly have a devastating effect on their everyday life. Selection of patients for neurosurgical treatment of their epilepsy ideally requires that decisions are made on the basis of the individual's clinical history, EEG and neuroimaging findings, and the results of neuropsychiatric and neuropsychological assessments. The latter should attempt to identify any indication that the not-to-be-operated-upon temporal lobe would be unable to support an adequate degree of memory, meaning that the person would be likely to suffer severe postoperative memory difficulties. This is done through an evaluation of the extent to which neuropsychological test results are consistent with what else is known about the lateralisation and localisation of the likely epileptic focus (Oxbury, 1997). Oxbury (1997) has indicated that the aims of neuropsychological assessment in epilepsy surgery programmes also include the prediction of other likely postoperative cognitive difficulties, as well as their contribution towards psychosocial and educational issues. In addition neuropsychological assessment is used to evaluate the actual effect of surgery on cognitive abilities, at different follow-up intervals.

Recent attempts have been made to determine whether preoperative neuropsychological assessment results can be used to predict postoperative seizure control (Sawrie *et al.*, 1998) and also to derive regression equations that can predict the degree of postoperative memory change that the person may experience following surgery (Baxendale, 1998). An estimation of the likely extent of cognitive change resulting from epilepsy surgery is information that should be available to prospective surgical candidates, to enable them to make an informed decision about the risks of surgery, especially as expectations concerning the outcome of surgery tend to centre on the likelihood of becoming seizure free (Wheelock *et al.*, 1998) or on practical expectations (such as driving, increased employment opportunities, new physical activities; Wilson *et al.*, 1998) rather than on cognitive factors.

Rehabilitation after Epilepsy Surgery — Life Without Seizures

Although seizure cessation is the desired outcome following epilepsy surgery, people for whom this is achieved may experience some difficulty in adjusting to their new seizure free life (Bladin, 1992; Wilson *et al.*, 1998). No longer having the disorder which proved a limiting factor in everyday life may lead to altered family and other interpersonal relationships, altered expectations as to future activities and a reformulation of the person's identity. All of these may pose considerable stress, even though psychosocial outcome following neurosurgery for epilepsy has been reported to be best for those in whom total seizure control is achieved (Seidman-Ripley *et al.*, 1993). Bladin (1992) suggests that for some individuals successful surgery may produce a sense of grief, in that the operation is perceived as having been undertaken too late for them to achieve the type of lifestyle they might have had, if surgery had been possible when they were younger.

Of course poor surgical outcome can also lead to psychological difficulties, in particular because of the disappointment created by a failure to produce complete seizure control. Patients with expectations that surgery will affect practical aspects of their lives (e.g. their ability to drive or gain employment) are more likely to feel satisfied with the outcome of their operation than those who expect it to improve their quality of life in rather non-specific ways (Wilson *et al.*, 1998). Thus, in addition to careful preoperative counselling about the range of likely outcomes of surgery, it may well be important to examine patients' expectations of surgery outcome. Assisting with patients' formulation of realistic post-operative outcomes might be a way in which clinical psychologists can help them deal with the various scenarios that might follow from surgery. The patients' own definition of surgery as successful should not in any case be taken as synonymous with having achieved complete seizure relief (Wilson *et al.*, 1998) but it appears that both postoperative seizure frequency and psychosocial difficulties will, together with preoperative expectations, influence patients' judgement of the operation's success. Clinicians might also want to consider possible differences in expectations of surgery between patients and their significant others (Wheelock *et al.*, 1998) when examining the source of psychosocial difficulties following surgery, especially as seizure reduction does not produce the same degree of improvement in psychiatric and psychosocial status as does seizure abolition (Blumer *et al.*, 1998; Wheelock *et al.*, 1998). Wheelock *et al.*, (1998) usefully suggest that clinicians explore with their patients how seizure reduction rather than elimination might nonetheless improve their quality of life, so that the former might not be perceived as a negative surgical outcome.

Neuropsychological Rehabilitation

Although there is a growing field of knowledge relating to the remediation of neuropsychological deficits, in particular memory, (Wilson *et al.*, 1994; Glisky, 1995; Cockburn and Evans, 1997; Hunkin *et al.*, 1998), relatively little work of this kind has been undertaken with people with epilepsy. Thompson (1997) indicates the value that memory training might have for patients who have to attend hospital appointments and give accurate reports of their seizure occurrence, information which will determine whether changes are made to drug treatments. She suggests that patients with epilepsy might in fact be better candidates for memory training than people who have sustained severe head injuries producing marked amnesias, since people with epilepsy will usually have insight into their difficulties and will have less severe memory problems, which may therefore be more amenable to treatment. It may be worthwhile considering however whether self-reported memory impairments reflect a degree of neuroticism, especially if everyday memory complaints cannot be substantiated on formal testing (Vermeulen *et al.*, 1993).

Thompson (1997) reviews work reported by Aldenkamp and Vermeulen (1993) describing a memory group for adults with epilepsy, run for six, fortnightly sessions and which produced small improvements in memory functioning. She also describes the development and use of a self-help memory manual, which appeared to be of most use for individuals with moderate as opposed to severe memory difficulties, and for those who were not depressed. In addition to outlining a range of memory training techniques that might be applied to people with seizures, she describes the potential use of a range of memory management strategies with individual patients to assist their recollection of things they have done and talked about. Memory retraining (successfully using a range of cueing techniques) with an individual who had developed a dense amnesia after suffering post-traumatic status epilepticus, has been described (Kime *et al.*, 1996).

While the application of memory retraining techniques to people with epilepsy is sparse, there is even less information on the application of other neuropsychological rehabilitation approaches, for example in the case of language or executive dysfunction (Goldstein and Cull, 1997). Yet guidance may well be available in the literature (von Cramon *et al.*, 1991; von Cramon & Matthes-von Cramon, 1994; Alderman, 1996), and is of relevance given the potential development of dysexecutive symptoms following epilepsy surgery (Goldstein *et al.*, 1993).

CONCLUSIONS

This chapter has indicated that there is a range of areas in which clinical psychologists can assist people with epilepsy, and their families, improve their quality of life or prevent the development of impairments or difficulties that would lead to a reduction in such quality. While some of the skills possessed by clinical psychologists can be used in an attempt to reduce the frequency with which seizures occur, others can be used to improve psychological state, assess the nature of and quantify cognitive impairment, assist in the rehabilitation of patients (both from a neuropsychological and psychosocial perspective) and deal with the challenges posed by either losing or continuing to experience seizures following epilepsy surgery. Given that the majority of clinical psychologists do not work in specialist epilepsy centres but will encounter patients who present to mental health services with, *inter alia*, epilepsy as one of their problems, their role in improving their patients' quality of life may not always focus heavily on the epilepsy. However, given the potential impact of epilepsy on the person's life, clinicians should consider the potential for the different types of intervention discussed above, when deciding how best to assist the patient with their difficulties.

References

Alderman, N. (1996) Central executive deficit and response to operant conditioning methods. *Neuropsychological Rehabilitation* **6**, 161–186.

Aldenkamp, A.P., Vermeulen, J. (1993) Neuropsychological rehabilitation of memory function in epilepsy. *Neuropsychological Rehabilitation* **1**, 199–214.

Andrews, G. (1990) The diagnosis and management of pathological anxiety. *Medical Journal of Australia* **152**, 656–659.

Appolone, C., Gibson, P. (1980) Group work with young adult epilepsy patients. *Social Work in Health Care* **6**, 23–32.

Baker, G.A. (1997) Psychological responses to epilepsy. In: Cull C., Goldstein L.H. (eds.), *The Clinical psychologist's Handbook of Epilepsy. Assessment and Management.* London: Routledge, 96–112.

Baker, G.A., Jacoby, A., Chadwick, D.W. (1996) The associations of psychopathology in epilepsy: a community study. *Epilepsy Research* **25**, 29–39.

Baxendale, S.A. (1998) *The Neuropsychology of Temporal Lobectomy: Preoperative Correlations and Postoperative Predictions.* University of London: Unpublished PhD Thesis.

Baxendale, S.A., van Paesschen, W., Thompson, P.J., Connelly, A., Duncan, J.S., Harkness, W.F., Shorvon, S.D. (1998) The relationship between quantitative MRI and neuropsychological functioning in temporal lobe epilepsy. *Epilepsia* **39**, 158–166.

Beck, A.T., Rush, J., Shaw, B., Emery, G. (1979) *Cognitive Theories of Depression.* New York: Wiley.

Betts, T. (1992) Epilepsy and stress. Time for proper studies of the association. *British Medical Journal* **305**, 378–379.

Binnie, C.D. (1993) Significance and management of transitory cognitive impairment due to subclinical EEG discharges in children. *Brain and Development* **15**, 23–30.

Binnie, C.D., Marston, D. (1992) Cognitive correlates of interictal discharges. *Epilepsia* **33** (Suppl. 6), S11–17.

Bladin, P.F. (1992) Psychosocial difficulties and outcome after temporal lobectomy. *Epilepsia* **33**, 898–907.

Blumer, D., Wakhlu, S., Davies, K., Hermann, B. (1998) Psychiatric outcome of temporal lobectomy for epilepsy: Incidence and treatment of psychiatric complications. *Epilepsia* **39**, 478–485.

Callias, M. (1980) Teaching parents, teachers and nurses. In: Yule W., Carr J. (eds.) *Behaviour Modification for the Mentally Handicapped.* London: Croom Helm, 175–200.

Carroll, D. (1992) Employment among young people with epilepsy. *Seizure* **1**, 127–131.

Chalder, T. (1996) Non-epileptic attacks: A cognitive behavioural approach in a single case with a four-year follow-up. *Clinical psychology and Psychotherapy* **3**, 291–297.

Chaplin, J.E., Yepez, R., Shorvon, S., Floyd, M. (1992) National General Practice study of epilepsy: the social and psychological effects of a recent diagnosis of epilepsy. *British Medical Journal* **304**, 1416–1418.

Chaplin, J.E., Floyd, M., Lasso, R.Y. (1993) Early psychosocial adjustment and the experience of epilepsy: Findings from a general practice survey. *International Journal of Rehabilitation Research* **16**, 316–318.

Cockburn, J., Evans, J.J. (1997) Research digest. Approaches to amelioration of memory impairment. *Neuropsychological Rehabilitation* **7**, 259–266.

Cockerell, O.C., Moriarty, J., Trimble, M., Sander, J.W., Shorvon, S.D. (1996) Acute psychological disorders in patients with epilepsy: A nation-wide study. *Epilepsy Research* **25**, 119–131.

Cooper, M. (1995) Employment and epilepsy — employers' attitudes. *Seizure* **4**, 193–199.

Corcoran, R., Thompson, P. (1993) Epilepsy and poor memory. Who complains and what do they mean? *British Journal of Clinical psychology*, **32**, 199–208.

Cull, C. (1997) Assessment and management of behaviour problems in children. In: Cull C., Goldstein L.H. (eds.), *The Clinical psychologist's Handbook of Epilepsy. Assessment and Management.* London: Routledge, 167–183.

Cull, C., Goldstein, L.H. (eds.) (1997) *The Clinical psychologist's Handbook of Epilepsy. Assessment and Management.* London: Routledge.

Dahl, J. (1992) *Epilepsy. A Behaviour Medicine Approach to Assessment and Treatment in Children. A Handbook for Professionals Working with Epilepsy.* Göttingen: Hogrefe and Huber.

Dahl, J., Brorson, L-O., Melin, L. (1992) Effects of a broad-spectrum behavioural medicine treatment program on children with refractory epileptic seizures: An 8 year follow-up. *Epilepsia* **33**, 98–102.

Dahl, J., Melin, L., Leissner, P. (1988) Effects of a behavioral intervention on epileptic behaviour and paroxysmal activity: A systematic replication of three cases with intractable epilepsy. *Epilepsia* **29**, 172–183.

Dahl, J., Melin, L., Lund, L. (1987) Effects of a contingent relaxation treatment program on adults with refractory epileptic seizures. *Epilepsia* **28**, 125–132.

Dahl, J., Melin, L., Brorson, L-O., Schollin, J. (1985) Effects of a broad-spectrum behavioural medicine treatment program on children with refractory epileptic seizures. *Epilepsia* **26**, 303–309.

Dorwart, R.A. (1984) Psychotherapy and temporal lobe epilepsy. *American Journal of Psychotherapy* **38**, 286–294.

Espadaler-Medina, J.M., Espadaler-Gamissans, J.M., Seoane, J.L (1992) Reflex epilepsy. *Clinical Neurology and Neurosurgery* **94** (Suppl.), S70-S72.

Ferrari, M., Matthews, W.S., Barabas, G. (1983) The family and the child with epilepsy. *Family Process* **22**, 53–59.

Fiordelli, E., Beghi, E., Bogliun, G., Crespi, V. (1993) Epilepsy and psychiatric disturbance. A cross-sectional study. *British Journal of Psychiatry* **163**, 446–450.

Forehand, R., McMahon, R. (1981) *Helping the Non-compliant Child: A Clinician's Guide to Parent Training.* New York: Guilford Press.

Fowler, M. (1997) Neuropsychological and cognitive assessment of children with epilepsy. In: Cull C., Goldstein L.H. (eds.), *The Clinical psychologist's Handbook of Epilepsy. Assessment and Management.* London: Routledge, 149–166.

Gillham, R. (1990) Refractory epilepsy: An evaluation of psychological methods in out-patient management. *Epilepsia* **31**, 427–432.

Gillham, R., Cull, C. (1997) The role of anti-epileptic drugs. Their impact on cognitive function and behaviour. In: Cull C., Goldstein L.H. (eds.), *The Clinical psychologist's Handbook of Epilepsy. Assessment and Management. and* London: Routledge, 77–95.

Glisky, E.L. (1995) Acquisition and transfer of word processing skill by an amnesic patient. *Neuropsychological Rehabilitation* **5**, 299–318.

Goldstein, L.H. (1990) Behavioural and cognitive-behavioural treatments for epilepsy: A progress review. *British Journal of Clinical psychology* **29**, 257–269.

Goldstein, L.H. (1991) Neuropsychological investigation of temporal lobe epilepsy. *Journal of the Royal Society of Medicine* **84**, 460–465.

Goldstein, L.H. (1993) Behaviour problems. In: Greenwood R., Barnes M.P., McMillan T.M., Ward C.D. (eds.) *Neurological Rehabilitation.* Edinburgh: Churchill Livingstone, 389–401.

Goldstein, L.H. (1997a) Effectiveness of psychological interventions for people with poorly controlled epilepsy. *Journal of Neurology, Neurosurgery and Psychiatry* **63**, 137–142.

Goldstein, L.H. (1997b) Psychological control of seizures. In: Cull C., Goldstein L.H. (eds.), *The Clinical psychologist's Handbook of Epilepsy. Assessment and Management.* London: Routledge, 113–129.

Goldstein, L.H. (1997c) Neuropsychological assessment. In: Cull C., Goldstein L.H. (eds.), *The Clinical psychologist's Handbook of Epilepsy. Assessment and Management.* London: Routledge, 18–34.

Goldstein, L.H. (2000) Psychologic methods. In: Oxbury J.M., Polkey C.E., Duchowny M. (eds.). *Intractable Focal Epilepsy: Medical and Surgical Treatment.* London: W.B. Saunders Ltd, *in press.*

Goldstein, L.H., Cull, C. (1997) The way forward. In: Cull C., Goldstein L.H. (eds.), *The Clinical psychologist's Handbook of Epilepsy. Assessment and Management.* London: Routledge, 203–212.

Goldstein, L.H., Polkey, C.E. (1992) Everyday memory after unilateral temporal lobectomy and amygdalo-hippocampectomy. *Cortex* **28**, 189–201.

Goldstein, L.H., Bernard, S., Fenwick, P.B.C., Burgess, P.W., McNeil, J. (1993) Unilateral frontal lobectomy can produce strategy application disorder. *Journal of Neurology, Neurosurgery and Psychiatry* **56**, 274–276.

Grasso, G., Bailo, P., Crivelli, E. (1992) Mental development integration in dynamic psychotherapy of an adolescent with partial seizures. *Giornale di Neuropsichiatria dell'Eta Evolutiva* **12**, 271–290.

Hoare, P., Kerley, S. (1992) Helping patients and children with epilepsy cope successfully: The outcome of a group programme for parents. *Journal of Psychosomatic Research* **36**, 759–767.

Hunkin, N.M., Squires, E.J., Aldrich, F.K., Parkin, A.J. (1998) Errorless learning and the acquisition of word processing skills. *Neuropsychological Rehabilitation* **8**, 433–449.

Jacoby, A. (1995) Impact of epilepsy on employment status: Findings from a UK study of people with well-controlled epilepsy. *Epilepsy Research* **21**, 125–132.

Kiesel, K.B., Lutzker, J.R., Campbell, R.V. (1989) Behavioural relaxation training to reduce hyperventilation and seizures in a profoundly retarded epileptic child. *Journal of the Multihandicapped Person* **2**, 179–190.

Kime, S.K., Lamb, D.G., Wilson, B.A. (1996) Use of a comprehensive programme of external cueing to enhance procedural memory in a patient with dense amnesia. *Brain Injury* **10**, 17–25.

Kingdon, D., Tyrer, P., Seivewright, N., Ferguson, B., Murphy, S. (1996) The Nottingham Study of Neurotic Disorder: influence of cognitive therapists on outcome. *British Journal of Psychiatry* **169**, 93–97.

Laaksonen, R. (1983) The patient with recently diagnosed epilepsy — psychological and sociological aspects. *Acta Neurologica Scandinavica* **93** (Suppl.), 52–59.

Lessman, S.E., Mollick, L.R. (1978) Group treatment of epileptics. *Health and Social Work* **3**, 105–121.

Lindsay, S.J.E., Powell, G.E. (1994) Practical issues of investigation. In: Lindsay S.E., Powell G.E. (eds.). *The Handbook of Clinical Adult Psychology, 2nd Edn.* London: Routledge, 1–34.

Lothman, D.J., Pianta, R.C. (1993) Role of child-mother interaction in predicting competence of children with epilepsy. *Epilepsia* **34**, 658–669.

McMillan, T.M., Powell, G.E., Janota, I., Polkey, C.E. (1987) Relationship between neuropathology and cognitive functioning in temporal lobectomy patients. *Journal of Neurology, Neurosurgery and Psychiatry* **50**, 167–176.

Manning, J.J., Hooke, G.R., Tannenbaum, D.A., Blythe, T.H., Clarke, T.M. (1994) Intensive cognitive behaviour group therapy for diagnostically heterogeneous groups of patients with psychiatric disorder. *Australian and New Zealand Journal of Psychiatry* **28**, 667–674.

Mathers, C.B.B. (1992) Group therapy in the management of epilepsy. *British Journal of Medical Psychology* **65**, 279–287.

Mendez, M.F., Doss, R.C. (1992) Ictal and psychiatric aspects of suicide in epileptic patients. *International Journal of Psychiatry in Medicine* **22**, 231–237.

Miller, L. (1994a) Psychotherapy of epilepsy: Seizure control and psychosocial adjustment. *Journal of Cognitive Rehabilitation* **12**, 14–30.

Miller, L. (1994b) The epilepsy patient: Personality, psychodynamics and psychotherapy. *Psychotherapy* **31**, 735–743.

Milne, D., Britton, P., Wilkinson, I. (1990) The scientist-practitioner in practice. *Clinical psychology Forum* **December**, 27–30.

Mogg, K., Bradley, B.P., Millar, N., White, J. (1995) A follow-up study of cognitive bias in generalised anxiety disorder. *Behaviour Research and Therapy* **33**, 927–935.

Murray, J. (1993) Coping with the uncertainty of uncontrolled epilepsy. *Seizure* **2**, 167–178.

Newsom-Davis, I., Goldstein, L.H., Fitzpatrick, D. (1998) Fear of seizures: An investigation and treatment. *Seizure* **7**, 101–106.

Oxbury, S. (1997) Assessment for surgery. In: Cull C., Goldstein L.H. (eds.), *The Clinical psychologist's Handbook of Epilepsy. Assessment and Management.* London: Routledge, 54–76.

Paladin, F., Cantele, P., Pinkus, L., Mattarollo, L. (1989) ESES: Multidisciplinary approach to a case of focal cortical dysplasia. *Archivo di Psicologia Neurologia e Psichiatria* **50**, 613–627.

Perini, G.I., Tosin, C., Carraro, C., Bernasconi, G., Canevini, M.P., Canger, R., Pellegrini, A., Testa, G. (1996) Interictal mood and personality disorders in temporal lobe epilepsy and juvenile myoclonic epilepsy. *Journal of Neurology, Neurosurgery and Psychiatry* **61**, 601–605.

Pershad, D., Siddiqui, R.A. (1992) Psychosocial dysfunction in adults with epilepsy. *International Journal of Rehabilitation Research* **15**, 258–261.

Psenska, T.M., Holden, K.R. (1996) Benign familial neonatal convulsions: Psychosocial adjustment to the threat of recurrent seizures. *Seizure* **5**, 243–245.

Puskarich, C.A., Whitman. S., Dell, J., Hughes, J., Rosen, A.J., Hermann, B.P. (1992) Controlled examination of progressive relaxation training of seizure reduction. *Epilepsia* **33**, 675–680.

Reisner, A D. (1990) A case of rapid reduction of panic symptoms: An eclectic approach. *Phobia Practice and Research Journal* **3**, 87–93.

Reiter, J., Andrews, D., Janis, C. (1987) *Taking Control of Your Epilepsy. A Workbook for Patients and Professionals.* Santa Rosa: The BASICS Publishing Company.

Rousseau, A., Hermann, B., Whitman, S. (1985) Effects of progressive relaxation on epilepsy: Analysis of a series of cases. *Psychological Reports* **57**, 1203–1212.

Sanders, P.T., Bare, M.A., Lesser, R.P. (1995) It is not harmful for patients with epilepsy to view their own seizures. *Epilepsia* **36**, 1138–1141.

Sawrie, S.M., Martin, R.C., Gilliam, F.G., Roth, D.L., Faught, E., Kuzniecky, R. (1998) Contribution of neuropsychological data to the prediction of temporal lobe epilepsy surgery outcome. *Epilepsia* **39**, 319–325.

Seidman-Ripley, J.G., Bound, V.K., Andermann, F., Olivier, A., Gloor, P., Feindel, W.H. (1993) Psychosocial consequences of postoperative seizure relief. *Epilepsia* **34**, 248–254.

Spector, S., Foots, A., Goldstein, L.H. (1995) Reduction in seizure frequency as a result of a group intervention for adults with epilepsy. *Epilepsia* **36**(Suppl. 3), S130.

Spector, S., Goldstein, L.H., Cull, C.A., Fenwick, P.B.C. (1994) Precipitation and inhibiting epileptic seizures: A survey of adults with poorly controlled epilepsy. Presented at a meeting of the International League Against Epilepsy, May, London.

Tan, S-Y., Bruni, J. (1986) Cognitive-behaviour therapy with adult patients with epilepsy: A controlled outcome study. *Epilepsia* **27**, 225–233.

Tancredi, R., Guerrini, R. (1992) Aggressiveness and libido in early psychotherapeutic work of a child with partial epilepsy. *Giornali di Neuropsichiatria dell'Eta Evolutiva* **12**, 261–269.

Taube, S.L., Calman, N.H. (1992) The psychotherapy of patients with complex partial seizures. *American Journal of Orthopsychiatry* **62**, 35–43.

Thompson, P.J. (1997) Epilepsy and memory In: Cull C., Goldstein L.H. (eds.), *The Clinical psychologist's Handbook of Epilepsy. Assessment and Management.* London: Routledge, 35–53.

Thompson, P.J., Upton, D. (1992) The impact of chronic epilepsy on the family. *Seizure* **1**, 43–48.

Troxell, J. (1997) Epilepsy and employment: The Americans with Disabilities Act and its protection against employment discrimination. *Medicine and the Law* **16**, 375–384.

Upton, D., Thompson, P.J. (1992) Coping with epilepsy: An intervention study. *Seizure* **1**, 11–23.

Vermeulen, J., Aldenkamp, A.P., Alpherts, W.C.J. (1993) Memory complaints in epilepsy: Correlations with cognitive performance and neuroticism. *Epilepsy Research* **15**, 157–170.

von Cramon, D.Y., Matthes-von Cramon, G. (1994) Back to work with a chronic dysexecutive syndrome? (A case report). *Neuropsychological Rehabilitation* **4**, 399–417.

von Cramon, D.Y., Matthes-von Cramon, G., Mai, N. (1991) Problem-solving deficits in brain-injured persons: A therapeutic approach. *Neuropsychological Rehabilitation* **1**, 45–64.

Wheelock, I., Peterson, C., Buchtel, H.A. (1998) Presurgery expectations, postsurgery satisfaction and psychosocial adjustment after epilepsy surgery. *Epilepsia* **39**, 487–494.

Whitman, S., Dell, J., Legion, V., Eibhlyn, A., Statsinger, J. (1990) Progressive relaxation for seizure reduction. *Journal of Epilepsy* **3**, 17–22.

Wilson, B.A., Baddeley, A., Evans, J., Shiel, A. (1994) Errorless learning in the rehabilitation of memory impaired people. *Neuropsychological Rehabilitation* **4**, 307–326.

Wilson, S.J., Saling, M.M., Kincade, P., Bladin, P.F. (1998) Patient expectations of temporal lobe surgery. *Epilepsia* **39**, 167–174.

Chapter 18

THE CONTRIBUTION OF THE NURSE

Anne Sweeney

EVOLUTION OF THE EPILEPSY NURSE SPECIALIST ROLE

The concept of the nurse specialist evolved in the UK during the 1970s, initially in chronic conditions such as diabetes and asthma. The first epilepsy nurse specialist post was created in Doncaster in 1988, by the King Edward's Fund for Primary Care Development to provide a community liaison service for people with epilepsy. Initially funded for 18 months, the post had become permanent by 1992 and had expanded to include two epilepsy nurse specialists. In 1992, the Epilepsy Specialist Nurse Association (ESNA) was founded by a group of seven nurses working with people with epilepsy and specialising in paediatrics, learning disability and care of older people. They came together with a common aim and interest, to support each other and share ideas about how to improve care and education of people with epilepsy and increase awareness of epilepsy generally. ESNA continues to expand rapidly and its current membership is approaching 300.

The continued development of nurse specialist posts in epilepsy is dependant mainly on recognition of their value in improving services by neurologists, neuropsychiatrists, paediatricians and general practitioners (GPs). To date funding has come from a variety of sources including NHS Trusts, individual charitable foundations such as the Roald Dahl Foundation and British Epilepsy Association. The latter organisation, in conjunction with the pharmaceutical company, Glaxo Wellcome, was responsible for the initiation of the Sapphire Nurse scheme, which has proved a highly successful venture funding currently 35 posts. However, this is short-term funding only. Individual trusts have to pick up the costs after a period of between 12 months to two years.

ESNA has representation on a number of epilepsy-related organisations in the UK including the Epilepsy Task Force, the Joint Epilepsy Council, British Epilepsy Association, the Joint Committee of Nurses, Midwives and Health Visitors, the National Society of Epilepsy and the Department of Health Epilepsy Advisory Board. This gives the epilepsy nurse specialist an audible voice in influencing epilepsy care, services and standards.

ESNA also has a standards working party, which to date, has produced five standards including on record keeping, documentation, information and education. These standards are set in order to ensure that the care received by people with epilepsy from ESNA members around the UK is based on agreed benchmarks. ESNA locality groups aim to meet the needs of its members at the local level. Other current developments include special interest groups (e.g. paediatrics, learning disabilities) and a working party looking at information in other languages.

KEY ELEMENTS OF THE NURSE SPECIALIST ROLE

In addition to basic nursing qualifications, specialist qualifications in paediatrics, learning disability or mental health are needed . Along with a working knowledge of epilepsy, the skills required of the epilepsy nurse specialist are those of the clinician counsellor, co-ordinator, teacher and researcher. The nurse specialist needs to adopt a holistic approach to epilepsy management, requiring consideration of the following:

- Active development of the nurse/patient/carer relationship in order to provide individualised information, support, counselling
- Accessibility to patients and their families, via a telephone link or 'drop in' service, complemented by contact through home, school or work visits
- Medication monitoring, including observing the efficacy of medication and any problems with compliance. Concerns regarding toxicity can then be communicated with the patient's doctor who may then instigate a change in medication. Drug information sheets detailing potential side effects and addressing comments and concerns such as what to do if a dose of medication is missed, can also be given to the patient
- Service co-ordination to ensure that all those involved with the care of patients with epilepsy are kept informed of any changes concerning its management. The link between primary care and secondary care is vital to good management and should provide a channel of communication and a shared care philosophy which will promote continuity of care
- Education, both of professionals and non-professionals — the timely combination of information and education can lead to a greater

understanding of the condition. The treatment of epilepsy should be based on current research evidence; important information can be delivered in a variety of ways. Information packs are now available for the child, adolescent or adult with epilepsy, directing them to other relevant sources of information and guiding them to some of the facts they should have about their epilepsy. Similar information packs are available for parents, other carers, both formal and informal, and schools.

SETTING UP AN EPILEPSY SERVICE

The epilepsy specialist nurse may be expected to take a central role in setting up epilepsy services, perhaps as service co-ordinator. Before developing a new service, the existing service, if any, has to be reviewed. Questionnaires can be used to ascertain current levels of knowledge, among those involved in service delivery, of epilepsy classification, syndromes, types of seizures, current medication, available literature and the epilepsy associations. The responses from the questionnaire help make the service co-ordinator aware of the educational/informational needs of members of the epilepsy team, as well as of service needs. It is important to involve all the members of the epilepsy team in development of the service.

It is important to monitor the effectiveness of any changes, and not just to assume that they constitute improvement. Any changes made to the epilepsy service can be evaluated through audit. Audit also provides valuable evidence on which to base future practice. The audit cycle should be repeated periodically in order to maintain continued improvement in the epilepsy service.

ADVANCING NURSING PRACTICE IN EPILEPSY

The nurse specialist role involves a number of areas of advanced nursing practice. For example, nurse led clinics aim to improve continuity of care for the patients and their families and other carers. Often such clinics reduce waiting time for follow-up appointments. Though the doctor should always be available to deal with any problems beyond the remit of the nurse specialist (e.g. unplanned medication changes), patients and their carers may be more at ease with the nurse. Some topics may be more easily addressed by the nurse (e.g. contraception, sexuality, fears and anxieties felt by the patient, parents or carers).

A second area of advanced nursing practice is that of nurse prescribing. This may help to streamline the service, but should only be undertaken by the nurse specialist with the full agreement and support of both the NHS Trust and the consultants with whom he or she works. Additional training should be given to ensure the specialist nurse's full competency in the use of the antiepileptic medication. Guidelines for the scope of nurse prescribing should be created and monitoring of this practice should be ongoing. A third example is that of triage of all patients referred to the neurologist or other consultant with a possible diagnosis of epilepsy. The nurse specialist will take a full detailed history from the patient, then, following discussion with the consultant concerned, arrange for the appropriate investigations to be carried out if the history and investigation results so indicate. The patient can then be 'fast-tracked' through the clinic.

EDUCATING THE PATIENT

It is vital that the information supplied to patients and their carers is understandable, appropriate to their needs, and available where and when required. If a person with epilepsy is to lead a happy, fulfilled and productive life, reaching their full potential, those involved in their care must ensure that they and their carers have an appropriate level of knowledge and understanding of their condition to make well-informed judgements and decisions. The diagnosis of epilepsy, treatment, and initial information should be given by a doctor with an interest and expertise in epilepsy. Ideally at the same time, the person with epilepsy will be introduced to the epilepsy nurse specialist, and supplied with appropriate literature, telephone contact numbers for the nurse specialist service and information relating to the epilepsy associations. The nurse specialist should arrange to see the patient within a few weeks of diagnosis, either in hospital or at home. The primary purpose of this visit is to begin answering the many questions that patients and carers will have in relation to living with epilepsy; at the same time, the nurse specialist will seek to develop further the family's knowledge and understanding of epilepsy. Issues which ESNA sees as important to cover are discussed below.

Clinical Issues

Patients and their families are likely to require information about the clinical aspects of epilepsy, including the type of their epilepsy and seizures. Specific information should be provided about the epilepsy syndrome and any associated problems, such as photosensitivity. Seizure management should be discussed along with the possibility of the keeping of a seizure diary, to monitor their condition. ESNA has produced a number of useful aids to management, including an 'Aid to Seizure Description' and guidelines about the management of seizures. Patients should also be provided with emergency helpline numbers (e.g. local Accident and Emergency Department number).

Medication

Patients and carers need to know that antiepileptic medication must be taken regularly for the period specified by the doctor managing the epilepsy and should not be stopped even though seizures are controlled, unless he or she confirms this course of action. It is helpful to patients if they know both the brand name and the generic name of their medication and any other relevant information, for example from a drug information sheet. Suggestions can be made to improve compliance including the use of colouring charts for younger children, dose set boxes, and prompt cards around the home.

Antiepileptic medication is often cited as the explanation for poor or unacceptable behaviour; but both patients and parents need to recognise that young children will have temper tantrums, and adolescents will strive for independence, independent of their epilepsy.

Contact With Other People With Epilepsy

Patients and carers often find it helpful to talk to other people in a similar situation to themselves; and the nurse specialist is often the person best-placed to facilitate such a meeting. He or she is also in a good position to make patients and carers aware of the existence and activities of the various epilepsy associations, and the valuable support they can offer through their fieldworkers, helpline, literature and local support groups.

Lifestyle

Very simple everyday events can create a great deal of anxiety for both patients and carers. The epilepsy specialist nurse should therefore help them to devise strategies for continuing with their normal activities with as little risk as possible. This is likely to involve consideration of: the level of seizure control, the precise nature of the activity or event in which the patient wishes to participate, and what constituted an appropriate level of supervision for such an activity. Legal aspects of epilepsy must also be considered (such as the rules about driving and employment).

THE ESNA CHECK LIST

ESNA has developed a checklist to help patients and carers voice their concerns and anxieties about managing epilepsy (Appendix 1). The checklist also helps to structure time spent with the nurse specialist, since in the experience of ESNA members, key questions are often forgotten due to stress, especially if the meeting is in the hospital. Home visits are far less stressful and families are often more relaxed in familiar surroundings and therefore can more readily voice their concerns.

CONCLUSION

My own experience as a nurse specialist in paediatric epilepsy over the past six years leads me to the conclusion that we must give patients and carers relevant and appropriate support and, most importantly, act as a point of contact for them. By providing a service in this way, epilepsy nurses can help patients and carers through the early stages of their condition, a task which is essential to their subsequent adjustment. The epilepsy nurse specialist plays a key part in supporting patients and enabling them to reach their maximum potential, and in so doing helps to make life with epilepsy easier to deal with and the quality of that life better.

APPENDIX 1 ESNA INFORMATION CHECKLIST			
TOPIC	**PRIORITY H/L**	**DATES**	**ACTION TAKEN**
GENERAL INFO			
DIAGNOSIS/CAUSES			
INVESTIGATIONS			
TRIGGERS			
PHOTOSENSITIVITY			
GENETICS			
DIARY			
FREE PRESCRIPTION			
CULTURAL/RELIGIOUS ISSUES			
LIFESTYLE			
SAFETY			
DRIVING			
SWIMMING/SPORT			
EDUCATION			
ALCOHOL			
SLEEPING			
TRAVEL			
EMPLOYMENT			
DIET			
TREATMENTS			
MEDICATION/SIDE EFFECTS			
COMPLIANCE			
ALTERNATIVE THERAPIES			
SURGERY			
VAGAL NERVE STIMULATION			
RELATIONSHIPS/REPRODUCTION			
CONTRACEPTION			
PRECONCEPTUAL			
PREGNANCY			
PARENTHOOD			
MENOPAUSE			
OTHER			
CONTACT NO			
ASSOCIATION INFO			
LEARNING DISABILITIES			

Chapter 19

THE ROLE OF THE SOCIAL WORKER

Patricia A. Gibson

It has long been recognized that the social, psychological and behavioural problems that frequently accompany epilepsy can be more handicapping than the actual seizures (Livingston, 1977). Unfortunately, in many countries, even the more developed, addressing the social needs and concerns of people with epilepsy and their families is not always of high priority. While a social worker would ideally be a part of every treatment team for epilepsy, in reality, this professional is not always included. Funding is quite often the issue since in many situations social workers do not directly charge for their services and often depend on institutional support.

HISTORY OF SOCIAL WORK

It is hard to know just where the first origins of 'social work' began. Most likely there have always been those in any group of people who felt compelled to look out for the less fortunate, who were more sensitive to social needs. In the United States, the early beginnings of organized charity were based on models of social care in England. The Almshouse or poor farm was the major helping resource in colonial America. In the 1800s friendly visiting by volunteers who worked to establish a personal relationship with the needy, became a major model for dealing with the urban poor. Associations for improving the condition of the poor were formed in the 1840s. These associations concentrated mostly on the conditions that created poverty. These charitable societies are considered forerunners of modern social casework. The settlement movement was the forerunner of group social work. Hull House, the best known settlement house in America, was established in 1889 by Jane Addams. The settlement houses directed their attention more to working conditions and economic reform. Overall, social work in America during these early years focused primarily on protecting and raising the standard of living (Levy Simon, 1998).

Dr. Richard Cabot introduced medical social services at Boston's Massachusetts General Hospital in 1905 to contribute to the development of preventive medicine. Dr. Cabot recognized the importance of continuity of care and therefore included social workers as home visitors in his clinic. Ida Cannon was hired as the first medical social worker. Social work provided an enlarged understanding of social conditions that may contribute to the client's distress (Gibelman, 1995).

With the development of psychiatric social work around 1908, social workers began to deal with universal problems of mental health and emotional adjustment rather than with the narrower problems of economic dependence and relief.

DEFINING SOCIAL WORK

Mary Richmond wrote *Social Diagnosis* in 1917 in which she defined social case work as consisting of 'those processes which develop personality through adjustments consciously effected, individual by individual, between men and their social environment' (Richmond, 1917). Richmond had a deeply held belief that if you gathered all the information about a person, the solution to his or her problem would become evident (Haynes, 1998).

Throughout the years obtaining a consensus on the nature of social work has been difficult. In spite of the large number of different methods, theoretical approaches, and specialized fields of practice, six steps in the social work process applicable to all methods and approaches can be distilled from the vast literature:

1. Intake and establishing contact
2. Assessment, diagnosis, and problem identification
3. Goal identification, service planning and basis for contract
4. Service treatment and intervention
5. Evaluation of outcomes
6. Feedback and application of results in future practice

The following definition of social work was adopted by the National Association of Social Workers (NASW) in 1970 and has become generally accepted in the United States: 'Social work is the profession of helping individuals, groups, or communities enhance or restore their capacity for social functioning and creating societal conditions favorable to this goal' (Gibelman, 1973). This definition includes clarification about the nature of social work practice as consisting of:

> the professional application of social work values, principles, and techniques to one or more of the following ends: helping people obtain tangible services;

> counselling and psychotherapy with individuals, families, and groups; helping communities or groups provide or improve social and health services; and participating in legislative processes. (Gibelman, 1973)

In the performance of social work roles, NASW (1981) identified 12 essential skill areas, including the ability to:

1. listen to others with understanding and purpose
2. elicit information and assemble relevant facts to prepare a social history, assessment, and report
3. create and maintain professional helping relationships
4. observe and interpret verbal and nonverbal behavior and use knowledge of personality theory and diagnostic method
5. engage clients, including individuals, families, groups, and communities, in efforts to resolve their own problems and to gain trust
6. discuss sensitive emotional subjects supportively and without being threatening
7. create innovative solutions to 'clients' needs
8. determine the need to terminate the therapeutic relationship
9. conduct research or interpret the findings of research and professional literature
10. mediate and negotiate between conflicting parties
11. provide interorganizational liaison services
12. interpret and communicate social needs to funding sources, the public or legislators (NASW, 1981).

Social work is a diverse profession with fluid boundaries. There is much greater public understanding of what physicians, nurses, psychologists, and even lawyers do than is the case with social workers. According to Gibelman, this phenomena results partly from the expansive and expanding boundaries of social work and the difficulty of providing succinct, encapsulated descriptions of a complex and multifaceted profession (Gibelman, 1995).

SOCIAL WORK'S ROLE IN EPILEPSY

In a 1997 survey by the International Professionals in Epilepsy Care (IPEC), it was found that social workers have widely varied roles in the treatment of epilepsy around the world (Brown, R., *personal communication*). Social workers were found to be providing patient education, counselling at the level of the individual, family and group, coordinating epilepsy monitoring units, monitoring drug studies, administering a variety of programmes and services in epilepsy, advocating for patients and their families, and holding education and research positions. Thus, from setting to setting the role changes.

Social workers are found in almost all hospital settings in the United States. They may or may not be specifically assigned to providing services to the epilepsy population. Except in special centres of excellence, most cover many population areas in the hospital and do not have special expertise in epilepsy. Much of their work is directed toward exploring financial assistance or discharge planning for patients.

Social workers provide services in a variety of other practice settings and at various levels. For example, social workers deliver services in private practice, epilepsy associations or foundations, institutions, school systems, clinics or centres, and correctional facilities. The range of practice settings is broad. Working in these many areas, social workers deal with social issues that cut across the broad spectrum of problems that affect individuals, groups, and communities. These problems include civil and legal rights, economic problems and poverty, employment, rural and urban problems, transportation, and problems unique to epilepsy.

The functions performed by social workers often overlap with the functions carried out by other helping disciplines. Our claim, as Stewart noted in 1984, is not to a monopoly of functions, but to 'uniqueness and distinctiveness in our view about human problems and their solutions and in our particular value and practice orientation' (Stewart 1984). While the role of social workers in epilepsy varies greatly, the following areas are the most common.

CASE MANAGEMENT

Case management is a procedure to plan, seek and monitor services from different agencies and staff on behalf of a client. Social workers are often involved as case managers with individuals with epilepsy who are unable to function independently. Effective case management requires continuity of care, emotional support, managerial interventions to address various needs, and enabling of client resourcefulness (Kanter, 1987). The tasks range from assessing client's needs and planning service to therapeutic intervention, monitoring and evaluation of the client's progress. The case manager is a broker and an advocate for the person with epilepsy.

PREVENTIVE COUNSELLING

An important part of the social care of epilepsy is preventive counseling. Preventive counselling should begin shortly after diagnosis and involve the client, family members and any others involved in the care of the client. Clients and family members need to ventilate their fears, worries and concerns. Observing a seizure, especially a tonic clonic seizure, in a loved one can be one of the most frightening experiences a person may have. Expressing these concerns is a beginning step in the process of dealing effectively with the psychosocial impact of epilepsy. Listening without interruption to the client and family's feelings and description of the event is extremely important. The social worker early on helps the client and family deal with irrational fears and crushed ambitions as well as other worries. During this early stage, groundwork can be laid to help parents realize the important role their attitude towards epilepsy plays in influencing how the child will begin to feel about him or herself. Parents need to understand how overprotecting can lead to emotional crippling. The disabling potential of epilepsy depends heavily upon the manner in which the family adjusts to the disorder and is able to help the child cope with the issues that are a part of epilepsy. Early intervention with counselling by the social worker can help prevent many of the social problems that frequently accompany the diagnosis of epilepsy.

INDIVIDUAL COUNSELLING

A chronic illness of any type has significant impact on the lives of people it touches and there are many social and psychological consequences when people don't cope well. For some, epilepsy may be looked upon as a minor inconvenience. They have a few seizures, are prescribed medicine, their seizures come under control and do not interfere with functioning. Others are not so lucky. For this group, epilepsy is a devastating diagnosis and looms large, colouring every aspect of their being. There are various emotional responses to any illness or disorder. While not everyone with epilepsy needs counselling, sometimes the emotional responses may be maladaptive and require intervention. The problems that a person with epilepsy faces are functions of a number of factors — the age of onset, severity of the disorder, how the patient/family system copes or responds to the seizures, and the quality of the interactions are among the many systems with which the client and family must deal. When problems begin to interfere with the client's functioning or quality of life, then individual counselling may be needed.

FAMILY COUNSELLING

The impact of having epilepsy can be significant medically, socially, psychologically, and financially. It upsets the equilibrium of the family system, affecting everyone in some way. It has the potential to break a family apart. Because epilepsy usually begins in childhood, the patient's formative years may be drastically altered by the reaction of the family, school and peer group to this disorder. When epilepsy develops in early childhood, much of the adjustment hinges on how the family adjusts to the disorder and is then able to help the young child cope with the ensuing issues and concerns. Certainly the severity of the seizure condition, presence of other handicapping conditions, the social, emotional, and financial stability of the family are all important variables. How disruptive the family perceives the disorder to be, regardless of whether or not that perception is accurate, is a key factor in their reaction. How the family functions prior to the diagnosis is important in how it copes with this situation. The family's adjustment in turn has a profound impact on how the child reacts. If the parents have a healthy attitude toward epilepsy and encourage normal function, then the child can grow up with epilepsy in its proper place — just one part of what makes up that person.

While seizures are the most visible part of the disorder, it is often the emotional and cognitive effects that devastate a child and his or her family. Epilepsy can affect the growing child's academic career, relationship with family and peers, and if not handled properly can destroy the child's self-esteem. According to Ziegler, the negative impact of epilepsy on a child's self-concept is one of the major long-term complications of childhood epilepsy. It is the family that manages the disorder and sets the stage for adjustment (Ziegler, 1981).

If the person diagnosed with epilepsy is a parent, then major issues about family role may present themselves. If the client is the father and can no longer drive or hold a job, this has major economic, social and psychological impact on the family. If the mother has epilepsy, then issues with child care, safety, transportation, and others are of concern. Early referral for family counselling should be made when the strains are first noticed.

GROUP COUNSELLING

Group counselling is an effective modality in dealing with social issues and concerns associated with epilepsy. It was not until after World War

II that group work moved solidly into rehabilitation settings. The big push for group work came from the thousands of soldiers and veterans who needed assistance for physical and emotional problems. By the 1950's group counselling was well established in a number of settings. In this era of cost containment and managed care, it is generally recognized that group services are more cost efficient than individual interventions (Toseland and Siporen, 1986).

In remedial groups the focus is on treatment of the individual through the use of a group method. In this group the social worker controls the formation and operation of the group. Group members are selected by the social worker who is guided by the goal of the group; members are usually selected because of similarities in presenting problems or target complaints. The most critical issue for success of remedial groups is group composition. For instance, grouping teenagers with seizures who are having difficulty accepting their diagnosis along with others who have made a successful adjustment is one example.

Klein in the early 70's pointed out that people may have difficulty functioning in various roles because they do not know what is expected. Some people are locked into 'sick roles'. Many of these persons are so locked into the sick role that access to other roles has been denied. Klein felt that a person can be taught about roles; an important task of groups is such re-education. The group functions as a microcosm of society, offering these clients experiences unavailable to them elsewhere. It provides an opportunity to practice behaviours, learn skills, gain insights, and build confidence necessary for the eventual assumption of different life roles (Klein, 1972). Many clients with epilepsy are in need of such opportunities to learn these skills.

Support groups for those with epilepsy and their families is a service sponsored by many epilepsy organizations or foundations (see Chapter 20). These groups offer an opportunity for persons with epilepsy to meet others, form friendships, and learn more about epilepsy and community resources. They provide a social outlet for those with limited opportunities for interaction and meetings may involve a social activity or outing. Support groups are usually open for inclusion and it is up to the client to choose to participate. These groups may or may not have professional leadership. In summary, the overall goal in counselling is to assess the problem and work with the individual, family, group or community in addressing and resolving it.

PATIENT EDUCATION

It is the responsibility of every professional working in the area of epilepsy to participate in the client's education about his/her disorder. The client and family must have a good understanding if treatment and habilitation is to be successful. Social workers teach clients early to become 'partners' with their medical professionals. The client's role and responsibility in his/her own care is stressed. When providing this education it is important to involve as many of the caretakers as possible — babysitters, grandparents, and so on. To be effective, patient education must be done on a continuous basis and needs to be presented on the level of the client. This may sound rather simple but communicating well is not always easy.

COMMUNITY EDUCATION

Many social workers provide epilepsy education to community professionals through one to one situations, workshops, seminars, conferences, or symposia. In the United States there are two nationwide telephone information lines for epilepsy education, both developed and managed by social workers. These lines provide a wide range of information on epilepsy to patients and their families, professionals and the public. In North Carolina, a major thrust of the Comprehensive Epilepsy Programme is on community education with educational programmes on epilepsy provided for approximately 5,000 to 8,000 professionals in the state each year.

ADVOCACY

Advocacy refers to the act of directly representing or defending others and seeks to champion the rights of individuals or communities through direct interventions or through empowerment. The National Association of Social Workers' Code of Ethics (NASW, 1994) identifies advocacy as a basic obligation of the profession and its members. Certainly, social workers in the field of epilepsy are in a good position to identify the needs of people with epilepsy and their families.

Legislative advocacy activity is centered on influencing the course or content of a legislative or regulatory measure. Efforts can be targeted to preventing harmful government actions or initiating or expanding new legislation; and may occur directly by using specific legislative advocacy tactics or indirectly by mobilizing community groups.

Advocacy has been a part of social work from the time of the charity movements in the 1870s (Edwards, 1995). An example of advocacy on behalf of people with epilepsy can be found in the states of North Carolina and Florida in the United States. In North Carolina, a social worker documented the need for medical care of indigent patients. She drafted legislation for the provision of free epilepsy clinics, a laboratory for blood levels, and an epilepsy medication fund. The epilepsy population, their physicians and other professionals were mobilized to lobby for passage of the legislation. The legislation was passed and these services became available in 1986. In Florida, advocacy efforts led to an even more extensive program of epilepsy services across the state. In Holland, social workers have been instrumental in setting up holidays for those with epilepsy who, perhaps, would not have such opportunities. There are many other examples of social work advocacy around the world.

SUMMARY

The profession of social work has much to offer the field of epilepsy. It was the vision of the United States Presidential Commission for the Control of Epilepsy and Its Consequences, headed by Dr. Richard Masland in 1975, that those with epilepsy be treated with a comprehensive approach that valued the contributions of a multidisciplinary group of professionals. The social worker would be a part of this team and would work with the client and family in an individualised way. This should be done in the manner described by Anthony Arangio in his position paper to the Commission, 'by communicating confidence, respect, consistency, humility, a desire to engage in team activity, and above all, an objective which insures client/families with epilepsy that all needed services will be available in order to maximise human dignity' (Arangio, 1977).

References

Arangio, A.A (1977) Systematic Examination of The Psychosocial Needs of Patients With Epilepsy: The Need for a Comprehensive Change-Approach. *Plan For Nationwide Action On Epilepsy*, Vol II, Part I, Sec I-VI DHEW, 385–396.

Edwards, R. (1995) Advocacy, In: *Encyclopedia of Social Work*, 19th ed., Vol 1, National Association of Social Workers (NASW) Press, 95–100.

Gibelman, M. (1973) *Standards For Social Service Manpower*, NASW Press, 4–5.

Gibelman, M. (1995) *What Social Workers Do*, NASW Press, 131.

Haynes, K. (1998) The One Hundred-Year Debate: Social Reform Versus Individual Treatment, *Social Work* **43** (60), 501–509.

Kanter, J. (1987) Mental Health Management: A Professional Domain. *Social Work* **32**, 461–462.

Klein, A.F. (1972) *Effective Group Work*. Follett Publishing, 103–106.

Levy Simon, B. (1998) The Profession of Social Work. In: *The Foundation of Social Work Practice*, 2nd edition, eds: Mark Mattini, Christine Lowery, Carol Meyer, NASW Press, 313–315.

Livingston, S. (1977) Psychosocial aspects of epilepsy. *Journal of Clinical Child Psychiatry* **6**, 6–10.

NASW (National Association of Social Workers) (1981) *NASW Standards For The Classification Of Social Work Practice*. NASW Press, 17–18.

Richmond, M. (1917) *Social Diagnosis*. Russell Sage Foundation.

Stewart, R. (1984) From The President, *NASW News*, Nov, 2.

Toseland, R., Siporen, M. (1986) When To Recommend Group Treatment: A Review Of The Clinical And Research Literature. *International Journal of Group Psychotherapy* **36**, 171–201.

Ziegler, R.G. (1981) Impairments Of Control And Competence, In: Epileptic Children And Their Families, *Epilepsia* **22**(3), 339-346.

Chapter 20

SUPPORT GROUPS FOR PEOPLE WITH EPILEPSY

Philip Lee

Support groups for epilepsy — for people with the condition, their families and carers — might be stimulated by a variety of different reasons but are invariably a spontaneous creation. Sometimes they are prompted by professionals working in the field — social workers, doctors, nurses and care workers — but more commonly they occur as a means of self-help, people affected by epilepsy doing it for themselves.

Why such groups have developed, why they continue to exist and why more and more of them are coming into being can be explained by two different factors. Firstly, they are symptomatic of a failure of the established health care and other systems to provide people with what they need. Support groups are set up to fill the gaps. Secondly, they are a manifestation of people affected by epilepsy taking positive action. By realising that they can play an influential role in the management of epilepsy, groups provide people with the opportunity to regain at least some control over their lives which it has taken away.

FILLING THE GAPS IN CARE

The principal motivation behind the formation of most groups is the frustration people feel from trying to use a health and social care system which has either failed to provide them with what they need or which has proved to be inaccessible and irrelevant to them. Self-help initiatives start and continue because there is often nothing else available that works. Having said this, it is unusual in the UK today to find a situation where the system has failed so completely that self-help is the only option. Self-help is in fact complimentary, filling the gaps in an under performing service, rather than providing a comprehensive alternative.

Surveys by British Epilepsy Association consistently indicate significant levels of dissatisfaction among people with epilepsy, not only with their medical care and treatment but also with the services provided by Education and Social Services (BEA, 1990; 1996). The lack of any real cohesion between the statutory providers of care and services and the complex systems which they operate prevent many people from satisfying what are, in reality, very often simple and uncomplicated needs. This can be as basic as just sitting down with someone who has time to listen. It is these simple needs that self-help is often so good at serving.

From lists published by the national epilepsy organisations, we can estimate that in 1999 there were at least 200 self-help or support groups for epilepsy located all over the UK (National Society for Epilepsy (NSE) 1995; BEA, 1999). Some are entirely independent local groups but most are linked in some way to one of the large national or regional epilepsy organisations, which they use as a resource for their training, epilepsy information and other support materials. Whatever their affiliation, all of the groups are a local response to a locally perceived need.

The primary organiser of local groups is British Epilepsy Association (BEA) with more than 120 under its umbrella. BEA is a voluntary health organisation of 21,000 members that represents people with epilepsy and others with an interest in the condition. It is a registered charity that exists to meet the identified needs of people with epilepsy by: raising awareness of the condition, providing advice and information, improving understanding of epilepsy, campaigning for change in service provision, and undertaking research and raising funds. The Association is in effect a national support group. It was founded in 1950 on the principles of self-help. It was created by and for people whose needs were not being fulfilled by anyone or anything else. Many of the pioneers of the early Association had their roots in local epilepsy support groups and simply extended the self-help principle, with the encouragement of interested professionals, to create a national organisation.

Traditionally the early groups were run mainly as social clubs providing, in many cases, the only social contact that people with epilepsy might have. They organised regular meetings and group holidays, providing a forum for the exchange of personal experiences for people to support each other. The provision of basic facts about epilepsy and personal support remain key components of many groups today.

TAKING POSITIVE ACTION

Epilepsy was then and still can be a tremendously isolating condition. The stigma which so many people with the condition attach to themselves, as well as the prejudice displayed by others towards them, cannot readily be addressed or corrected by medication, however effective it might be at controlling seizures. The opportunity to meet privately with others who have had very similar experiences can be reassuring, enlightening and give hope. Reducing isolation by providing contact opportunities in a non-threatening, sympathetic and understanding environment continues to be a valuable contribution that support groups can make.

The contrasting environment which groups offer is especially significant for people who are having frequent seizures. A person having a seizure at a support group (as long as it is not serious or prolonged or causes any physical damage) is treated with care and familiarity by group members. Seizures at groups can also be a valuable educational experience. Many people who have seizures themselves may never actually have seen someone else having a seizure.

Most groups will operate a regular cycle of meetings, but support can and does expand outside of meetings, typically with phone calls, visits, letters, newsletters, social and other special events. All of these activities help to involve people, further reducing isolation, and conveying not only a sense of belonging but also a sense of ownership.

Group activities can also help people to develop skills in caring, organising, administration, promotion, fundraising and book-keeping. Groups give people a chance to actively challenge the limitations they have set themselves and which they believe the condition imposes upon them. In this way they can give a terrific boost to peoples' confidence and low self-esteem.

Not surprisingly, many people affected by epilepsy want as much information about their condition as they can get. All too often this is very hard to obtain from a GP, hospital clinic, social worker or teacher (Buck *et al.*, 1996). This is a crucial gap which support groups fill admirably. They not only increase access to information, they also provide an alternative and possibly challenging view. Not only do they give advice and information themselves but they are also an important signpost to other sources of help and a valuable entry point to the wider network of community support that is available.

A lot of groups maintain a library of epilepsy information (leaflets, books and even videos) and invite guest speakers to attend meetings. With more relevant information and understanding of their condition, people are able to make a more informed choice about their care and treatment. This creates the potential for real empowerment, with better informed people becoming more effective partners in their own healthcare. However, the givers and receivers of information need to guard against the danger of both information overload and self-diagnosis.

Increasingly, groups are providing information to their wider communities. Many see it as a vital part of their work to educate the wider general public about the facts about epilepsy, particularly first aid procedures. Equally, professionals in health, education and social services stand to benefit from the information groups provide for them.

Typically a support group will include people with epilepsy of all ages, their family members and other carers. Sometimes, interested professionals will lend their assistance as well. Groups are consequently a useful partnership activity, helping to link the recipients and providers of care together and offering a positive joint activity that a carer and a person with epilepsy can do together.

For carers and family members as well as people with epilepsy, groups can be a vital way to reduce stress, to allow honest comments, to learn about coping strategies and at times to simply release pent up emotions like guilt, frustration and anger. Epilepsy has the potential to change the lives not just of those with the condition, but also of their friends and family; and sometimes it helps just to discuss this.

At an individual level, there are clearly benefits which people can derive from a support group. However it's important to recognise that there are limitations to what a group can offer and achieve. To be successful, these limitations have to be acknowledged by those running the group and those seeking help from it.

How active a group will be, what it does and how well it responds to the needs of local people will largely depend on the situations of its members; how much time they have and what skills and abilities they possess. Enthusiasm is rarely a problem, at least not at the beginning, but members' demands will often outweigh the group's abilities and capacity to help. Funding is always a constraint on group activity. Groups rely on voluntary fundraising to support their work and need to devote a lot of energy to raising the money they need. This can sometimes divert groups from their more direct support work. However effective the fundraising, there is rarely enough money to meet all the objectives of the group.

There are of course practical obstacles to attending a group including lack of public transport, distance, tiredness, seizure frequency, lack of awareness of a group's existence, antipathy to groups and the pressure of other commitments such as caring for a family or working. Transport in particular is a common limitation, ever more so with the decline in public transport services, especially in rural areas. For people still experiencing frequent seizures, public transport is essential for mobility and concessionary bus travel for people with epilepsy is not universally guaranteed. Commonly, groups therefore tend to draw their support from within a tight radius of up to 10 miles.

Support groups have been criticised for labelling epilepsy. Some people will not attend simply to avoid the label they feel is attached to membership. The self-imposed stigma of epilepsy and a reluctance to accept a diagnosis of the condition is a frequent barrier to participation. Equally, groups are not to everyone's taste. Many people will attend just one meeting and never return, either because they have found what they wanted or because the group or the self-help concept is not attractive to them. For whatever reason, it is clear that not everyone is comfortable in a group setting and some people prefer a more personal or private relationship. It is worth noting that a third of the 30,000 calls a year to BEA's telephone helpline are made anonymously. In response to this and as a supplement to its group work, BEA has for several years been running a pen friend service, linking together individuals with epilepsy and families of people with epilepsy. Another development is BEA's Accredited Volunteer scheme, through which trained volunteers, often linked to groups, provide a personal one-to-one service, outside of the group setting.

THE DEVELOPING POLITICAL ROLE OF THE SUPPORT GROUP

In 1999, there is still a demand for the traditional range of group support and activity based on providing social contact, providing basic facts about epilepsy and educating the wider general public. However, since the mid-1990's new trends have been developing reflecting emerging technology, changes in needs and expectations and changes in society as a whole.

New technology is opening up avenues for self-help via internet Websites and chat rooms. Websites especially bring into sharp relief some of the potential drawbacks of self-help. Large numbers of presumably well intentioned people have set up epilepsy Websites all over the world. These range from the genuinely informative and helpful to the outright dangerous in their mis-information and mis-direction. Epilepsy and self-help are therefore no different to any other subject on the Net, but this does require the 'surfer' to display an educated filter to whatever they pick up. In truth, unregulated self-help, and perhaps by definition there is no other type, has always needed to be treated with some degree of caution by the recipient.

The traditional support group format is broadly based, drawing in all types of interested people. However, because of their generality, not everyone is able to find exactly what they want. One outcome of this has been the recent development of more specialised groups that either differentiate between carers and people with epilepsy or which are focused on a particular aspect of the condition. Examples include BEA's *PACE* groups for parents of children with epilepsy. Other groups have been founded for people with particular epileptic syndromes and for people undergoing certain types of treatment such as brain surgery or vagal nerve implant surgery.

The emergence in the 1990's of the support group *Epilepsy Bereaved?* exemplifies the way that groups as a whole have diversified. *Epilepsy Bereaved?* began as a small group of bereaved relatives and carers who had lost a family member as a result of an epilepsy related death. They could not find the support and care they particularly wanted from any existing source, including from the existing voluntary organisations for epilepsy, and were appalled at the lack of information and knowledge about epilepsy related death in general. To get what they wanted and needed these people had to largely support themselves and from this has grown a national charity with a distinctive identity and agenda. In concert with others, but primarily as a result of *Epilepsy Bereaved?*'s work, the Department of Health commissioned in 1999 the UK's first ever audit into epilepsy related death.

This is a radical example of what a support group can achieve. It also highlights an emerging role that groups are taking on as they grow in self-confidence and respond to changes in society. Increasingly, people are encouraged to view themselves as consumers of healthcare and other services rather than as patients or passive recipients. As consumers they are being encouraged to take an active role in their condition, to be more demanding with higher expectations and to be better informed about their options. This is happening at a time when the pressures on the NHS have never been greater and its ability to respond is severely restricted. The current Government's emphasis on partnership in healthcare and their desire to see 'joined up' services linking health, education and social welfare is creating a new environment which places the person with epilepsy and their carers at its heart.

Support groups are already proving to be effective vehicles for organising this involvement and influence, whether at local level through small groups, at regional level through alliances of groups, or at national level through organisations like British Epilepsy Association and *Epilepsy Bereaved?*.

To play this new and demanding role requires different skills and perceptions to those once associated with a support group. Horizons have been widened beyond that of the group itself simply filling gaps left by an inadequate system. Now groups are learning how the systems work, pinpointing why they are failing and discovering the levers to pull to make things better. Consequently groups are evolving into much more political organisations.

As groups have become more sophisticated and aware of the power they have to change and influence things, their representations have caused improvements in local services. For example, in the late 1990's there has been huge growth in the number of clinical nurse specialists in epilepsy and local epilepsy clinics as a direct result of the intervention of support groups. In Huddersfield, for example, the support group campaigned for and won the appointment of both a local neurologist and a clinical nurse specialist in epilepsy. In Kent, local groups worked together to put a similar case for an epilepsy specialist nurse and to raise the pump priming money to ensure the appointment could be made. Elsewhere group members have joined Community Health Councils and local health and social services planning teams to ensure that epilepsy is included in local planning and that commissioners and providers of care are aware of their needs.

Ironically the success of support group lobbying and campaigning for better services has impacted to some degree on their traditional activities. As services and access have improved, people are better able to find the basic facts they want about epilepsy, without the support group providing them. This may have partly removed one of the original driving forces for the formation of some groups, but they continue to have a role to play. Looking to the future one can see groups acting increasingly as local consumer watchdogs on their services and holding the statutory providers to account. Despite this, it is hard to see a time when the system will be so perfect that it leaves no gaps at all. These gaps are all the incentive people need to jump in and fill them with self-help.

As mentioned earlier, groups have been criticised by their own members and other observers for 'ghettoising' epilepsy. There may have been some justification for this in the past, when much of the activity was insular and introverted. However, as groups become more outward looking through their campaigning and lobbying activity, the criticism becomes less justified. Far from secluding epilepsy, groups are realising that they can more easily improve the quality of the services they need by being as public as possible. Having said this, having the courage to do this and stand up and declare for epilepsy is not easy in a society which still discriminates against the condition.

CONCLUSION

In conclusion, support groups for epilepsy are not unlike support groups for any other condition. They have evolved out of a lack of support from statutory providers and as a consequence of individuals not being prepared to accept this and being willing to do something about it themselves. From providing basic direct services themselves, such as advice and information, groups are evolving into sophisticated articulators of the needs of local people and a powerful pressure group to ensure that those needs are better met.

The gap between need and provision in epilepsy care and support is slowly closing, but services are still fragmented and patchy around the country and where necessary self-help will continue to provide as best it can. There is often no other alternative. There is also one support service which groups are uniquely placed to deliver. That is the need to simply meet and talk to someone else in a similar situation, to learn from their experience and take comfort and hope from their example.

Do support groups influence peoples' quality of life? Undoubtedly, at a national level, organisations like BEA have made a major contribution over many years and will continue to do so in the future. The Association's influence is now actively sought by policy and decision makers across the widest range of issues from driving license regulations to national policy on health, education and social welfare.

At an individual level, there is no definitive answer. The benefit a person obtains from attending a local group can range from nothing at all to a hugely positive life changing experience. Many people ascribe their group with giving them the confidence to apply for and hold down employment, to go out more and develop social skills leading to friendships and relationships inside and outside the group, to break free from well meaning but over-protective parents, or to sign up for higher education courses. Membership of an epilepsy support group may thus confer benefits in a number of different ways, which may ultimately contribute to improvements in a person's quality of life.

References

BEA (1990) *Towards a New Understanding, A Charter for People with Epilepsy.* Leeds: BEA.

BEA (1996) *A Patient's Viewpoint.* Leeds: BEA.

BEA (1999) *Epilepsy Today,* March Issue No. 46, Leeds: BEA.

Buck, D., Jacoby, A., Baker, G.A., Graham-Jones, S., Chadwick, D.W. (1996) Patients' experiences of and satisfaction with care for their epilepsy. *Epilepsia* **37**(9), 841–49.

NSE (1995) *Epilepsy Review,* Spring Issue No. 16, Bucks: NSE.

CONCLUSIONS

Chapter 21

IMPROVING QUALITY OF LIFE: THE NEXT STEPS

Gus A. Baker and Ann Jacoby

All chronic conditions present important quality of life challenges to those affected by them and to those concerned with their treatment. Because of the clinical complexities surrounding its definition, diagnosis and management and the cultural-historical legacies surrounding its present-day social reality, it seems to us that epilepsy presents more challenges than most. In the preceding chapters, our various contributors have tried to summarise current understanding of how a diagnosis of epilepsy impinges on a person's quality of life and how its impact can be minimised through optimal clinical management, provided by a multi-disciplinary team. In this last chapter, we speculate on how current and future developments in the treatment and delivery of services for epilepsy may impinge on the quality of life of people receiving them. We also focus on how theoretical and methodological developments in the science of quality of life assessment will influence future quality of life research.

TECHNOLOGICAL ADVANCES IN THE TREATMENT OF EPILEPSY

The New Genetics

Advances in the sciences of molecular biology and genetics have dramatically increased understanding of the basis of seizures and epilepsy and begun to unravel the vexed question of why some patients and not others develop epilepsy which is pharmaco-resistant (Regesta and Tanganelli, 1998). Genetic research has been directed both at elucidating the inherited basis of some epilepsies and at clarifying the role of specific genes in response to, or consequent upon, seizure activity (Mamelak and Lowenstein, 1998). Several 'epilepsy genes' have already been discovered, others will be identified in the near future (Nance *et al.*, 1998). It is currently estimated that genetic factors may be implicated in up to 50% of all epilepsies (Smith *et al.*, 1998); and this percentage may increase as work in this field progresses. Genetic counselling is likely therefore to become an increasingly important element of the management of people with epilepsy, with affected individuals needing information and support to make informed decisions, particularly with regard to genetic testing and future reproductive behaviour (Anderson *et al.*, 1998). The ways in which the new genetics will influence clinical management of people with epilepsy facing such screening decisions, for example in relation to the use of decision aids (O'Connor *et al.*, 1999), and the resultant impact on their quality of life can only be a matter of speculation at this stage.

Advances in Pharmacological Treatment of Epilepsy

Until fairly recently, choice of antiepileptic medication was limited, the majority of patients being prescribed one of the four standard drugs, whose mechanisms were relatively poorly understood (see Chapter 2). Over the last two decades, novel antiepileptic drugs have been developed that target specific mechanisms underlying epileptic events (Dichter, 1998). For example, vigabatrin and tiagabine both alter the action of GABA, the former by inhibiting its metabolism, the latter by inhibiting its re-uptake after synaptic release (Dichter, 1998; and see Chapter 2). The search for even more effective and less toxic drugs continues and it has been suggested that new agents will be aimed not just at treating the symptoms of epilepsy (i.e. the seizures) but at curing the condition itself (Sankar and Weaver, 1998). In this area too, the importance of advances in genetics will be felt, since understanding of the genetic basis of abnormal processes in the brain will enable the development of agents to prevent or reverse the epileptic process (Meldrum, 1998). It remains to be seen whether any of these so-called 'designer' drugs prove to be the *magic bullet* that stops seizures without producing unacceptable side-effects. As for the standard drugs, a comprehensive assessment of these novel compounds should not rely only on standard clinical parameters, but also examine those issues identified by patients themselves as most pertinent in terms of their quality of life.

Neurosurgical Advances

Though the majority of people with epilepsy will continue to be treated for their condition with pharmacological agents, developments in neuro-imaging, diagnosis, long-terming monitoring and surgical techniques will also present important new treatment possibilities. The number of people with epilepsy undergoing surgery tripled between 1985 and 1990 (Engel *et al.*, 1998) and many different surgical procedures are now on offer, including resection, disconnection and selective removal of discrete lesions. The ultimate aim of surgery is improved QoL and the general assumption has been that this will inevitably follow from improved clinical outcome. Recently, however, the results of a number of studies have challenged that assumption. Hermann *et al.*, (1992) showed that the most significant predictor of post-operative psychosocial adjustment was, in fact, the adequacy of patients' pre-operative adjustment. Bladin (1992) reported that around two-thirds of patients in whom surgery had apparently been successful (in as much as they were rendered seizure-free) nonetheless experienced post-operative psychiatric problems, including anxiety, depression and psychosis. This finding links with research into the role of patients' expectations of the outcome of surgery. Wilson *et al.*, (1998) found that among patients rendered seizure-free by surgery, those who saw their operation as successful had very clear and concrete goals; whereas those who judged it unsuccessful had broader and less clearly defined ones. Similarly, Wheelock *et al.*, (1998) showed that patients who failed to acknowledge the possibility of continuing seizure activity post-operatively and who did not achieve complete control reported little improvement in their quality of life. Consideration of this element of treatment for epilepsy alone serves to emphasise the importance of a comprehensive assessment of outcome which goes beyond simply counting seizures.

Vagal Nerve Stimulation

Another new non-pharmacological treatment for epilepsy whose quality of life impacts are as yet largely undocumented is the vagal nerve stimulator (Schachter, 2000). Vagal nerve stimulation (VNS) involves implantation of a battery-powered pulse generator into the upper left chest; the pulses being conveyed to the left vagus nerve by means of two electrodes. In two recent studies which followed implanted patients for 12 weeks, the efficacy of VNS was demonstrated by the finding that seizure frequency was reduced by both high and low stimulation. VNS appears to be safe and generally well tolerated, but adverse effects such as hoarseness, throat pain, voice alteration and cough are reported both short and longer term. One important quality of life question this raises is whether such VNS-specific effects are seen as generally more or less acceptable to the recipients of the device than the CNS effects typically experienced by those treated with pharmacological agents.

The message from all of this is that technological advances are rapidly increasing our understanding of the processes and mechanisms that constitute epilepsy and the means of treating it. Such developments are exciting for the clinician and basic scientist and clearly important. However, past experience suggests it is unlikely that only benefits will accrue from these developments. The possible costs and negative impacts of such 'high-tech' approaches on their recipients, including increased anxiety and the demands of more complex decision-making cannot be disregarded. Documenting the ways in which such technological innovations affect those at the receiving end at the level of their quality of life will be critical to understanding their real impact.

SERVICE PROVISION FOR PEOPLE WITH EPILEPSY

In the United Kingdom, a series of government sponsored reports on the provision of services for people with epilepsy have been published over the past 40 years (Thompson, 1990), the most recent being the report of the Clinical Standards Advisory Group (CSAG, 2000). CSAG was set up to advise on standards of clinical care and access and availability of services to patients. Among its major recommendations are that:

- a network of neurologist-led epilepsy centres be established, to act as a link between primary care facilities and regional or supra-regional neurological facilities
- a network of paediatric epilepsy clinics also be established, again with formal links to regional paediatric neurologists
- regional implementation groups be set up to facilitate the establishment of these networks and strengthen primary care services for epilepsy

CSAG also recommended a number of changes to the clinical process. These include:

- making services more receptive to the views of patients and carers and more responsive to the needs of specific patient subgroups
- providing more equitable and easy access to services
- strengthening of the epilepsy surgery services
- improved services for learning disabled people with epilepsy
- access to regional and supra-regional services for people with complex epilepsy

Many of these recommendations are in line with those made in previous reports. Only time will tell whether they will have more impact on the organisation of services for epilepsy than has previously been the case and whether the changes wrought improve the quality of life of the recipients.

The Role of the Primary Care Physician

In its report, CSAG recognises the pivotal role the primary care physician plays in managing people with epilepsy in the UK, both by providing clinical care and acting as gatekeeper for referral to secondary and tertiary care. In the US too, current emphasis is on the primary care physician managing people with stable epilepsy, with minimal recourse to secondary care. Schachter and Alsgaard (1999) make the point however, that this can only be effective if primary care physicians, who are not necessarily expert in epilepsy, are given appropriate tools and proper guidelines about diagnosis, management and treatment. Recently, a number of such guidelines have been published (SIGN, 1997; Wallace *et al.*, 1997), though it should be said that many are consensus statements rather than being evidence-based.

It is interesting that in such research as has been done into patient preferences for epilepsy care, people with epilepsy tend to see primary care physicians as having greater interpersonal skills than hospital physicians, but as lacking the required expertise to manage epilepsy effectively. In the CSAG project, improved physician knowledge about epilepsy was commonly cited by the people with epilepsy surveyed as key to improving the quality of their primary care. In our own study of patient satisfaction with epilepsy care (Buck *et al.*, 1996) and the Doncaster study described by de Groot in Chapter 16, patients receiving care from both sources were more likely to feel their views were taken into account by their primary care physician, but also less likely to believe that the primary care physician was well informed about epilepsy. Hopefully, dissemination of such findings will speed acceptance of the message that primary care physician-related barriers to optimal care must be addressed. De Groot suggests a number of ways in which this could happen.

The Role of the Nurse Specialist

A key role in the provision of care for people with epilepsy has also been suggested for the epilepsy nurse specialist (Schachter and Alsgaard, 1999; CSAG, 2000). A number of possible tasks have been identified, in line with the description provided by Sweeney in Chapter 18. While we support the principle behind this development, it is salutary that the few studies examining the effectiveness of the specialist nurse have produced results which are not wholly convincing. The overall message appears to be that despite improvements in the level of information given to people about their epilepsy and their subsequent satisfaction with care, other outcomes are largely unaffected. For example, Mills and colleagues (1999a, b) found that patients who used a primary care based epilepsy specialist nurse service complied less well with treatment regimes and perceived more negative effects of their condition on their functioning and quality of life. Likewise, Warren *et al.*, (1998) reported that patients receiving care from a hospital based nurse specialist had higher levels of knowledge about their condition and were more satisfied with their care, but performed less well in terms of clinic attendance and medication adherence and showed no improvements in psychosocial functioning. It is important in our view that the cost savings shown in Warren's study are not allowed to overshadow the relative lack of evidence of benefits in other directions. The epilepsy specialist nurse is certainly not the panacea for all the current ills in epilepsy care.

Information and Choice

Most people with chronic conditions appear to want information (Deber, 1994) and to want all that is available (Blanchard *et al.*, 1988); but health professionals appear not always fully attuned to this need (Waitzkin, 1985). Repeatedly, research has shown that lack of information is a source of concern to a significant proportion of people with epilepsy (Buck *et al.,* 1996; Ridsdale *et al.*, 1996; Mills *et al.*, 1997). This is an important gap, given that we know that possession of accurate information is significantly related to level of well-being and quality of life. Hills and Baker (1992) found that people with epilepsy who were more informed about the management and treatment of their condition perceived themselves as being in more control and subsequently had significantly better psychological profiles than those who were less informed. Our own recent European-wide study confirms this earlier finding. People with higher levels of knowledge about their condition tended also to score higher on measures of adjustment to epilepsy and lower on measures of epilepsy impact and stigma (Baker *et al., in press*). In the last section of this book, our various contributors have argued eloquently the case for their inclusion in the multidisciplinary team. It is clear that the hospital-based neurologist may not be best placed to provide information to patients in a form and setting conducive to meeting their needs. Other members of the team, whether it be the clinical psychologist, specialist nurse or social worker, have a key role to play here, as highlighted in the relevant chapters.

Even when they prefer the clinician to assume the role of primary decision maker, patients often actively seek information about their condition. Though the link between information provision, improved well-being and overall quality of life may be tenuous, there is little doubt that increasing information leads to increased overall satisfaction with health care. Increased satisfaction with care has, in turn, been shown to be related to other important outcomes including compliance with treatment and clinic re-attendance (Fitzpatrick, 1984). Physicians are likely to find it easier to work with well-informed patients, who understand the risks and benefits of the various treatment options available to them (Schachter and Alsgaard, 1999). There is also now a political agenda behind increased information provision (Coulter, 1999). People with chronic conditions like epilepsy are increasingly required to be co-participants in their care and to actively self-manage their condition. They can only do so if well enough informed about all the available alternatives and possibilities.

A Political Voice for Epilepsy

Chadwick (1990) has suggested that one explanation for the poor and fragmented services provided to people with epilepsy in the developed world is that the negative attitudes held by the lay public are also held by health professionals and service providers. This has resulted in a relatively low priority being given to epilepsy care and, as a consequence, a lack of financial commitment. Another important element in this scenario has been the absence of an effective political lobby for epilepsy. In the UK, the situation appears to be changing for the better. Philip Lee, in his chapter, has documented the ways in which patient groups such as British Epilepsy Association have moved from a support role at the level of the individual to a campaigning role at both local and national level, with the aim of influencing professionals and policy makers.

In producing this text we are conscious, both as editors and contributors, of its focus on epilepsy as defined clinically and socially in the developed world. We are only too well aware of how much more difficult the position is for people with epilepsy living in developing countries, where epilepsy remains a highly stigmatising disorder and where treatment options are minimal or non-existent. It is for this reason that campaigns at the international level, such as the Global Campaign, a joint initiative of the International Bureau for Epilepsy, the International League Against Epilepsy and the World Health Organisation, are important. The Global Campaign has as its major objective to persuade the WHO General Assembly that epilepsy be recognised as a global health priority. As part of the campaign, demonstration projects are being conducted in selected developing countries with a view to reducing the QoL and economic burdens of epilepsy and improving education, training and health care delivery. Central to both the Global Campaign and the work of national organisations such as BEA is the need to improve public awareness and attitudes towards epilepsy and so reduce the level of stigma and discrimination, at whatever level it operates.

THE CONTINUING ROLE OF QoL ASSESSMENT

Since both epilepsy *per se* and treatments for epilepsy have the potential to profoundly affect quality of life, assessment of their effects will continue to be an important research priority. Our various contributors have amply illustrated the value of quality of life research applied descriptively, within the context of clinical research, and even at the level of individual patient care. We would suggest that among future research priorities should be:

1. *Exploration of the process of adjustment to epilepsy.* To date, there have been almost no longitudinal studies in epilepsy, particularly of newly diagnosed patients. Thus, it has been difficult to disentangle the various factors promoting or detracting from the ability of a person so affected to cope with and adjust to their condition. Without understanding the direction of relationships between factors, it is difficult to design effective educational and management strategies for people with epilepsy or to identify those people who will benefit most from them.
2. *Studies of the longer term impact of treatment for seizures and epilepsy.* Most studies of the outcomes of treatment for epilepsy confine themselves to measurement of short-term outcomes only. Drug trials, for example, are generally of fairly short duration, typically 16 to 20 weeks. Many QoL domains will be unaffected in the short term by changes in clinical status or may even by affected negatively (Berzon, 1998). Longer term follow up will therefore allow for more meaningful assessments of the impact of treatment on QoL.
3. *Studies of the role of the complimentary therapies.* The possibility of non-pharmacological treatment of seizures, including through the

use of complimentary therapies, has been raised by a number of authors. Kloster *et al.,* (1999) examined the effect of acupuncture on seizure frequency in patients with intractable epilepsy, but were unable to show any beneficial effects. Their study was, however, limited by small sample size and the lack of a group of patients with more benign epilepsies which might have been more responsive to treatment. There have been similar limitations in a number of other studies addressing this topic. On a more positive note, an audit of the use of aromatherapy to treat seizures by Betts *et al.,* (1999) suggests that in a significant group of patients, better seizure control can be achieved. Given that they may have marked benefits over conventional treatments for seizures, such therapies require more robust assessments which include quality of life outcomes.

4. *Evaluations of differing systems of delivering care.* As the studies by Mills and Warren show, new services and systems of delivering care for people with epilepsy require careful evaluation of their costs and benefits. Changes currently proposed for the UK should, if implemented, be carefully monitored and their impact on patient satisfaction and wider quality of life documented.

RESOLVING UNRESOLVED ISSUES

As is clear from the review by von Steinbuchel and colleagues in Chapter 5, considerable progress has been made in the development of epilepsy-specific QoL measures for adults. Assessment of QoL issues for children is less advanced (a situation in no way unique to epilepsy), though a number of new measures have been devised (Austin *et al.,* 1991, Austin and Huberty, 1993; Hoare and Russell, 1995; Carpay *et al.,* 1996; Cramer *et al., in press*). These have begun to address the limits of previous work relating to children, in as much as several are intended for completion by children themselves (often with parent-completed parallel measures) and are age-specific. There is still however, in our view, the need for more systematic, theory-driven developmental work relating to this group. At the opposite end of the life cycle, Tallis points out that to be of value, QoL assessments in older people must also be age-specific, taking into account any differences in the clinical features of epilepsy, health status and life circumstances associated with older age. Further work is also clearly justified in this area. Likewise, as Espie and Kerr highlight, assessment of quality of life for people with learning disability remains something of a methodological minefield, presenting enormous challenges to the QoL researcher. What appears evident from the arguments our various contributors make is that to be meaningful, QoL assessments need to be target-group specific, measuring domains that are of real relevance and importance to those at whom they are aimed and grounded in their experience.

Another difficulty raised by Espie and Kerr in relation to learning disabled people but equally applicable to other patient subgroups is the degree to which QoL assessments reflect low expectations based on previous life experience of having epilepsy. This phenomenon of response shift — where individuals facing a significant health challenge 'experience a change in their internal standards of expectations for optimal functioning' (Schwartz and Laitin, 1998) — may mean that QoL comparisons over time are invalid and cloak the real effects of treatments under scrutiny (or, indeed, the lack of them). This is a relatively new area of investigation but methods are being developed to address it (see, for example, Nieuwkerk *et al.*, 1999).

A third important issue, particularly within the context of clinical trials, is that of the cross-cultural applicability of QoL measures. Hunt (1998) points out that the socio-cultural circumstances in which a person with a chronic illness such as epilepsy is placed largely determine such relevant attributes as their customary behaviours, relationships and social interactions, the values they place on these, their expectations about and perceptions of health and ill health and their use of language to describe such phenomena. It therefore cannot be assumed that a QoL measure developed for one cultural or social setting will be readily transferable to another. We have already acknowledged the emphasis in this book on the clinical and social reality of epilepsy in the developed world. Currently available QoL measures for epilepsy are similarly biased, in that almost all are the product of QoL research efforts in the UK and US. Even if rigorous translation rules are applied, they may still lack cultural applicability, raising the question of whether their use indicates that, in Hunt's words, 'enthusiasm has outrun common sense'! We agree with her about the range of difficulties over development and application of QoL measures cross culturally which must be addressed if the claims made for them are to be seen as scientifically credible.

Lastly, we turn to the question of whether it is realistic to aim for a 'gold standard' QoL measure for epilepsy. To some extent, this has already happened in relation to generic QoL measures, with the SF-36 (Ware and Sherbourne, 1992) currently occupying pride of place, supported by a wealth of data on its psychometric properties (including in relation to people with epilepsy; see Jacoby *et al.*, 1999). In epilepsy the picture is, at least for the present, less clear-cut. There is, as yet, relatively little evidence about the responsiveness of the various epilepsy-specific measures (see Chapter 5) and no one measure clearly out-performs the others with regard to the issues of validity and reliability. For this reason, we think it will be some time before any of those available consistently finds favour. However, we agree with Hays (1995) that what is most needed now is consolidation of efforts to evaluate the various measures already in existence, rather than proliferation of further measures.

CONCLUSION

For us as editors of this text, the case for QoL assessment in epilepsy remains unquestioned. The level of attention now given to the topic suggests that there is widespread acceptance in the epilepsy research and clinical communities that data on seizure frequency alone are insufficient to provide a full picture of the position for people with epilepsy. QoL measures have an important place in elucidating the real outcomes of epilepsy care, or illuminating ways in which that care should be targeted, and they should not be seen simply as paying lip service to a particular political tenet of the moment. While we admit Betts' claim in Chapter 10 that some physicians have always given consideration to QoL issues, we do not accept that this has universally been the case. The early work to promote QoL assessment grew out of studies by social scientists that described the experience of chronic illness and so illuminated its 'particular predicaments'. In doing so, such studies also highlighted the ways in which the perspectives of people with chronic illness can differ markedly from those of the health professionals responsible for their care.

The clinical and social complexities implicit in the term 'epilepsy' make it an unceasingly fascinating topic for physicians and social scientists alike. Rapid developments in basic, clinical and quality of life science mean that its fascination is unlikely to diminish. Hopefully they will also mean that the management of people with epilepsy will move closer to the optimal. This combined with a good therapeutic relationship, supportive family and friends and an empathic community should allow people with epilepsy to make a positive adjustment to their condition and so enjoy as good a quality of life as those without.

References

Anderson, V.E., Andermann, E., Hauser, W.A. (1998) Genetic counselling. In: Engel, J Jr., Pedley, T.A. (eds.) *Epilepsy: A Comprehensive Textbook*. Vol. I. Philadelphia: Lippincott-Raven, 225–232.

Austin, J.K., Huberty, T.J. (1993) Development of the Child Attitude Toward Illness Scale. *Journal of Paediatric Psychology* **18**,467–80.

Austin, J.K., Patterson, J.M., Huberty, T.J. (1991) Development of the Coping Health Inventory for children. *Journal of Paediatric Nursing* **6**(3),166–74.

Baker, G.A., Jacoby, A., De Boer, H., Doughty, J., Myon, E., Tiaeb, C. (2000) Knowledge of epilepsy: A European study. Interim findings. *Epilepsia* in press.

Berzon, R.A. (1998) Understanding and using health-related quality of life instruments within clinical research studies. In: Staquet, M.J., Hays, R.D., Fayers, P.M. (eds.) *Quality of Life assessment in Clinical trials*. Oxford: Oxford University, 3–18.

Betts, T., Jackson, V., Howes, L. (1999) Audit of the use of aromatherapy in an epilepsy clinic. *Seizure* **8**, 377 (Abstract).

Bladin, P.F. (1992) Psychosocial difficulties and outcome after temporal lobectomy. *Epilepsia* **33**(5), 898–907.

Blanchard, C.G., Labreque, M.S., Ruckdeschel, J.C., Blanchard, E.B. (1988) Information and decision making preferences of hospitalised adult cancer patients. *Social Science and Medicine* **27**, 1139–1145.

Buck, D., Jacoby, A., Baker, G.A., Graham-Jones, S., Chadwick, D. (1996) Patients experiences of and satisfaction with care for their epilepsy. *Epilepsia* **37**, 841–849.

Carpay, H.A., Arts, W.F.M., Vermeulen, J., Stroink, H., Brower, O.F., Peters, A.C.B., van Donselaar, C.A., Aldenkamp, A.P. (1996) Parent-completed scales for measuring seizure severity and severity of side-effects of antiepileptic drugs in childhood epilepsy: development and psychometric analysis. *Epilepsy Research* **24**, 173–81.

Chadwick, D.W. (1990) Chairman's introduction. In: Chadwick, D.W. (ed.) *Quality of life and quality of care in epilepsy* Royal Society of Medicine Round Table Series No. 23. London: RSM, 3–6.

CSAG (Clinical standards advisory group) (2000) *Epilepsy: a report of the clinical standards advisory group*. London: HMSO.

Coulter, A. (1999) Paternalism or partnership? Patients have grown up — and there's no going back. *British Medical Journal* **319**, 719–20.

Cramer, J.A., Westbrook, L., Devinsky, O., Perrine, K., Camfield, C., Hermann, B., Abremson, H. (2000) Evaluation of an instrument to assess quality of life in epilepsy for adolescents (QOLIE-AD). *Epilepsia, in press.*

Deber, R.B. (1994) Physicians in healthcare management: the patient physician partnership: changing roles and the desire for information. *Journal of the Canadian Medical Association* **151**, 171–176.

Dichter, M.A. (1998) Overview: The neurobiology of epilepsy. In: Engel, J Jr., Pedley, T.A. (eds.) *Epilepsy: A Comprehensive Textbook*. Vol. I. Philadelphia: Lippincott-Raven, 233–236.

Engel, J. Jr., Wieser, H.G., Spencer, D. (1998) Overview: surgical therapy. In: Engel, J Jr., Pedley, T.A. (eds.) *Epilepsy: A Comprehensive Textbook*. Vol. II. Philadelphia: Lippincott-Raven, 1673–1676.

Fitzpatrick, R. (1984) Satisfaction with healthcare. In: Fitzpatrick, R., Hinton, J., Newman, S., Scambler, G., Thompson, J. (eds.) *The experience of illness*. London: Tavistock, 154–175.

Hays, R.D. (1995) Directions for future research. *Quality of Life Research* **4**, 179–80.

Hermann, B.P., Wyler, A.R., Somes, G. (1992) Preoperative psychological adjustment surgical outcomes are determinants of post-operative psychosocial status after anterior temporal lobectomies. *Journal of Neurology, Neurosurgery and Psychiatry*; **55**, 491–496.

Hills, M.D. and Baker, P.G. (1992) Relationships among epilepsy, social stigma, self esteem and social support. *Journal of Epilepsy* **5**, 231–238.

Hoare, P., Russell, M. (1995) The quality of life of children with chronic epilepsy and their families: preliminary findings with a new assessment measure. *Developmental Medicine and Child Neurology* **37**, 689–96.

Hunt, S.M. (1998) Cross cultural issues in the use of quality of life measures in randomised control trials. In: Staquet, M.J., Hayes, R.D., Feyers, P.M. (eds.) *Quality of life assessment in clinical trials*. Oxford University Press, 51–68.

Jacoby, A., Baker, G.A., Steen, N., Buck, D. (1999) The SF36 as a health status measure for epilepsy: a psychometric assessment. *Quality of Life Research* **8**, 351–364.

Kloster, R., Larsson, P.G., Lossius, R., Nakken, K.O., Dahl, R., Xiu-Ling, X., Wen-Xin, Z., Kinge, E., Rossberg, E. (1999) The effect of acupuncture in chronic intractable epilepsy. *Seizure* **8**, 170–74.

Mamelak, A.N., Lowenstein, D.H. (1998) Regulation of gene expression. In: Engel, J Jr., Pedley, T.A. (eds.) *Epilepsy: A Comprehensive Textbook*. Vol. I. Philadelphia: Lippincott-Raven, 291–306.

Meldrum, B.S. (1998) Current strategies for designing and identifying new antiepileptic drugs. In: Engel, J Jr., Pedley, T.A. (eds.) *Epilepsy: A Comprehensive Textbook*. Vol. II. Philadelphia: Lippincott-Raven, 1405–1416.

Mills, N., Bachmann, M.O., Harvey, I., Hine, I., McGowan, M. (1999a) Effect of a primary care based epilepsy specialist nurse service on quality of care from the patients' perspective: quasi-experimental evaluation. *Seizure* 8, 1–7.

Mills, N., Bachmann, M.O., Harvey, I., Hine, I., McGowan, M. (1999b) Effect of a primary care based epilepsy specialist nurse service on quality of care from the patients' perspective: results at two-year follow-up. *Seizure* 8, 291–296.

Mills, N., Bachmann, M.O., Hanesy, I., McGowan, M., Hine, I. (1997) Patients experience of epilepsy in health care. *Family Practice* **14**(2), 117–123.

Nance, M.A., Hauser, W.A., Anderson, V.E. (1998) Genetics diseases associated with epilepsy. In: Engel, J Jr., Pedley, T.A. (eds.) *Epilepsy: A Comprehensive Textbook*. Vol. I. Philadelphia: Lippincott-Raven, 197–210.

Nieuwkerk, P.T., Gisolf, E.H., Sprangers, M.A.G. (1999) Measuring change in quality of life (QoL): retrospective versus prospective measures. *Quality of Life Research* 8, 620 (Abstract).

O'Connor, A.M., Rostrom, A., Fiset, V., Tetroe, J., Entwistle, V., Llewellyn-Thomas, H., Holmes-Rovner, M., Barry, M., Jones, J. (1999) Decision aids for patients facing health treatment or screening decisions: systematic review. *British Medical Journal* **319**, 731–34.

Regesta, G., Tangeanelli, P. (1998) Clinical aspects and biological bases of pharmacoresistant epilepsy. *Epilepsia* **39** (Suppl 2), S46.

Ridsdale, L., Robbins, D., Fitzgerald, A., Jeffrey, S., McGee, L. (1996) Epilepsy monitoring and advice recorded: general practitioners views, current practice and patients preferences. *British Journal of General Practice* **46**, 11–14.

Sankar, R., Weaver, D.F. (1998) Basic principles of medicinal chemistry. In: Engel, J Jr., Pedley, T.A. (eds.) *Epilepsy: A Comprehensive Textbook*. Vol. II. Philadelphia: Lippincott-Raven, 1393–1404.

Schachter, S.C. (2000) Vagal nerve stimulation. In: Schmidt, D. and Schachter, S.C. *Epilepsy: Problem solving in clinical practice*. London: Martin Dunnitz, 439–456.

Schachter, S.C., Alsgaard, K. (1999) The management of epilepsy in managed healthcare. In: Mallarkey, G., Palmer, K.J. (eds.) *Issues in epilepsy*. Aukland: Addis International, 13–27.

Schwartz, C.E., Laitin, E.A. (1998) Using decision theory in clinical research: applications of quality adjusted life years. In: Staquet, M.J., Hayes, R.D., Feyers, P.M. (eds.) *Quality of life assessment in clinical trials*. Oxford: Oxford University Press, 119–142.

SIGN (Scottish Intercollegiate Guidelines Network; 1997) SIGN Guideline No. 21: *Diagnosis and management of epilepsy in adults*. Edinburgh: SIGN.

Smith, D.F., Appleton, R.E., MacKenzie, J.M., Chadwick, D.W. (1998) *An atlas of epilepsy*. New York: Parthenon.

Thompson, P. (1990) The Cohen report onwards. In: Chadwick, D. (ed.) *Quality of life and quality of care in epilepsy*. Royal Society of Medicine Round Table Series. No. 23. London: RSM, 7–15.

Waitzkin, H. (1985) Information giving in medical care. *Journal of Health and Social Behaviour* **26**, 8

Wallace, H., Shorvon, S.D., Hopkins, A., O'Donoghue, M. (1997) Adults with poorly controlled epilepsy. London: Royal College of Physicians.

Ware, J.E., Sherbourne, C.D. (1992) The MOS 36 item short-form health survey (SF36) I: Conceptual framework and item selection. *Medical Care* **30**(6), 473–483

Warren, E., Baker, G.A., Campion, P., Chadwick, D.W., Jacoby, A., Luker, K. (1998) *An evaluation of a nurse specialist/case manager intervention in the management of epilepsy.* Report for the North West Regional Health Authority. R & D Directorate.

Wheelock, I., Peterson, C., Buchtel, H.A. (1998) Presurgery expectations, post surgery satisfaction and psychosocial adjustment after epilepsy surgery. *Epilepsia* **39**(5), 487–494.

Wilson, S.J., Saling, M.M., Kincade, P., Bladin, P.F. (1998) Patient expectations of temporal lobe surgery. *Epilepsia* **39**(2), 167–174.

International League Against Epilepsy

Executive Office:

Irene Kujath
Epilepsie-Zentrum Bethel
Klinik Mara I
Maraweg 21
D-33617 Bielefeld
Germany
Tel: +49 521 144 4897 or 144 3686
Fax: +49 521 144 4637
Email: *ILAE-secretariat@mara.de*

International Bureau for Epilepsy

Executive Office:

PO Box 21
2100 AA Heemstede
The Netherlands
Tel: +31 23 523 7411
+31 23 529 1019 direct line
Fax: +31 23 547 0119
Email: *ibe@xs4all.nl*

INTERNATIONAL BUREAU FOR EPILEPSY CHAPTERS

Argentina
Associacion de Lucha contra la Epilepsia
Tucuman 3261
CP 1189 Buenos Aires
Tel: +54 114 8620 440
Fax: +54 114 8634 350

Australia
National Eilepsy Association of Australia
Suite 2B, 44–46 Oxford Street
PO Box 879
Epping

NSW 2121
Tel: +61 298 698 444
Fax: +61 298 694 122
Email: *epilepsy@nectar.com.au*

Austria
Epilepsie Selbsthilfegruppen Osterreichs
Haupstr. 44/2/2
2344 Ma Enzersdorf

Belgium
Les Amis de la Ligue Nationale
Belg Contre L'Epilepsie
Avenue Albert 135
Brussels 1060
Tel: +322 344 3263
Fax: +322 346 1193

Canada
Epilepsy Canada
1470 Peel Street
Suite 745
Montreal
Quebec H3A ITI
Tel: +1 514 845 7855
Fax: +1 514 845 7866
Email: *epilepsy@epilepsy.ca*
Website: *www.epilepsy.ca*

Chile
Liga contra la Epilepsia de Valparaiso
Alvares 1532
Casilla 705 (Hospital G. Fricke)
Vina del Mar
Fax: +56 2699 4084
Email: *liche@entelchile.net*

Colombia
Liga Colombiana contra la Epilepsia
Cap de Bolivar
Barrio Ternera
calle la El Eden

Y 5007 Cartagena
Tel: +57 566 18 107
Fax: +57 566 18 111
Email: *fandino@cartagena.cetcol.net.co*

Croatia
Croatian Association for Epilepsy
Department of Paediatrics
Division of Neuropediatrics
University Hospital Center Rebro
Kispaticevia 12
10 000 Zagreb
Tel: +385 121 3087
Fax: +385 121 0900

Cuba
Cuban Chapter IBE
Sociedad de Neurociencias de Cuba
Seccion de Epilepsia
Hospital Psiquiatrico de la Habana
Ave Independcia No 26520
Rpio Mazorra Ap 9
Boyoros, Cuidad de la Habana
CP 19220
Tel: +537 451 688
Fax: +537 451 512
Email: *Irrivera@ffa.giron.sld.cu*

Czech Republic
Czech Epilepsy Association
Spolecnost 'E'
Novodvorska 994
CZ 14221 Prague
Tel/Fax: +4202 4404 1557
Email: *elitera@iol.cz*

Denmark
Dansk Epilepsiforening
Dr Sellsvcj 28
DK 4293 Dianalund
Tel: +45 5826 44 66

Fax: +45 5826 44 51
Email: *epilepsi@get2net.dk*

Ecuador
Asociacion de Padres de Ninos con Epilepsia
Isla Marchena 300 y Los Granados
PO Box 17-15-221 C
Quito
Fax: +593 246 9141
Email: *gbpesantez@puceuio.puce.edu.ec*

Finland
Epilepsialiitto
Malmin Kauppatie 26
FIN-00700 Helsinki
Tel: +358 9350 82 320
Fax: +358 9350 82 322
Email: *epilepsialiitto@epilepsia.fi*
Website: *www.epilepsia.fi*

France
AISPACE
11 Avenue Kennedy
F-59800 Lille
Tel: +33 320 926 533
Fax: +33 320 094 124
Email: *info@aispace.asso.fr*

Germany
Deutsche Epilepsie Vereinigung
Zillestraße 102
10585 Berlin
Tel: +49 30 342 4414
Fax: +49 30 342 4466

Ghana
Ghana Epilepsy Association
c/o PO Box M230
Accra

Greece
Greek National Association against Epilepsy
Aghia Sophia Children's Hospital
Department of Neurology/Neurophysiology
Athens 11527
Tel: +30 177 516 37
Fax: +30 177 057 85
Email: *graaepil@otenet.gr*

Hungary
Hungarian Epilepsy Association (HALE)
1028 Budapest
Hidegkuti ut 71
Tel/Fax: +36 1393 288 29

Iceland
The Epilepsy Association of Iceland
PO Box 5182
126 Reykjavik
Tel: +354 551 4570
Fax: +354 551 4580/+354 561 8070
Email: *jonsg@itn.is*

India
Indian Epilepsy Association
No 8, Palam Marg
Vasant Vihar
New Delhi 110 057
Fax: +91 124 350 035

Indonesia
PERPEI
Jl. Jelita Utara No. 11
Rawamangun
Jakarta 13220
Fax: +62 21 797 0533

Iran
Iranian Epilepsy Association
PO Box 15655/199
Tehran
Fax: +98 75 33 847

Ireland
Brainwave The Irish Epilepsy Association
249 Crumlin Road
Dublin 12
Tel: +3531 455 7500
Fax: +3531 455 7013
Email: *brainwve@iol.ie*

Israel
EYAL Israel Epilepsy Association
4 Avodat Yisrael St
PO Box 1598
Jerusalem 91014
Tel: +972 2537 1044
Fax: +972 2653 5508

Italy
Associazione Italiana contro l'Epilessia (AICE)
via T. Marino No 7
20121 Milano
Tel: +3902 809 299
Fax: +3902 809 799

Japan
The Japan Epilepsy Association
5F Zenkokuzaidan Building 2-2-8
Nishiwaseda
Shinjuku-ku
Tokyo 162
Tel: +81 332 025 661
Fax: +81 332 027 235

Kenya
Kenya Association for the Welfare of Epileptics
PO Box 60790
Nairobi
Tel: +254 257 0885
Email: *kawe@iconnect.co.ke*

Korea
Korean Epilepsy Association/Rose Club
#157-1 Saejong-ro
Jongro-ku
Seoul 110-021
Tel: +822 394 2375
Fax: +822 394 7169
Email: *RoseClub@hitel.net*

Malaysia
Persatuan Epilepsi Malaysia
Neurology Department
Hospital Kuala Lumpur
Jalan Pahang 50586
Kuala Lumpur
Malaysia
Tel: +603 292 3123
Fax: +603 291 1186

Mexico
Groupo 'Aceptacion' de Epilepticos
Amsterdam 1928 No. 19
Colonia Olimpica-Pedregal
Mexico 04710 DF
Fax: +525 575 3250

The Netherlands
Epilepsie Vereniging Nederland
PO Box 270
3990 GB Houten
Tel: +31 306 344 063
Fax: +31 306 344 060
Email: *evn@epilepsiefonds.nl*

New Zealand
Epilepsy Association of New Zealand Inc
PO Box 1074
Hamilton
Tel: +64 7834 3556
Fax: +64 7834 3553
Email: *epilepsy@wave.co.nz*

Norway
Norsk Epilepsiforbund
Storgt. 39
0182 Oslo
Tel: +47 2220 6021
Fax: +47 2211 5976
Email: *nef@epilepsi.no*

Peru
Peruvian Association of Epilepsy
Castilla 678-E 101
Lima 32
Fax: +51 1466 0063
Email: *acmhma@colmed.org.pe*

Poland
Polskie Stowarzyszenie
Ludzi Cierpiacych na Padaczke
15-482 Bialystok
Ul. Fabryczna 57 (XIp)
Tel/Fax: +48 8575 4420

Portugal
Liga Portuguesa contra a Epilepsia
Rua S da Bandeira 162-1 o
4000 Porto
Fax: +351 233 22 121
Email: *fjpinto@ip.pt*
Website: *www.lpce.pt*

Scotland
Epilepsy Association of Scotland
48 Govan Road
Glasgow
G51 1JL
Tel: +44 141 427 4911
Fax: +44 141 419 1709
Email: *admin@epilepsyscotland.org.uk*

Senegal
Ligue Senegalaise contra l'Epilepsie
Commission Socio-Educative
Clinique Neurologique
Centre Hospitalo-Universitaire de Fann
BP 5035
Dakar-Fann
Tel: +221 825 3678
Fax: +221 825 9227
Email: *neurofan@telecomplus.sn*

Singapore
Singapore Epilepsy Foundation
2 Finlayson Green #16/05
Asian Insurance Building
Singapore 049247
Tel: +65 222 8291
Fax: +65 222 3041
Email: *gnrlsh@sgh.gov.sg*

Slovenia
Liga Proti Epilepsiji Slovenije
Institute of Clinical Neurophysiology
Hospital of Neurology
Medical Centre
SI-1525 Ljubljana
Tel: +38 661 131 3206
Fax: +38 661 302 771
Email: *dusan@uikn.mf.uni-lj.si*

South Africa
South African National Epilepsy League
SANEL PO BOx 73
Observatory 7935
Cape Town
Tel: +27 214 473 014
Fax: +27 214 485 053
Email: *sanel@mweb.co.za*

Sri Lanka
Epilepsy Association of Sri Lanka
10 Austin Place
Colombo 8
Tel: +94 1696 283

Sweden
Svenska Epilepsiforbundet
PO Box 9514
102 74 Stockholm
Tel: +46 866 943 06
Fax: +46 866 915 88
Email: *susanne.lund@epilepsi.se*

Switzerland
Schweizerische Liga Gegen Epilepsie
Dorfstrasse 2
Postfach 233
8712 Stafa/ZH
Zurich
Switzerland
Tel: +411 926 8971
Fax: +411 926 8972
Email: *SLgE@bluewin.ch*

Taiwan
Taiwan Epilepsy Association
c/o Division of Epilepsy
Department of Neurology
Chang Gung Memorial Hospital
199 Tun-Hwa N. Road
Taipei 105
Tel: +88 633 281 200 ext 2249
Fax: +88 633 281 320
Website: *www.epilepsyorg.org.tw*

Tunisia
Tunisian Association against Epilepsy
Neurological Department
EPS Charles Nicolle
Tunis 1006
Tel: +2161 562 834
Fax: +2161 562 777/834

UK
British Epilepsy Association
New Anstey House
Gateway Drive
Yeadon
Leeds LS19
Tel: +44 113 210 8800
Fax: +44 113 391 0300
Email: *epilepsy@bea.org.uk*
Website: *www.epilepsy.org.uk*

USA
Epilepsy Foundation
4351 Garden City Drive
Landover Maryland 20785
Tel: +1 301 459 3700
Fax: +1 301 577 2684
Email: *postmaster@efa.org*
Website: *www.epilepsyfoundation.org*

Yugoslavia
Jugoslovensko Drustvo za Epilepsiju
Yugoslav Society for Epilepsy
Slobodana Penezica-Krcuna 23
Beograd
Belgrade
Tel: +381 1168 6155 ext 137
Fax: +381 1168 6656
Email: *yusepi@rhc.ztp.co.yu*

Zimbabwe

Epilepsy Support Foundation
PO Box A104 Avondale
Old General Hospital
Mazoe Street
Harare
Tel: +263 472 4071

INDEX

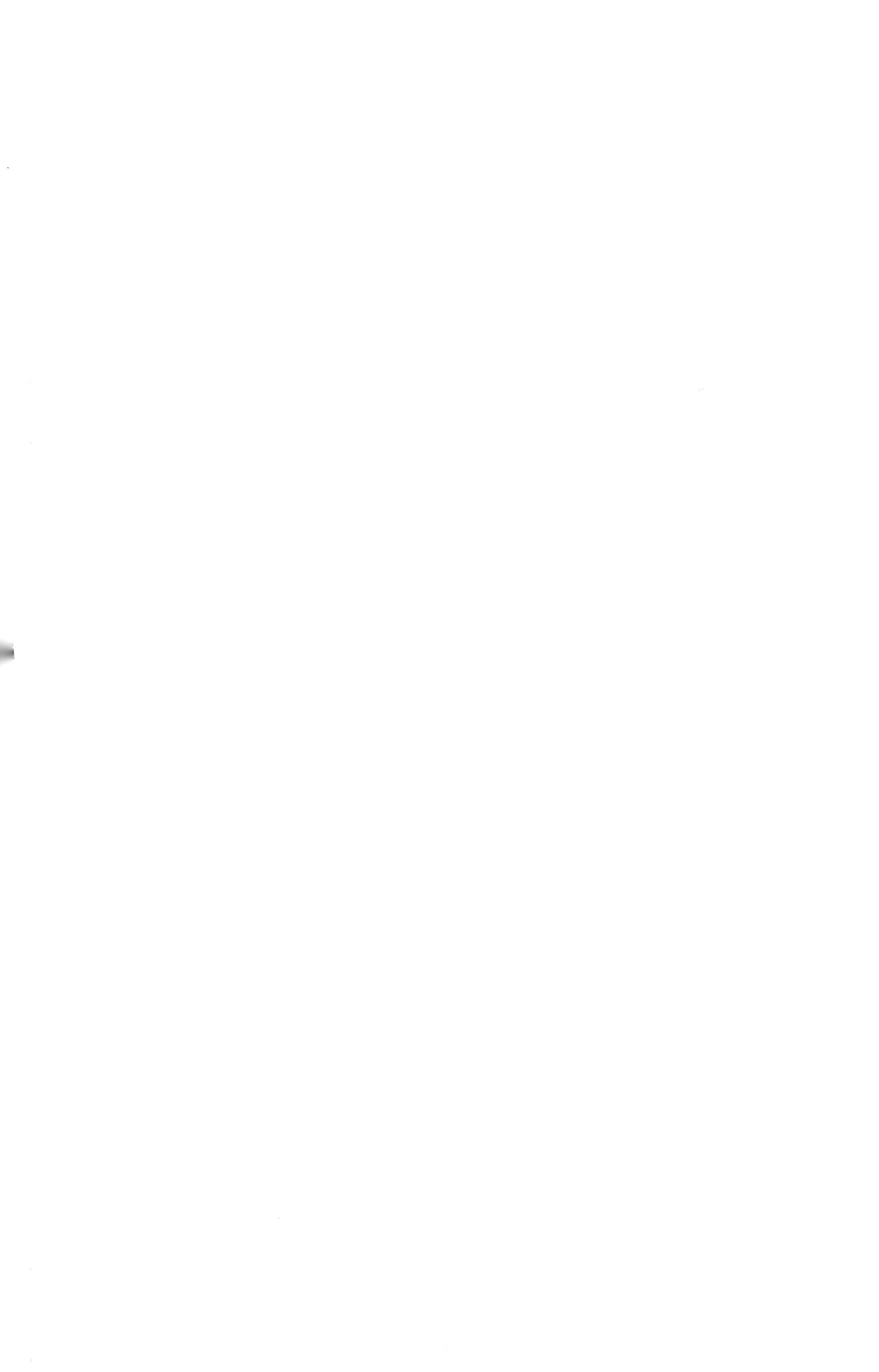